Vaccines for Veterinarians

Vaccines for Veterinarians

IAN R. TIZARD, BVMS, PhD, DACVM (HONS), DSc (HONS)

University Distinguished Professor Immunology Emeritus
Department of Veterinary Pathobiology
The Texas Veterinary Medical Center
Texas A & M University
College Station, Texas
USA

ELSEVIER

For additional online content visit ExpertConsult.com

Elsevier
3251 Riverport Lane
St. Louis, Missouri 63043

VACCINES FOR VETERINARIANS

ISBN: 978-0-323-68299-2

Library of Congress Control Number: 2019949241

Content Strategist: Jennifer Catando
Content Development Specialist: Nani Clansey
Project Manager: Umarani Natarajan
Publishing Services Manager: Shereen Jameel
Design Direction: Ryan Cook
Illustration Manager: Teresa McBryan
Marketing Manager: Bergen Farthing

Printed in China

Last digit is the print number: 9 8 7 6 5 4 3 2 1

Working together
to grow libraries in
developing countries

www.elsevier.com • www.bookaid.org

DEDICATION

This book is dedicated to the memory of my former graduate student, Dr. Monie Singh Bhogal, who was murdered in Somalia in January 1999 while supervising the Rinderpest vaccination program for the Italian aid agency, Terra Nuova.

Vaccines are among the world's greatest medical advances. Despite ill-informed and irrational resistance to their use, vaccination has brought most major infectious diseases under control and massively increased human longevity. Vaccines have had similar beneficial effects on livestock production, eliminating animal plagues, and making intensive livestock production possible. Companion animals and wildlife have also benefited enormously from the proper application of vaccination. The great triumphs of smallpox and rinderpest eradication would not have been possible without vaccines. They are the most cost-effective methods of preventing infectious diseases ever conceived.

We cannot, however, rest on past achievements. Emerging diseases, difficult organisms, antibiotic resistance, and a constant need to improve both the safety and efficacy of vaccines ensure that research and development must continue. In addition, unlike some human vaccines, the production of veterinary vaccines is subject to significant economic constraints. Although vaccination of companion animals is regarded as a responsibility to protect a beloved pet, especially in developed and prosperous countries, the drivers of vaccine use in livestock and poultry and also in less developed countries are economic. Animal vaccines are commodities made for the purposes of improving animal productivity and health. They will not be commercially produced if they do not generate significant revenue. They will not be used if they do not reduce disease costs. It does not matter that the science behind these new vaccines is incredibly elegant and sophisticated. If they cannot be produced or used profitably, they will not be manufactured. In general, governments and taxpayers will not subsidize animal vaccine production. Some exceptions may be made for zoonotic or wildlife diseases such as rabies.

The importance of vaccine profitability ensures that animal vaccines must be easy to manufacture, cheap to produce and store, and have a market size that ensures a reasonable return on investment.

But vaccine production is not static. The technologies of the past 100 years, although incredibly successful, are no longer adequate. Driven by the three big exceptions, tuberculosis, AIDS, and malaria, in addition to the emerging diseases such as Ebola and Zika, human vaccine production processes are changing. Reverse vaccinology driven by computational methods and vaccinomics is radically altering the way in which vaccines are developed. A meningitis vaccine developed by these computational methods is already on the market. A Zika virus vaccine went from inception to the clinic in 6 months. Veterinary vaccines are not far behind. The first commercially available DNA-plasmid vaccine was for West Nile disease in horses. Several animal replicon RNA vaccines have been licensed. Chimeric vaccines are now available against West Nile virus and porcine circovirus. Animals also have their exceptionally difficult problem diseases such as porcine reproductive and respiratory syndrome (PRRS), foot and mouth disease, influenza, and especially African swine fever. These remain enduring threats, although progress in developing new or more effective vaccines is being made here too.

Human and animal vaccinologies are also diverging. In humans, serious discussions are under way regarding the production of individualizing vaccines to match a person's specific immune system. In animals, especially livestock and fish, economics still rule. Mass production and a significant cost/benefit ratio are critical.

We must not forget that antivaccine advocates are vocal, not only in the human area, but also in Veterinary Medicine. The effective control of infectious diseases and the development of herd immunity have reduced the prevalence of many infectious diseases to very low levels. As a result, owners often remain ignorant of the threats posed by these infections. The best, really the only, defense against ill-informed and conspiracy theory–based antivaccine sentiment is to promote evidence-based vaccinology. Hopefully this text will provide a baseline for the rational use, promotion, development, and improvement of veterinary vaccines.

This text is therefore designed to be a comprehensive review of currently available animal vaccines and vaccination. It brings together the science and technology of vaccine production. It examines the issues associated with the use of animal vaccines. Safety is a critical issue in this age of antivaccination sentiment and social media. Regulations and assessment of vaccine efficacy and safety are major contributors to the costs of producing a vaccine and must also be considered. The second half of the text reviews the major vaccines used in each species, their risks, benefits, and interesting immunologic features. It is not intended to be a comprehensive catalog of all such products, nor does it discuss new vaccine research in detail. After all, many experimental vaccines never reach the marketplace. New vaccine administration methodologies are also discussed, especially with respect to the mass vaccination of poultry, pigs, fish, and wildlife. Finally, consideration is given to newly available vaccines against parasites and the increasingly successful field of cancer immunotherapy.

I must express my appreciation to my colleagues, John August, Luc Berghman, Stacy Eckman, Jill Heatley, Jeffrey Musser, Susan Payne, and Darrel Styles, who reviewed and corrected chapters for me. All errors and omissions are mine alone.

College Station, TX
December 2018

Many acronyms in the discipline of vaccinology relate not just to immunology but also to the regulatory networks that oversee their production and licensure. Here are some that are widely employed throughout this text.

AABP	American Association of Bovine Practitioners
AAEP	American Association of Equine Practitioners
AAFP	American Association of Feline Practitioners
AAHA	American Animal Hospital Association
AIDS	acquired immune deficiency syndrome
APC	antigen-presenting cell
APHIS	Animal and Plant Health Inspection Service (USDA)
AVMA	American Veterinary Medical association
BCG	bacillus Calmette-Guérin *(Mycobacterium bovis)*
BCR	B cell (antigen) receptor
BoLA	bovine leukocyte antigen
BPL	beta-propiolactone
CDC	Center for Disease Control and Prevention
CMI	cell-mediated immunity
CpG	cytosine-phosphate-guanosine nucleotide motif
CVB	Center for Veterinary Biologics (USDA)
CVMP	Committee for Medical Products for Veterinary Use
CFR	code of federal regulations
DAMP	damage-associated molecular pattern
DC	dendritic cell
DIVA	differentiate infected from vaccinated animals
ELISA	enzyme-linked immunosorbent assay
Fab	antigen-binding fragment
FAO	Food and Agriculture Organization
Fc	crystallizable fragment (of immunoglobulin)
FeLV	feline leukemia virus
FMDV	foot and mouth disease (virus)
FPT	failure of passive transfer
GLP	good laboratory practice
GMO	genetically modified organism
GMP	good manufacturing practice
FIV	feline immunodeficiency virus
HA	hemagglutinin
HDN	hemolytic disease of the newborn
HI	hemagglutination inhibition (test)
ID	intradermal
IFN	interferon
Ig	immunoglobulin
IL	interleukin
IM	intramuscular (route)
IN	intranasal (route)
ISCOM	immune-stimulating complex

ISG	immune serum globulin
IU	international unit
kb	kilobase (one thousand base pairs) of DNA
LPS	lipopolysaccharide
MAb	monoclonal antibody
MAP	*Mycobacterium avium paratuberculosis*
MHC	major histocompatibility complex
MCS	master cell stock
MLV	modified live virus (or vaccine)
MSV	master seed virus
OIE	Originally the Office International des Epizooties but currently the World Organization for Animal Health.
Omp	outer membrane protein
OMV	outer membrane vesicles
O/W	oil-in-water emulsion
PAMP	pathogen-associated molecular pattern
PCR	polymerase chain reaction
PF	protective fraction
PRR	pattern-recognition receptor
PRRS(V)	porcine respiratory and reproductive system (virus)
R_0	basic reproductive number
S19	strain 19 *Brucella abortus* vaccine
SC	subcutaneous (route)
TCR	T cell (antigen) receptor
TLR	toll-like receptor
Th cell	helper T cell
TK	thymidine kinase
TNF	tumor necrosis factor
Treg	regulatory T (cell)
ts	temperature sensitive (mutant)
USDA	United States Department of Agriculture
VLP	virus-like particle
WHO	World Health Organization
W/O	water-in-oil emulsion
WSAVA	World Small Animal Veterinary Association

CONTENTS

A Brief History of Veterinary Vaccines

Vaccination is the most efficient and effective method of controlling infectious diseases ever developed. The enormous improvements in human health through the twentieth century and beyond have been, in large part, a result of the development of effective vaccines. Likewise, many of the improvements in animal health, especially the great increases in productivity resulting from effective disease control are a direct result of vaccine use. The eradication of smallpox in humans as well as the elimination of rinderpest in cattle are both directly the result of effective vaccination campaigns.

The early history of veterinary vaccines can be divided into four stages. The first stage was the discovery of variolation against human smallpox and its eventual evolution into vaccination. The second stage was launched by the discoveries of Louis Pasteur and his colleagues that led to the early production of numerous effective vaccines against predominantly bacterial diseases. The third stage, typified by the development of the canine distemper vaccines, was a process of progressive improvement of these vaccines and resulted from a growing knowledge about viruses and their behavior. Finally, the sophisticated use of vaccines has led to the elimination of two major diseases, smallpox and rinderpest, and the near eradication of others.

Variolation and Vaccination

The earliest record of protective immunity dates from 430 BCE, when the Greek historian Thucydides describing the plague of Athens (of unknown cause) observed "… for no one caught the disease twice, or, if he did, the second attack was never fatal."

Sometime before the fifteenth century, the Chinese also observed that those individuals who recovered from an attack of smallpox never suffered from it a second time. It was a small step therefore to attempt to protect children from the disease by deliberately infecting them. Initially the process involved blowing dried scab powder up the nose of infants. Eventually however, improved results were obtained by placing the dried scabs in a small incision in the arm. The resulting local disease was less severe and mortality correspondingly lower. Descriptions of this technique spread westward along the Silk Road until it eventually reached the Ottoman Empire—modern Turkey. It was widely employed across the Middle East.

Reports of this technique called "variolation," eventually reached England in the early 1700s. One such example came in 1714 by way of a letter from a physician, Dr. Emanuel Timoni, who practiced medicine in Constantinople. In addition, first-hand reports from Lady Mary Montagu,

1

the wife of the English Ambassador to Constantinople impressed the people who mattered. Lady Montagu arranged to have her own son successfully variolated through Dr. Timoni. Voltaire described her as "[a] woman of so fine a genius, and endued with as great a strength of mind, as any of her sex in the United Kingdom." These reports were taken seriously because the Prince of Wales (the future King George II) and his wife were terrified that smallpox would attack their grandchildren. As a result, the process was investigated by variolating prisoners in London's Newgate Prison. When this "Royal Experiment" proved to be successful, variolation was rapidly adopted in England. Around the same time (1721) variolation was successfully used by Dr. Zabdiel Boylston in Boston who had read Timoni's letter. Although the technique worked, it was still accompanied by significant morbidity and some mortality, so it was not universally adopted in the American colonies. Some believed that diseases such as smallpox were God's punishment for sins so that variolation was obviously in conflict with God's will and thus inappropriate. Variolation clearly worked; however, nobody at that time had any concept as to how it might induce immunity to smallpox. Nevertheless, attempts were made to replicate the technique in other diseases. The most significant of these attempts resulted in the discovery of vaccination.

EDWARD JENNER

In 1768, John Fewster, a physician in Gloucestershire, in the west of England, and his colleagues began to inoculate their patients against smallpox. They found however that many patients did not react to variolation. Upon inquiry, Fewster found that these patients had previously been infected with cowpox. Fewster reported his observations to the local Medical Society, but he did not fully recognize its significance and never published his findings. Among the Society's members was a young apprentice called Edward Jenner. In 1774 an English farmer, Benjamin Jesty, performed the first documented substitution of cowpox for smallpox. He obtained the scab material from a cow of a neighbor and inoculated his wife in the arm under her elbow. He never wrote an account of this and he did not determine if she was immune. The widespread acceptance of this method did not come for another 24 years. In the 1790s, Edward Jenner was still working as a physician in the west of England, and he remembered Fewster's observation. He also recognized that deliberate inoculation of cowpox could confer immunity against smallpox.

Cowpox, otherwise known as vaccinia (*vacca* is Latin for cow), is a virus-mediated skin disease of cattle. Affected animals generally develop a large weeping ulcer on hairless skin such as the udder. When these infected cattle are hand milked, the vaccinia virus can readily enter cuts or abrasions on the milker's hands. Humans infected by this virus develop a localized weeping lesion that scabs over and heals within a few weeks. We now know that the cowpox virus triggers a powerful immune response. Most importantly, however, vaccinia virus is closely related to smallpox virus to such an extent that these individuals also develop immunity to smallpox.

Edward Jenner began a systematic study of the protective effects of vaccination and published his results in 1798. The scientific method was not well established in the late eighteenth century. Thus Jenner published a series of case reports on vaccination. This drew immediate attention because the method worked well and was clearly very much safer than variolation (Box 1.1). Despite some initial opposition, the principal physicians and surgeons of London supported Jenner, and, as a result, vaccination was rapidly adopted in Europe and the Americas, whereas variolation was discontinued (Fig. 1.1). Jenner quite properly received credit for publishing the vaccination process, but his biographer invented a myth that Jenner alone had discovered the process by talking to a dairymaid. In fact, this protective effect of vaccination was independently recognized in several other English and European communities.

It must be emphasized that Jenner had no concept of microbiology, viruses, or immunity. For example, he did not know where smallpox came from. He noted, however, that the disease occurred in farms where there were both cattle and horses. The same workers looked after

BOX 1.1 ■ Thomas Jefferson and Edward Jenner

Thomas Jefferson was an enthusiastic amateur scientist. When he was informed about Jenner's discovery, Jefferson sent him a letter:

Washing, Dec 25, 1800

Sir,

    I received last night, and have read with great satisfaction, your pamphlet on the subject of the kinepock, and pray you to accept my thanks for the communication of it.

    I had before attended to your publications on the subject in the newspapers and took much interest in the result of the experiments you were making. Every friend of humanity must look with pleasure on this discovery, by which one evil more is withdrawn from the condition of man; and must contemplate the possibility, that future improvements and discoveries may still more and more lessen the catalogue of evils. In this line of proceeding you deserve well of your country; and I pray you accept my portion of the tribute due to you, and assurance of high consideration and respect, with which I am, Sir

    Your most obedient, humble servant,

    Thomas Jefferson

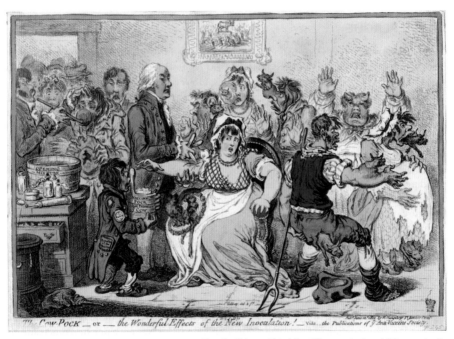

Fig. 1.1 Antivaccination sentiment is not new. The English satirist John Gilray caricatured this vaccination scene in 1802. The central figure is likely not Edward Jenner, but George Pearson, an enthusiastic advocate of vaccination. If this happens to you, seek immediate medical attention. (From the British Museum. With permission.)

both, and he suggested that they transmitted cowpox from horses to cattle. Jenner therefore believed that the skin disease of horses colloquially called "the grease" was the source of cowpox. He likely confused this disease with horsepox. However, he clearly believed that horses were the original source of cowpox, and as a result he obtained some of his vaccine material from horses. Horsepox, which like other poxviruses caused multiple skin lesions, was a common disease of horses at that time. Jenner continued to believe in "equination," and in later years tended to prefer the use of equine material to cowpox.

Subsequent to Jenner's discovery, the British government decided to vaccinate all their soldiers. The contract to produce this vaccine was given in 1801 to a Dr. John Loy who used material from horses exclusively. In 1803 an Italian physician, Dr. Luigi Sacco, read a book by Dr. Loy and also used equine "grease" with great success in children. Although cowpox was the preferred material for vaccination through the nineteenth century, equine material was used on occasion. It is likely that at least some of the vaccinia stocks used in humans were of equine origin. Vaccinia virus as currently used differs significantly from circulating cowpox virus strains. Although horsepox has become almost extinct, it has been possible to examine the genome of a Mongolian strain of horsepox. This is also related to but distinct from vaccinia. Several horsepox genes are present in different vaccinia strains, whereas some vaccinia strains appear to be more closely related to horsepox than to cowpox.

Although physicians (and veterinarians) were totally unaware of how vaccinia worked, it did not stop them from seeking to use this methodology to prevent other diseases. Many believed vaccinia to be an effective treatment for unrelated diseases in humans including the plague and cholera.

CATTLE PLAGUE

Cattle plague (rinderpest) was a major devastating disease in Europe until the end of the nineteenth century when it was eliminated by movement control and slaughter. We now know it was caused by a morbillivirus related to human measles. However, in the eighteenth century many of those who encountered cattle plague considered that it was very similar to smallpox. Thus once variolation (inoculation) was introduced into Europe in 1717, numerous individuals attempted to prevent cattle plague by inoculating healthy cattle with material from plague-affected cattle. One such method involved making an incision in the dewlap and inserting a piece of string that had been soaked in nasal or ocular discharge. This was removed after 2 to 3 days. It was claimed that animals sickened and then recovered. A booklet was published in 1757 recommending this procedure, and it was widely adopted in England. However, it was eventually recognized that all such attempts were not effective and killed a lot of cattle. Despite this, widespread attempts to inoculate cattle against rinderpest were conducted in Denmark, the Netherlands, and what is now Germany. By 1770 most had been abandoned.

In 1774, an adaptation of the vaccination procedure was tested in the Netherlands by Geert Reinders, a farmer from Groningen. He had noticed that calves from recovered cows appeared resistant to reinfection. This may have been the first recognition of the phenomenon of maternal immunity. Reinders made use of this resistant period to inoculate 6- to 8-week-old calves with nasal material from recovered cows. He also observed that he got better results if he repeated the inoculation of these calves two more times. Reinders was criticized by those who believed that disease was a manifestation of God's will. More importantly, his was not a practical procedure and fell into disuse.

Reinders success encouraged others to pursue other methods of inoculation against cattle plague and it was widely employed across northern Europe. In 1780 the Amsterdam society for the Advancement of Agriculture reported that of more than 3000 animals inoculated, 89% had survived as opposed to 29% survival in uninoculated animals. As a result, more than half the cattle were inoculated in some regions of the Netherlands. As the results of inoculation gradually improved, an argument developed between those that believed inoculation to be the solution to the cattle plague problem and those who believed that prompt slaughter was a more effective control procedure. Over the course of the nineteenth century, slaughter gradually superseded inoculation as a control method in Europe.

CONTAGIOUS BOVINE PLEUROPNEUMONIA

This disease was a major problem in Europe through the nineteenth century and inoculation was first attempted in England and Germany at that time. However, credit is usually given to Louis Willems of Hasselt in Belgium, who in the early 1850s inoculated lung fluid from affected animals into the tail of recipient cattle. He used a large lancet dipped in the fluid and used this to make two to three incisions at the tip of the tail. It caused large abscesses, the animals sickened and recovered, the tail commonly fell off (the Willems reaction), but the animals became immune (Fig. 1.2). Several European governments formed commissions to look into Willems claims and confirm its effectiveness. The Dutch reported that untreated cattle had 35% mortality. In vaccinated animals 8% to 10% had severe reactions with 1.1% mortality. Use of this vaccine became widespread, but it was eventually replaced with modern live attenuated vaccines, which can also cause severe reactions.

A similar process was independently developed in sub-Saharan Africa long before European colonization. It is speculated that the technique was developed following the introduction of

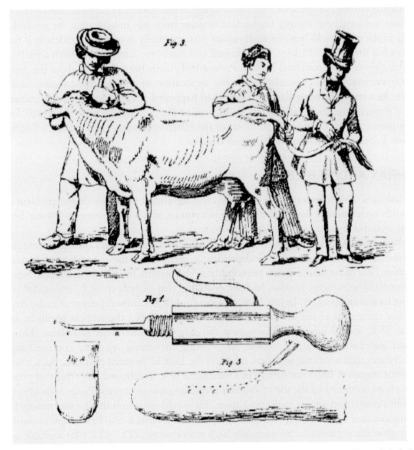

Fig. 1.2 The correct way to vaccinate cattle against contagious bovine pleuropneumonia. (From C.A. Spinage: "Cattle plague: a history," Kluwer; "The tail method of inoculation for pleuropneumonia" and the reference is Keulen, 1854. With permission.).

variolation by Saharan nomads. In this case, material from pleuropneumonia lesions was inoculated subcutaneously to cattle through an incision on the bridge of the nose. The inflammatory reaction produced exostoses on the nasal bone and at one point Dr. de Rochebrune reported that he had discovered a new species of bovine, *Bos triceros*. Postvaccinial reactions were severe but the surviving animals were strongly immune. A similar technique may have previously been used in Iran for the prevention of caprine pleuropneumonia in goats.

Louis Pasteur

During the latter half of the nineteenth century the new science of microbiology led inexorably to the recognition that many significant diseases were caused by microorganisms, especially bacteria. The French chemist and microbiologist Louis Pasteur was one of the pioneers of microbiology and the microbial theory of infectious diseases. As such he collected and investigated any bacteria that appeared to be pathogenic. In 1879 he received a bacterial sample from Jean Toussaint (1847–1890), a professor at the Toulouse Veterinary College. This bacterium, now called *Pasteurella multocida*, is the cause of fowl cholera. Inoculation of this bacterium into chickens causes lethal disease. During the course of his studies, Pasteur's assistant Émile Roux inadvertently allowed a culture of *P.multocida* to age in the laboratory cupboard for several weeks. (This may not have been entirely inadvertent because Roux was investigating the survival of the bacteria in the culture). When this aged culture was eventually injected into chickens it failed to sicken or kill them. The chickens were retained and sometime later injected with a fresh culture of the bacterium. They remained healthy. Pasteur had clearly been thinking about the process of smallpox vaccination and speculating on the application of this process to other infectious diseases. As a result, he recognized that what had happened with the aged bacterial culture was, in many respects, similar to vaccination. Pasteur called the procedure *vaccination* as well. In 1880 Pasteur presented his results to the members of the National Academy in a treatise "Of Infectious Diseases, Especially the Disease of Chicken Cholera."

ANTHRAX AND RABIES

Fowl cholera, although important, was not the most significant infectious disease problem affecting French agriculture at that time. Anthrax, in contrast, was a major issue so Pasteur began to develop a vaccine against anthrax (*Bacillus anthracis*).

In the years 1880 and 1881 three investigators, William Greenfield in London, Pasteur in Paris, and Toussaint in Toulouse, had independently recognized the importance of microbial attenuation (loss of virulence) and its relationship to vaccination. In 1878, John Burdon-Sanderson and Greenfield working in London had demonstrated that anthrax could be attenuated without affecting its immunogenicity. In July 1880, a report from Toussaint was presented to the Academy describing the results of his vaccine trials. He had simply killed the anthrax bacilli by heating them at 55°C for 10 minutes. This vaccine effectively protected dogs and sheep. This result surprised and bothered Pasteur because his working hypothesis regarding the mechanism of immunity was that a vaccine somehow depleted the host of essential nutrients. As a result, the pathogenic organism could not survive in a vaccinated host. It followed from this that protection could only be conferred by the use of vaccines containing live organisms. Pasteur was skeptical of Toussaint's results and set out to disprove them. He would not admit that he was wrong. Pasteur thus concentrated his efforts on attenuating *B. anthracis* so that it could no longer cause disease. Pasteur grew the organism at an unusually high temperature (42°C–43°C) for multiple generations. This worked, but the early results were erratic and inconclusive.

In March 1881, Pasteur reported that his vaccine was working. This report provoked a challenge for a public trial by a group of local veterinarians, a challenge that Pasteur accepted. In

May 1881, Pasteur put on a public demonstration of his anthrax vaccine at Pouilly-le-Fort outside Paris. He used two groups of animals (Fig. 1.3). The vaccinated group, 24 sheep, 1 goat, and 6 cattle, received two doses of the vaccine at a 15-day interval. The unvaccinated group received nothing. On May 31, thirty days after the first dose, all were challenged with a live anthrax culture. On June 2 more than 200 interested observers came to see the results. All the unvaccinated animals were dead or dying, whereas all the vaccinated animals survived. It was a major media event and a triumph. The publicity given to this experiment made Pasteur famous and introduced the public to the great potential of vaccines in combatting infectious disease. Pasteur claimed publicly that he had used a live attenuated vaccine. Only he and his colleagues knew that he had killed the bacteria in the vaccine with potassium bichromate. Toussaint, who received no credit, published only two more papers before having a mental breakdown and dying at the age of 43.

Subsequently Pasteur and his colleague Louis Thuillier identified *Erysipelothrix rhusiopathiae* as the cause of swine erysipelas. Pasteur showed that its repeated passage through pigeons increased its virulence for pigs. In contrast, serial passage through rabbits significantly reduced its virulence in pigs. He therefore developed a vaccination process against swine erysipelas that consisted of a series of injections of bacteria that had been attenuated by repeated passage in rabbits followed by a series of injections of pigeon-passaged organisms. This study is notable because it was the first example of microbial attenuation by passage in an unusual species, a process that has been widely employed since.

Pasteur and Roux went on to develop a rabies vaccine. They infected rabbits with rabid brain tissue (they didn't know it was a virus). Once disease developed, they removed the rabbit's spinal cord and dried it for 5 to 10 days—thus attenuating the agent, and then prepared an emulsified injectable. By drying spinal cords for different time periods, Pasteur and Roux were able to produce rabies viruses with different degrees of attenuation. They could then inoculate dogs with a series of emulsified cords containing viruses of increasing virulence and demonstrate that they usually developed strong immunity to rabies. In preliminary studies they showed that they could protect a dog after it had received a rabid bite.

They had been working on this project for some time when in July 1885 a child, Joseph Meister, was brought to them. Meister had been badly savaged by a rabid dog. Under considerable pressure Pasteur vaccinated him. He gave Meister 13 injections over 10 days using spinal

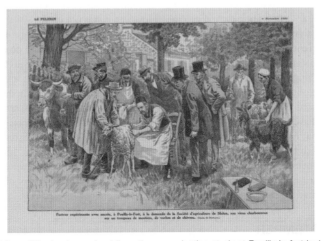

Fig. 1.3 A depiction of Pasteur's great public anthrax vaccination study at Pouilly-le-fort in 1881. It received enormous positive publicity and launched the science of immunology. (From The Pasteur Institute/Musee Pasteur. With permission.)

cord emulsions beginning 3 days after the bites. He began with the driest and eventually proceeding to fresh infected cord. Meister survived to become the gate-porter of Pasteur's grave and committed suicide rather than permit German troops to open the crypt in 1940. In July 1886, a 7-year-old boy named Harold Newton Newell became the first person to receive Pasteur's rabies vaccine in the United States. He only received the first four inoculations, but his fate is unknown.

DEAD VACCINES

Although Pasteur was highly successful in developing practical vaccines, he had no concept as to how they worked. In 1880, he had put forward a tentative hypothesis that the vaccine organism consumed a necessary nutrient when it first invaded the body. Accordingly, this implied that vaccines only worked if they contained living organisms. This of course was completely wrong. However once news of his vaccine discoveries was published, others took up the cause very rapidly. By December 1880, Dr. Daniel Salmon could report, "At present, the attention of USDA investigators is still, for the most part turned to methods of prevention, and chief among these is inoculation by means of a mitigated virus." In 1886, Daniel Salmon and Theobald Smith were able to protect pigeons by inoculating them with a heat-killed culture of "hog cholera virus," now known as *Salmonella choleraesuis*. Thus killed vaccines also worked. This eventually led to the rapid development of a great diversity of killed bacterial vaccines.

Other advances soon followed. In 1888, Émile Roux and Alexandre Yersin at the Pasteur Institute showed that a bacterium-free filtrate of a diphtheria culture contained the bacterial exotoxin. In 1890, Emil von Behring, working with Shibasaburo Kitasato, immunized guinea pigs and rabbits with killed tetanus or diphtheria broth cultures. They demonstrated that the serum of these immunized animals contained an "antitoxin" that could neutralize their toxins. This antitoxic activity could be passively transferred to nonimmune animals. They called these antitoxic substances, antibodies. In 1894, Emil Roux successfully treated 300 children with diphtheria using antidiphtheria serum. In 1896, this was regarded as "the most important advance of the century in the medical treatment of acute infective disease."

Vaccination and Antiviral Vaccines

Pasteur and his successors succeeded in laying the foundations of modern immunology and in developing numerous new antibacterial vaccines. However, it was not until 1898 that Loeffler and Frosch showed that the agent of foot-and-mouth disease could pass through a bacteria-proof filter. In 1905 Henri Carré showed that the agent of canine distemper could do the same. Thus he could filter nasal discharges or pericardial effusions through a fine porcelain filter. Although the filtrate contained no bacteria, it could still cause disease and death in susceptible dogs. This discovery was ignored for 20 years. British and American investigators firmly believed that the disease was caused by *Bordetella bronchiseptica*. It was not until 1926 that Carré's claims were verified by Laidlaw and Duncan. There was a great reluctance by bacteriologists to abandon the methodology that had yielded such great results. This did not just apply to distemper. For many years, scientists clung to the notion that influenza was caused by a bacterium. Indeed, both distemper and influenza are characterized by secondary bacterial invasion. As a result, it is by no means difficult to isolate multiple bacteria from the tissues and body fluids of affected animals. Bacteriologists had no shortage of alternative candidate agents to investigate.

CANINE DISTEMPER

Throughout the nineteenth and early twentieth century, distemper was a devastating disease of dogs. It does not appear to have been present in the United Kingdom before the 1790s. It was of special concern because it affected foxhounds and thus foxhunting by the upper class. Its cause was unknown, but that did not prevent attempts at immunization. Jenner had studied this disease and had shown that it was infectious but not transmissible to humans. Thus Edward Jenner vaccinated the Earl of Berkley's foxhounds with cowpox without success. Nevertheless, the vaccination was employed for many years, like so many other vaccinations for other diseases. One ardent fan of giving vaccinia to his dogs to prevent distemper was General George Custer. Custer even wrote a letter to an English hunting magazine encouraging the use of vaccinia for this purpose. As late as 1902, a Dr. Brown from Cambridge, England, reported, "For a number of years I have inoculated puppies…with vaccine lymph, and with the best results. During my time I have never heard of a case of distemper arising after inoculation." This was not a commonly held view.

Arthur Senner was the first to describe bacteria in association with distemper lesions and fluids in 1875. He isolated a "short and narrow bacillus" and a micrococcus from blood, lungs, and other organs, and concluded that the bacillus was the causal agent. Other investigators followed, each claiming that their bacterium was the cause of distemper. In 1890, a Dr. Millais isolated a bacillus from a distemper case. He heated a culture of this organism to 60°C for 10 minutes and administered this heated culture subcutaneously to ten puppies. He subsequently challenged them intranasally and claimed that all were protected. In 1901 a Dr. Copeman produced a similar vaccine (heated broth culture—60°C for 30 minutes, plus phenol preservative). There was considerable debate about the efficacy of Copeman's vaccine. Many claimed it was useless, whereas others such as His Grace, the Duke of Beaufort, thought it was great, stating, "If we go on with the same results, it will be the greatest boon that has ever been brought out."

Later in 1901, a Dr. Physalix reported on the isolation of the causal agent of distemper—*Pasteurella canis*. He developed a vaccine using this organism. Physalix claimed that he had induced typical distemper when a pure culture of *P. canis* was injected. He also reported on the development of a vaccine containing an organism attenuated by repeated subculturing. As with other early vaccines of this nature there was a great deal of skepticism regarding the effectiveness of Physalix's vaccine. A Committee of Veterinary Surgeons, established in 1903, reported that the vaccine failed to confer any immunity to distemper. Despite this, Professor Lignières produced a new polyvalent vaccine against *P. canis* in 1903. It consisted of a mixture of different strains attenuated by several hundred subcultures. It too didn't work.

In 1912, an American veterinarian, Dr. Ferry, produced a polyvalent, polymicrobial distemper vaccine. In fact Dr. Ferry had discovered *Bordetella bronchiseptica*. His vaccine contained a mixture of *B. bronchiseptica, Staph. pyogenes,* and *Strep. pyogenes.* This vaccine was widely used and regarded as useful. Nevertheless, over several years, enthusiasm for Ferry's vaccine waned. Ferry himself acknowledged this in 1923 when he suggested that the dose employed was far too low. We now recognize that *B. bronchiseptica* is a causal agent of kennel cough, and it is likely therefore that his vaccine prevented some such cases. Nevertheless, in 1926 Hardenbergh showed that a pure culture of this organism could not protect dogs against distemper.

It is probable that the first effective distemper vaccine was produced by a professor at the University of Rome, Dr. Vittorio Puntoni, in 1923. He succeeded in serially passaging distemper by intracerebral inoculation. Subsequently he made a suspension of the brain of an infected dog and added formalin 1:10,000. After two days he administered this subcutaneously to dogs. He boosted this with live attenuated material or with additional doses of the inactivated material and apparently obtained significant protection. In 1927, Lebailly, a French investigator, demonstrated that infected dog spleens contained large amounts of virus. Therefore he took infected spleens, ground them up, added formalin, and produced an effective vaccine.

In England, studies in dogs were initially discouraged by antivivisectionist sentiment. As a result, distemper vaccine studies moved slowly until it was shown that ferrets were also highly susceptible to this disease. Patrick Laidlaw and George Duncan initially produced a formalized killed vaccine derived from a ferret spleen extract. Field trials in 1928, especially on foxhounds, showed significant protection. As a result, they published a detailed methodology and made the vaccine freely available for commercial development. Unfortunately, the newly released vaccine caused some side effects including postdistemper encephalitis. These appear to be in part caused by rushing the vaccine to market without adequate safety testing. In 1930, the killed vaccine was withdrawn and replaced with an antiserum-virus product. This mixture was less effective than the killed vaccine, but results improved greatly when the virus was injected first, followed several hours later by the antiserum. Subsequent developments included adapting the virus to growth in eggs and eventually to tissue culture.

By the beginning of the Second World War, vaccine technology was firmly established. Many important infectious diseases had been controlled by effective vaccines. The subsequent development of vaccines centered on previously uncontrolled diseases such as polio, on improving unsatisfactory vaccines such as those against foot-and-mouth disease, and on reducing adverse effects. The development of Salk's inactivated polio vaccine after passage in cultured monkey kidney cells was the first step in the development of the modern cell-culture-based vaccine industry. Because of the risks associated with modified live organisms, investigators began to create vaccines based on individual viral components or subunits. Although safer, these subunit vaccines tend to be less immunogenic. Polysaccharide and virus-like particle vaccines began to be produced in the 1980s. As a result of these impressive advances, most major infectious diseases remain relatively well controlled—thanks to vaccines. There is however room for improvement and a continuous push for improved safety. Additionally, the appearance of new infections such as porcine epidemic diarrhea and Hendra virus, as well as the inexorable spread of others into new geographic areas, continues to fuel the demand for new improved veterinary products.

The Eradication of Rinderpest

Rinderpest is caused by a morbillivirus closely related to human measles virus. Indeed, the two viruses probably diverged from a common precursor about 10,000 years ago when people and cattle first lived in close proximity. This disease affected cattle, buffalo, and yaks. A short incubation period was followed by a prodromal phase of depression and inappetence. Eventually ulcers appeared on mucus membranes. These spread and coalesced leading to respiratory distress, massive diarrhea, dehydration, and death.

The first recorded probable epidemic of rinderpest occurred between 376 and 386 AD. The disease was likely brought to Europe by invaders from Central Asia, the Huns and the Mongols, as they gathered large herds of cattle as spoils of war. As time passed these raids were transformed into trading partnerships. From the seventeenth century on, the disease was repeatedly introduced into Western Europe by organized cattle trading, mainly from Russia; at that time it was known as the "Russian disease." Bernardino Ramazzini, Professor of Medicine at Padua University, wrote the first clinical description in 1712. However, in 1711 Johann Karol in Prussia recognized that rinderpest was transmissible and that cattle that recovered from it were resistant to reinfection. As described previously, during the eighteenth century, numerous attempts were made to vaccinate animals, usually unsuccessfully. Major rinderpest outbreaks occurred throughout the eighteenth and nineteenth centuries across Europe, killing huge numbers of cattle. Indeed, so important was rinderpest that the French king's controller of finances gave funds to Claude Bourgelat in 1762 to found the first veterinary school in Lyons. Other countries soon followed. The graduates were needed to fight the cattle plague.

Rinderpest was introduced into sub-Saharan Africa in 1887 when infected cattle from India were imported into Ethiopia to feed Italian soldiers. The disease infected local cattle with 90% mortality, and over the next decade spread across the continent. This Great Rinderpest Pandemic caused major cultural, social, and economic upheaval. The disease raged uncontrolled across the

African continent, causing widespread famine, devastating communities, and wiping out huge numbers of domestic and wild ungulates. When it reached Natal in 1896, it killed more than 90% of all African-owned cattle. Thereafter the virus became endemic and circulated in the pastoral communities of East Africa. In 1902 Maurice Nicolle and Mustafa Adil Bey demonstrated that rinderpest was caused by a filterable agent; in other words, a virus.

The disease also came back to Europe in the 1920s when it was introduced by a herd of zebus being shipped from India to Brazil. They came into contact with some imported American cattle that were sold at Belgian markets and went on to infect cattle across Germany. This outbreak was controlled by restriction of cattle movement, immediate slaughter, and vaccination. As a result of this outbreak it was decided to create the Office International des Epizooties (OIE)—now known as the World Organization for Animal Health.

In 1897, the eminent microbiologist Robert Koch, working in South Africa, developed a vaccine containing bile from rinderpest-infected cattle that was administered subcutaneously. Koch had shown that the virus in bile was not usually infectious. Nevertheless, this was still a highly dangerous procedure. Koch also showed that immune serum gave short-term passive protection. But a vaccine containing hyperimmune serum and virulent virus produced prolonged strong immunity. This "serum-virus simultaneous" method was the most effective rinderpest vaccine for many years and helped eliminate the disease from Europe in 1928.

Various methods of inactivating rinderpest virus were studied in the 1920s because the serum-virus technique was complex and costly. Eventually a formalin-inactivated vaccine was developed and used with some success in Asia. Unfortunately, the duration of immunity conferred by these formalized vaccines was very short (6 months) and their large-scale production impractical.

Subsequently it proved possible to adapt the virus to growth in goats. Serial passage in goats clearly reduced their virulence for cattle although it was not completely innocuous. It caused fever and mild lesions in European cattle. This "caprinized" vaccine was developed in the 1920s, and after various improvements was widely employed until the 1950s. However, it could still cause severe reactions in cattle including significant weight loss. Meanwhile, efforts continued on adapting rinderpest virus to rabbits (lapinization). After more than 600 passages in rabbits, it was unable to cause disease in cattle and was widely adopted by affected countries.

In spite of limited success obtained using egg-adapted rinderpest, in 1959 Dr. Walter Plowright and his colleagues, working in Kenya, succeeded in growing rinderpest virus in bovine kidney cells. Although the virus in the initial cultures was virulent, this rapidly declined so that virus passaged 95 times no longer caused a fever in cattle and could induce prolonged strong immunity. This vaccine protected against all strains of rinderpest, induced lifelong immunity, and was remarkably free of side effects. This vaccine rapidly replaced both the caprinized and lapinized vaccines.

Beginning in 1960 a series of coordinated regional vaccination campaigns were mounted in an effort to control, and ideally eliminate, the disease. The first of these vaccination campaigns, called Joint Program 15 (JP-15) and organized by the Organization of African Unity, was very successful and clinical disease outbreaks were massively reduced. Seventeen out of the twenty-two countries involved were infected at the beginning of the campaign, and this had dropped to one by 1979. However, the money ran out, urgency was lost, surveillance systems failed to recognize covert infections in domestic and wild ungulates, vaccination programs were discontinued, and as a result, the disease reemerged across Africa. Similar efforts were launched across Asia beginning in Afghanistan, and by 1972, the disease was restricted to Lebanon. However, as in JP-15, success bred complacency and the disease reemerged in the 1980s.

A second round of control programs was instituted when in 1982 the Pan-African Rinderpest Campaign was instituted. This was so successful that in 1994 the goal of rinderpest eradication was established by the United Nations Food and Agriculture Organization (FAO) and the World Organization for Animal Health (OIE).

Several key factors were in place to make this program a success. Thus new highly sensitive diagnostic tests based on the identification of antirinderpest antibodies were developed. These tests based on enzyme-linked immunosorbent assays (ELISAs) were essential for monitoring the vaccination program. More importantly was the development of a thermostable Plowright vaccine. A major limitation of the original vaccine was the need to keep the vaccine cold—maintain the cold chain. However, by 1992 researchers at Tufts University had adapted the virus for growth in monkey kidney cells that resulted in a thermostable vaccine—ThermoVax, which had a shelf life of 30 days when unrefrigerated. This development made it much easier to deliver the vaccine to remote villages and thus reach many more animals. This innovation, together with others such as working with community elders who provided local intelligence, ensured that most of their cattle were vaccinated, generated significant community support, and assured the success of the program. Massive vaccination campaigns together with careful epidemiology, controls on animal movement, and focusing on a regional approach progressively reduced the number of infected countries. When disease reservoirs were identified, vaccination teams quickly moved in to contain the infection. Between April 1989 and July 1990, 24.1 million vaccine doses were administered. Fortunately, the disease in wild ungulates disappeared when the local cattle herds were vaccinated. The surviving wild ungulate populations were too small to sustain the infection, and herd immunity soon developed. By 1999, the campaign was intensified under the slogan "Seek, Contain, Eliminate." The disease was detected in Pakistan and Sudan for the last time in 2000. The last known cases of rinderpest occurred in Kenya in October 2001. It took some time to confirm that rinderpest was indeed finally exterminated, and vaccination continued until 2006. It was not until June 28, 2011, that the FAO and the WHO declared that the disease was eradicated. The destruction of the last remaining stocks of rinderpest virus held in the UK began in June 2019. The eradication of rinderpest was an incredible veterinary achievement and a triumph for the science of immunology.

Sources of Additional Information

Baron, M.D., Banyard, A.C., Parida, S., Barrett, T. (2005). The Plowright vaccine strain of Rinderpest virus has attenuating mutations in most genes. *J Gen Virol,* 86, 1093–10101.

Boylston, A.W. (2018). The myth of the milkmaid. *N Engl J Med,* 378, 414–415.

Bresalier, M., Worboys, M. (2014). 'Saving the lives of our dogs': the development of canine distemper vaccine in interwar Britain. *Br J Hist Sci,* 47, 305–334.

Esparza, J., Schrick, L., Damaso, C.R., Nitsche, A. (2017). Equination (inoculation of horsepox): An early alternative to vaccination (inoculation of cowpox) and the potential role of horsepox virus in the origin of the smallpox vaccine. *Vaccine,* 35, 7222–7230.

Hoenig, L.J., Jackson, A.C., Dickinson, G.M. (2018). The early use of Pasteur's rabies vaccine in the United States. *Vaccine,* 36, 4578–4581.

Lombard, M., Pastoret, P.P., Moulin, A.M. (2007). A brief history of vaccines and vaccination. *Rev Sci Tech,* 26, 29–48.

Mariner, J.C., House, J.A., Mebus, C.A., Sollod, A.E., et al. (2012). Rinderpest eradication: Appropriate technology and social innovations. *Science,* 337, 1309–1312.

Plotkin, S. (2014). History of vaccination. *Proc Natl Acad Sci USA,* 111, 12283–12287.

Roeder, P., Mariner, J., Kock, R. (2013). Rinderpest: the veterinary perspective on eradication. *Philos Trans R Soc Lond B. Biol Sci,* 368, 20120139.

Smith, K.A. (2012). Louis Pasteur, the father of immunology? *Front Immunol,* 3, 68.

Tizard, I. (1999). Grease, anthraxgate, and kennel cough: a revisionist history of early veterinary vaccines. *Adv Vet Med,* 41, 7–24.

Youde, J. (2013). Cattle scourge no more. The eradication of rinderpest and its lessons for global health campaigns. *Politics Life Sci,* 32, 43–45.

The Science Behind Vaccine Use

Both components of the immune system, namely innate immunity and adaptive immunity, are required to generate a strong, effective, protective response to vaccines. Thus the rapidly responding innate immune responses also promote the initial stages of adaptive immunity. We take advantage of this by adding adjuvants to vaccines to initiate these innate responses and so enhance their effectiveness. Innate immune responses are also essential in providing the rapid protective immunity that develops when we use vaccines containing modified live viruses.

There are two major arms of the adaptive immune system. Antibody- mediated responses are optimized for the elimination of extracellular invaders such as bacteria. They are preferentially induced by vaccines containing nonliving antigens. Vaccines can also activate the cell-mediated responses required to eliminate intracellular invaders such as viruses and some specialized bacteria. These cell-mediated responses are preferentially induced by vaccines containing live organisms, especially viruses. The persistence of vaccine-mediated protection is determined by the survival of memory cells that can respond very rapidly to subsequent microbial invasion.

Innate Immunity

All animals need to detect and eliminate microbial invaders as fast and as effectively as possible. This immediate defensive response is the task of the innate immune system. Many different innate defense mechanisms have evolved over time and they all respond rapidly to destroy invaders while minimizing collateral damage. Innate immune responses are activated when cells use their pattern recognition receptors to detect either microbial invasion or tissue damage. For example, cells can sense the presence of invading microbes by detecting their characteristic conserved molecules. These are called *pathogen-associated molecular patterns* (PAMPs). These cells can also sense tissue damage by detecting the characteristic intracellular molecules released from broken cells. These molecules are called *damage associated molecular patterns* (DAMPs).

The body employs sentinel cells whose job it is to detect PAMPs and DAMPs, and once activated, emit signals to attract white blood cells. The white cells converge on the invaders and destroy them in the process we call inflammation. In addition, animals make many different antimicrobial proteins, such as complement, defensins, and cytokines, that can either kill invaders directly or promote their destruction by defensive cells. Some of these antimicrobial molecules are present in normal tissues whereas others are produced in response to the presence of PAMPs or DAMPs—for example, the damage caused by an injected vaccine.

13

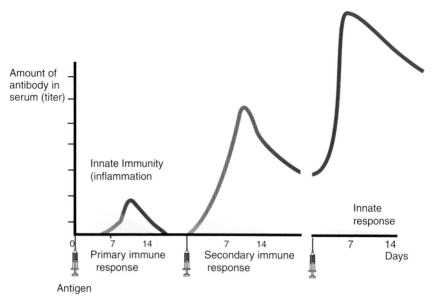

Fig. 2.1   The characteristic time courses of the innate (*blue*) and adaptive (*red line*) immune responses. Repeated administration of a foreign antigen results in massive enhancement of adaptive immunity. As a consequence, innate immune response intensity is reduced. Vaccination exploits these processes to induce prolonged strong immunity and generate long-lived memory cells.

The innate immune system lacks specific memory and, as a result, each episode of infection tends to be treated identically. The intensity and duration of innate responses such as inflammation therefore remain unchanged no matter how often a specific invader is encountered. These responses also come at a price; the pain of inflammation or the mild toxic effects of vaccines largely result from the activation of innate immune processes. More importantly however, the innate immune responses serve as one of the triggers that stimulate antigen-presenting cells to initiate the adaptive immune responses and eventually result in strong long-term protection (Fig. 2.1).

Adaptive Immunity

Adaptive immunity develops when foreign antigens bind to B cell or T cell antigen receptors and trigger strong defensive responses. Adaptive immune responses are the basis of successful vaccination. There is a growing tendency among immunologists to classify these adaptive immune responses into two types. Type 1, or cell-mediated immunity, is mediated by type 1 helper (Th1) cells. Type 1 responses are responsible for immunity to bacteria, viruses, protozoa, and fungi. They generate some antibodies, strong cytotoxic T cell responses, and also activate macrophages. Type 2 immunity in contrast is mediated by type 2 helper (Th2) cells. These cells promote antibody formation. Antibodies generated by type 2 responses are responsible for the destruction of extracellular bacteria and viruses, parasitic helminths and arthropods, and also for allergic reactions.

Note that antibodies and T cells have quite different functions. Thus antibodies are optimized to deal with the organism itself, such as free virus particles and bacteria. T cells, on the other hand, attack and destroy abnormal cells such as those that develop in virus infections or mutated cancer cells. T cells do not recognize free viruses or bacteria. Thus antibodies produced by B cells constitute the primary immune mechanism against extracellular organisms. On the other hand, viruses, bacteria, and protozoa that can live inside cells can only be controlled by T cells. The T cells can either kill the infected cell or release cytokines that inhibit microbial growth. Vaccine usage must take this major divide between antibodies and T cells into account. It is often necessary to design a vaccine that specifically stimulates a type 1 or type 2 response, depending on the nature of the infectious agent.

Adaptive immune responses can be considered to proceed in four major steps (Fig. 2.2). These are: Step 1: Antigen capture and processing; Step 2: Helper T cell activation; Step 3: B cell and/ or cytotoxic T cell mediated responses that eliminate the invaders; and Step 4: The generation and survival of large populations of memory cells. It is these memory cells that provide a vaccinated animal with the ability to respond rapidly and effectively to subsequent microbial infection. When designing an effective vaccine, consideration must be given to optimizing each of these four steps. This can be accomplished by careful selection of appropriate antigens and by the addition of adjuvants that enhance all stages of the process.

STEP 1: ANTIGEN CAPTURE AND PROCESSING

The induction of adaptive immune responses requires the activation of antigen-presenting cells, primarily dendritic cells. This activation is mediated by cytokines generated during the initial innate response. These activated dendritic cells are needed to capture and process exogenous antigens.

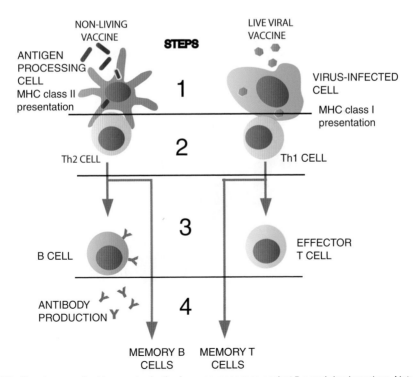

Fig. 2.2 The steps required to mount adaptive immune responses against live and dead vaccines. Note that antibody-mediated responses are induced by nonliving agents, whereas cell-mediated responses require infection by live organisms. *MHC,* Major histocompatibility complex.

Exogenous Antigens

One type of foreign antigen is typified by the invading bacteria that grow in the tissues and extracellular fluid. These live outside cells and so are called *exogenous antigens*. Exogenous antigens must first be captured, processed, and presented in the correct fashion to helper T cells if they are to be recognized as foreign. This is the responsibility of specialized antigen-processing cells.

The most important of these antigen-processing cells are dendritic cells (DCs). DCs have a small cell body with many long cytoplasmic processes known as dendrites. These dendrites increase the efficiency of antigen trapping and maximize the area of contact between DCs and other cell types (Fig. 2.3). Dendritic cells are found throughout the body and form networks in virtually every tissue. They are especially prominent in lymph nodes, skin, and mucosal surfaces, sites where invading microbes are most likely to be encountered.

The number of dendritic cells varies considerably among tissues. Thus DCs are present in high numbers within the dermis. As a result, intradermally administered vaccines are readily recognized. Likewise circulating DCs are common in well-vascularized muscles, the preferred site of injection for many vaccines. There are fewer DCs in the subcutis and adipose tissue, thus explaining why these are usually a less effective routes for vaccine administration.

When DCs encounter foreign antigens and are stimulated by "danger signals," such as DAMPs from tissue damage or PAMPs from infection or from a vaccine, they mature rapidly. This maturation and activation causes DCs to migrate toward the source of the antigen, either at the injection site or in the draining lymph node. (In the absence of these danger signals, DCs will not be activated. Most inactivated vaccines thus require adjuvants to generate the required danger signals.) The activated, mature DCs capture antigens by phagocytosis. If they ingest bacteria, they can usually kill them. The pH within the phagosomes of DCs is less acidic than in other phagocytic cells, and as a result the ingested microbial antigens are not totally degraded but fragments are preserved. These antigen fragments are bound to specialized receptors called major histocompatibility complex (MHC) class II molecules and expressed on the DC surface.

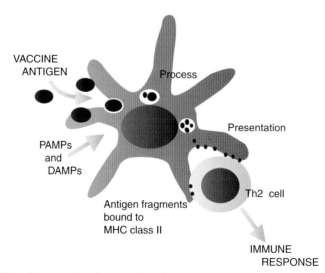

Fig. 2.3 Dendritic cells capture invading organisms, ingest them, and break them up into small fragments. These fragments bind to major histocompatibility complex class II molecules and are carried to the cell surface where they are presented to helper T cells. The process is enhanced by innate immune mechanisms driven by pathogen-associated molecular patterns and damage-associated molecular patterns. Thus innate responses promote adaptive immune responses. *MHC*, Major histocompatibility complex

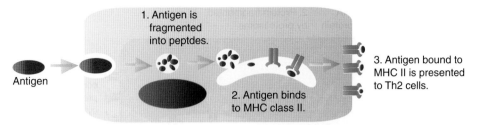

Antigen

1. Antigen is fragmented into peptdes.

2. Antigen binds to MHC class II.

3. Antigen bound to MHC II is presented to Th2 cells.

Fig. 2.4 The processing of exogenous antigens by an antigen-presenting cell. Ingested antigens are incorporated into endosomes where they are fragmented by proteases. The resulting peptides are then transported to the endosomal compartments where they are inserted into the antigen-binding grooves of major histocompatibility complex (*MHC*) class II molecules. These antigen-MHC complexes are then transported to the cell surface where they are presented to helper T cells.

The DCs carry these MHC-bound antigen fragments to lymph nodes where they are presented to helper T cells. The DCs embrace the T cells while the T cells palpate the DCs for the presence of MHC-bound antigen fragments. If the T cell antigen receptors can bind any of these presented fragments, the T cells will respond.

MHC class II molecules are dendritic cell surface receptors that bind processed peptide fragments from exogenous antigens. Exogenous antigen processing involves multiple steps (Fig. 2.4). First, the antigen must be endocytosed and taken into the cell. The ingested proteins are broken up by proteases into peptide fragments of varying length. The endosomes containing these peptide fragments then fuse with other endosomes carrying newly synthesized MHC class II molecules. Once an antigen peptide binds to an MHC molecule, the complex moves to the cell surface. When it reaches the cell surface, the MHC-peptide complex is exposed and made available for inspection by any passing T cell. It has been calculated that an antigen-processing DC contains about 2×10^5 MHC class II molecules that can present peptide fragments to T cells. If costimulation is provided, a single T cell can be activated by binding 200 to 300 of these peptide-MHC complexes. It is therefore possible for a single antigen-processing dendritic cell to present many different antigens to multiple T cells simultaneously. Only a few DCs are needed to trigger a strong T cell response, and one dendritic cell may activate as many as 3000 T cells.

Because helper T cells must recognize MHC-antigen complexes to respond to an antigen, MHC class II molecules effectively determine whether an animal can mount an immune response. Class II molecules can bind some, but not all, peptides created during antigen processing so they select those antigen fragments that are to be presented to the T cells. The response to vaccines is thus controlled by an animal's set of MHC genes—its MHC haplotype.

Endogenous Antigens

A second type of invading organism is typified by viruses that invade cells and force them to make new viral proteins. These "endogenous antigens" are processed by the cells in which they are synthesized.

The function of T cell–mediated immune responses is the detection and destruction of cells producing abnormal or foreign proteins. The best examples of such cells are those infected by viruses. Viruses take over the protein-synthesizing machinery of infected cells and use it to make new viral proteins. To control virus infections, cytotoxic T cells must be able to recognize a virus-infected cell by detecting the viral proteins expressed on its surface. T cells can detect these endogenous antigens, but only after they have been processed and bound to MHC class I molecules (Fig. 2.5).

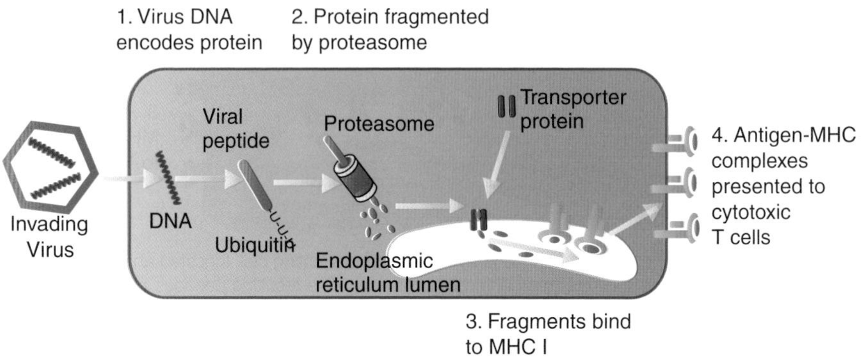

Fig. 2.5 The processing of endogenous antigens. Samples of newly synthesized cellular proteins are labeled with ubiquitin. As a result, they are broken into fragments by proteasomes. The peptides are then carried by transporter proteins to the lumen of the endoplasmic reticulum where they are bound by major histocompatibility complex (*MHC*) class I molecules. The peptide-MHC complexes are then carried to the cell surface where they are presented to cytotoxic T cells. If the proteins originate from a foreign source such as a virus, the infected cell may be killed.

Living cells continually break up and recycle the proteins they produce. As a first step, the protein is tagged with a small protein called ubiquitin. These ubiquinated proteins are recognized by proteasomes, powerful tubular complex proteases. Ubiquinated proteins are inserted into the inner channel of the proteasome, where they are broken into 8 to 15 amino acid peptides like a meat grinder. Some of these peptide fragments are rescued from further destruction by attachment to transport proteins. These fragments are then transported to a newly formed MHC class I molecule. If they fit the MHC antigen-binding site, they will be bound. Once loaded onto the MHC, the MHC-peptide complex is carried to the cell surface and displayed to any passing T cells.

A cell can express about 10^6 MHC-peptide complexes at any one time. A minimum of about 200 MHC class I molecules loaded with the same viral peptide is required to activate a cytotoxic T cell. Thus the MHC-peptide complexes can provide passing T cells with fairly complete information on virtually all the proteins being made by a cell. Analyses of peptide binding indicate that the binding groove of a class I molecule can bind over a million different peptides with various levels of affinity. The number is not unlimited, however, and binding is not always strong. As a result, not all of the antigens within a vaccine may induce a protective immune response. Thus these MHC molecules also determine whether an animal can respond to a specific antigen.

STEP 2: HELPER T CELL ACTIVATION

There are several populations of lymphocytes with antigen-binding receptors. These include helper and regulatory T cells that control immune responses, cytotoxic T cells that destroy abnormal cells, and B cells that produce antibodies. Each of these cell types will respond to any vaccine antigens that can bind to their receptors.

Helper T Cells

Helper T cells are found in follicles and germinal centers within lymph nodes. Each helper T cell is covered by about 30,000 identical antigen receptors. If these receptors bind sufficient antigen in the correct manner, the T cell will initiate an immune response. It does this by secreting multiple cytokines and expressing new cell surface molecules. The other antigen-responsive cell populations, B cells and cytotoxic T cells, cannot respond properly to antigens unless they too are stimulated by helper T cells. There are four major types of helper T cells. These are called: helper 1 (Th1), helper 2 (Th2), helper 17 (Th17), and regulatory (Treg) cells, and each is distinguished by the mixture of cytokines that they secrete as well as their functions. For vaccination purposes, the most important populations are the Th1 and Th2 cells.

T cell antigen receptors (TCRs) form a large diverse repertoire. Any foreign antigen that enters the body will probably encounter and be able to bind to the receptors on at least one T cell. Each T cell has receptors of a single specificity. T cell antigen receptors only recognize antigens attached to MHC molecules. They cannot recognize or respond to free antigen molecules.

The binding of an antigen-MHC complex to a T cell antigen receptor is usually not sufficient by itself to trigger a helper T cell response. Additional signals are needed for the T cell to respond fully. For example, adhesion molecules must bind the T cells and antigen-presenting cells firmly together and permit prolonged, strong signaling between them. TCR-antigen binding triggers the initial signaling steps. Receptors on antigen-presenting cells bind to their ligands on T cells and amplify these signals. T cells must also be stimulated by cytokines secreted by the antigen-presenting cells. These cytokines determine the way in which a T cell responds to antigen by turning on some pathways and turning off others.

When DCs present their antigen load to helper T cells, they generate three signals. The first signal is delivered when T cell antigen receptors bind antigen fragments attached to MHC class II molecules. The second signal provides the cells with additional critical costimulation through contact with other cell surface receptors such as adhesion molecules. The third signal determines the direction in which naïve helper T cells will develop and is provided by secreted cytokines. For example, some microbial antigens trigger DCs to secrete interleukin-12 (IL-12). These are called DC1 cells because their IL-12 activates Th1 cells and so triggers type 1 responses. Other microbial antigens can cause DCs to secrete IL-4, and IL-6. These cytokines stimulate Th2 differentiation and are produced by DC2 cells. They stimulate type 2 responses. It may also be that the same dendritic cell can promote a type 1 or a type 2 response, depending on the dose and type of antigen it encounters. The response may also depend on its location. For example, DCs from the intestine or airways seem to preferentially secrete IL-4 and thus promote type 2 antibody responses.

Because MHC molecules can bind many different antigenic peptides, any individual peptide will only be displayed in small amounts. T cells must be able to recognize these few specific peptide-MHC complexes among a vast excess of MHC molecules carrying irrelevant peptides. The number of MHC-peptide complexes signaling to the T cell is also important because the stimulus needed to trigger a T cell response varies. For example, at least 8000 TCRs must bind antigen for a helper T cell to become activated in the absence of a molecule called CD28, but only about 1000 TCRs need be engaged if CD28 is present. The duration of signaling also determines a T cell's response. In the presence of appropriate antigens, T cells need to bind DCs for less than 15 seconds. T cells can make 30 to 40 DC contacts within a minute. Sustained signaling is however required for maximal T cell activation. Thus during prolonged cell interactions, each MHC-peptide complex may trigger up to 200 TCRs. This serial triggering depends on the kinetics of TCR-ligand interaction. CD28, for example, reduces the time needed to trigger a T cell and lowers the threshold for TCR triggering. Adhesion molecules stabilize the binding of T cells to antigen-processing cells and allow the signal to be sustained for hours.

Naïve T cells have strict requirements for activation. They must receive a sustained signal for at least 10 hours in the presence of costimulation or for up to 30 hours in its absence. This level of costimulation can only be provided by dendritic cells, which supply high levels of costimulatory and adhesion molecules. This is relevant to vaccine usage because once primed, memory T cells become much more responsive to the same antigen.

STEP 3: B AND T CELL RESPONSES

B Cell Responses

As described earlier, the division of the adaptive immune system into two major components is based on the need to recognize two distinctly different forms of foreign invaders: exogenous and endogenous. Antibodies deal with the microbe. They attack bacteria and free virus particles and parasites. Antibodies also provide the first line of defense against organisms that can survive and grow within cells. However, once these organisms succeed in entering cells then cytotoxic T cells are needed to kill the infected cell, release cytokines that inhibit microbial growth, or prevent pathogen survival within cells.

In general, B cell responses are affected by the dose of antigen administered. At priming, higher antigen doses favor the induction of plasma cells over memory cells. Lower doses generally favor memory cell production. At revaccination, higher doses of antigen favor stronger responses. Thus increased doses of antigen, within limits, promote greater B cell responses. On the other hand, very high doses of antigen exert less selective pressure on B cell responses so that cells do not have to compete for limited amounts of antigen and hence lower affinity antibodies can be produced. Adjuvants, by providing the required "danger" signals reduce the dose of antigen needed to induce a protective response. Modified live vaccines that cause local inflammation are "naturally adjuvanted" and are thus more immunogenic than killed/inactivated vaccines. Very few killed vaccines can induce high, sustained antibody responses after a single dose.

B cells are activated within the lymph nodes draining the vaccine injection site. When a B cell encounters an exogenous antigen that binds its receptors, with appropriate costimulation it will respond by secreting these receptors into body fluids, where they are called antibodies. Each B cell is covered with about 200,000 to 500,000 identical antigen receptors (BCRs). Unlike the TCRs, however, BCRs can bind soluble antigens. Antibodies are simply BCRs released into body fluids; they all belong to the family of proteins called immunoglobulins.

Although the binding of antigen to a BCR is an essential first step, this alone is usually insufficient to activate B cells. Complete activation of a B cell also requires multiple costimulatory signals from helper T cells and their cytokines.

When helper T cells "help" B cells they start the process that leads to B cell division and differentiation into antibody-secreting cells. They stimulate B cell proliferation and survival. The "help" also triggers somatic mutation within B cells and thus results in an increase in antibody-binding affinity (Fig. 2.6).

To do all this, however, the helper T cells must themselves recognize the antigen. Helper T cells are essential for the induction of high-affinity antibodies and immune memory. A B cell can capture and process antigen, present it to a helper T cell, and then receive costimulation from the same T cell. B cells thus play two roles. They respond to antigen by making antibodies while at the same time acting as antigen-processing cells. The helper T cells stimulate the B cells using signals from cytokines as well as through interacting receptor pairs.

Bacterial polysaccharides can provoke antibody formation in the absence of helper T cells. These so-called T-independent antigens are usually simple repeating carbohydrate polymers such as *Escherichia coli* lipopolysaccharide, polymerized salmonella flagellin, or pneumococcal polysaccharide. T-independent antigens bind directly to B cell TLRs and cross-link multiple BCRs, thus providing a sufficient signal for B cell proliferation. Characteristically, T-independent antigens such as pure polysaccharide antigens only trigger B cell IgM responses and fail to generate memory cells. They are ineffective in vaccines because they are unable to trigger helper T cells.

When appropriately stimulated and costimulated, B cells divide. This division is asymmetric so that one daughter cell gets a lot of antigen, whereas the other daughter cell gets very little or none. The cell that gets lots of antigen then differentiates into an antibody-producing plasma cell. The cell that gets none continues the cycle of dividing and mutating and eventually becomes a

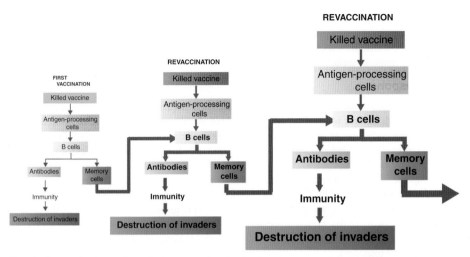

Fig. 2.6 In adaptive immunity on first exposure to a foreign invader or a vaccine, the immune system generates a primary immune response that destroys the invaders, while at the same time generating memory cells. On second exposure to that invader, or revaccination, these memory cells initiate much stronger immune responses that result in a much more efficient elimination of the invaders or stronger protection.

memory cell. The cells destined to become plasma cells develop a rough endoplasmic reticulum, increase their rate of synthesis, and secrete large quantities of immunoglobulins.

A key feature of B cell responses is the progressive increase in the affinity of antibodies for their antigens over time. This is especially important during following vaccination. These changes in antibody affinity take place within germinal centers in lymph nodes and spleen. B cells stimulated by antigen migrate to the germinal centers where they proliferate, while the genes encoding their antibody variable regions mutate. B cells divide every 6 to 8 hours so that within just a few days a single B cell develops into a clone of several thousand cells. During this phase of rapid B cell division, the BCR variable region genes (encoding the antigen-binding sites) mutate randomly on average, once per division. This repeated mutation ensures that the B cells have BCRs that differ from the parent cell. Once these cells have been clonally expanded, they are presented with antigen by the dendritic cells. Because of their mutations, some of these B cells bind the antigen with greater affinity, and others bind it less strongly. A process of selection then occurs. If a mutation has resulted in greater affinity for the antigen, this stimulates more B cell proliferation. If the affinity drops, then B cell stimulation is correspondingly reduced. Thus cycles of somatic mutation and selection lead to a rapid improvement in antigen binding—a process called affinity maturation. These antigen-selected B cells eventually leave the germinal center to form either plasma cells or memory B cells. In contrast, those B cells that have reduced antigen binding will die. Thus the B cell population that emerges from a germinal center is very different from the population of cells that entered it. Likewise the antibodies produced at the beginning of an immune response improve progressively as the response proceeds. In general, higher affinity antibodies are more bactericidal and better able to neutralize viruses and toxins.

Affinity maturation takes time and, in general, the highest affinity antibodies are produced when vaccine doses are well spaced out. This is because antigen concentrations decline over time. When antigen is limiting then it will preferentially stimulate those B cells that can bind it with the greatest affinity.

Antibodies alone can confer protection against many infections. These include diseases caused by microbial intoxication such as tetanus where antibodies neutralize toxins. Antibodies can also inhibit viral binding to susceptible cells and so limit viral spread. Antibodies can kill bacteria by activating complement or opsonizing them, and so reduce bacterial colonization. Oral or intra-nasal vaccines will induce secretory immunoglobin (Ig)A that limits microbial colonization and shedding on mucosal surfaces.

T Cell Responses

Not all invaders are found outside cells. As discussed earlier, all viruses and some bacteria grow inside cells at sites where antibodies cannot go. Antibodies are therefore of limited use in defending the body against such invaders. These intracellular organisms must be eliminated by two different cell-mediated processes. Either infected cells are killed rapidly by cytotoxic T cells so that the invader has no time to grow, or alternatively, infected macrophages develop the ability to destroy the intracellular organisms. In general, organisms such as viruses that enter the cell cytosol or nucleus are killed by T cell cytotoxicity, whereas organisms such as bacteria or parasites that reside within endosomes are destroyed by macrophage activation. T cells mediate both processes. The antigens that trigger these immune responses are endogenous. For this reason the use of live vaccines or vectors (or specialized adjuvants) is necessary for the induction of strong cytotoxic T cell responses.

If endogenous antigens bound to MHC class I molecules trigger a T cell's antigen receptors, it will respond. For example, when a virus infects a cell, T cells recognize the processed viral peptides expressed on the cell surface. The T cells that respond to these endogenous antigens carry the cell surface protein CD8. They use this CD8 to bind the MHC class I molecules on the infected cells, thus promoting cell attachment, intercellular signaling, and the killing of the infected cells.

Different levels of stimulation trigger different activation responses in CD8 T cells. As with helper cells, the duration of the stimulus is important. Although activated cytotoxic T cells can be triggered by brief exposure to antigen, naïve T cells need to be stimulated for several hours before responding. Once activated, naïve $CD8^+$ T cells undergo multiple rounds of division to generate large numbers of cytotoxic effector cells. Some calculations have suggested that they probably divide every 4 to 6 hours and undergo as many as 19 cell divisions in the week following antigen-exposure. These activated cells migrate to lymphoid organs and differentiate into effector and memory cells. Short-lived effector cells form the bulk of the population and these will mostly die once infections are cleared. Cells that may have received less stimulation survive and become long-lived memory cells. The differentiation into these two cell populations is probably due to asymmetric cell division.

Once fully activated, $CD8^+$ T cells leave lymphoid organs and seek out infected cells by themselves. When they recognize a foreign antigen expressed on another cell, the T cells will bind and kill their target. The density of antigen-MHC complexes on a target cell required to stimulate T cell cytotoxicity is much lower than that needed to stimulate cytokine production. Thus T cell recognition of a single antigen-MHC complex may be sufficient to trigger killing of the target. Cytotoxic T cells need to be highly sensitive to viral peptides so that they can kill all the infected cells as soon as possible. Within seconds after contacting a T cell, the target cell begins to undergo apoptosis, and is dead in less than 10 minutes. Cytotoxic T cells can disengage and then move on to kill other target cells within minutes. In addition, several cytotoxic cells can join in killing a single target. Within a few minutes of binding to a target cell, the T cell cytoplasmic granules fuse with the T cell membrane in such a way that their toxic granule contents are injected into the target cell. Cytotoxic T cell granules contain several lethal molecules, of which the most important are perforins, granzymes, and granulysin.

Macrophage Activation

When macrophages attack and ingest invading bacteria, they produce enzymes and oxidants that assist in the killing process. This response, however, may be insufficient to kill some invaders. For example, bacteria such as *L. monocytogenes*, *M. tuberculosis*, and *Brucella abortus*, and protozoa such as *Toxoplasma gondii,* can grow inside normal macrophages. Antibodies are ineffective against these organisms, so protection against this type of infection requires additional macrophage activation.

Macrophages are activated by T cell-derived gamma interferon (IFN-γ). Activated macrophages secrete proteases, cytokines such as interferons, vasoactive molecules, and complement components. They increase expression of MHC class II and promote antigen loading onto MHC molecules, so enhancing antigen presentation. These activated macrophages enlarge and show increased membrane activity, increased formation of pseudopodia, and increased uptake of fluid droplets. They move more rapidly in response to chemotactic stimuli. They contain increased amounts of lysosomal enzymes and respiratory burst metabolites, and they are more avidly phagocytic than normal cells. They produce greatly increased amounts of nitric oxide synthase. As a result, activated macrophages kill intracellular organisms or tumor cells by generating high levels of nitric oxide. The nitric oxide can destroy nearby tumor cells and intracellular bacteria such as *Listeria monocytogenes.*

STEP 4: MEMORY CELL GENERATION

Immunological memory is the ability of the immune system to respond in a faster and stronger manner when it re-encounters the same antigen. This is the basis for adaptive immunity and of vaccination. In addition to mounting an immediate defensive response when encountering antigen, both B cells and T cells set aside a new population of memory cells. These memory cells are able to respond more rapidly and effectively to antigens they re-encounter. The memory cells confer immediate protection and generate secondary immune responses that are much more rapid and effective than primary responses (Fig. 2.7).

Memory B Cells

One reason that the primary antibody response ends is that the responding B cells and plasma cells are short-lived and thus simply removed by apoptosis. If all these cells died, however, immunological memory could not develop. Clearly some B cells must survive as memory cells.

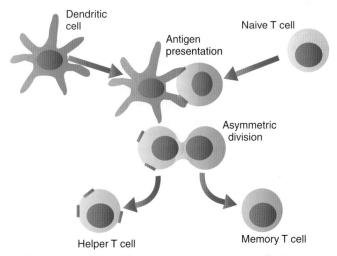

Fig. 2.7 The formation of memory cells. Following the interactions between T cells and antigen-presenting cells, the T cells divide asymmetrically. The pole of the cell that binds the antigen-presenting dendritic cell gives rise to effector cells. The opposite pole gives rise to memory cells. A similar process of asymmetrical cell division likely occurs with B cells as well.

These cells survive within the lymph nodes and bone marrow, where they proliferate, and form germinal centers. (Asymmetric division as described above likely accounts for these two different fates.) These cells persist under the influence of survival and rescue signals. For example, nearby T cells promote expression of *bcl*-2. *Bcl*-2 protects the B cells against apoptosis and allows them to survive. Memory cells thus form a reserve of long-lived antigen-specific stem cells to be called on next time they encounter an antigen.

There are two populations of memory B cell distinguishable by their antibody expression, their location, and their passage through germinal centers. One population consists of small, long-lived resting cells that look like generic lymphocytes. Their survival does not depend on antigen contact. Once re-exposed to antigen, they proliferate and differentiate into plasma cells without undergoing further mutation. It has been calculated that in a secondary immune response, the clonal expansion of these memory B cells results in 8- to 10-fold more plasma cells than in a primary immune response.

A second memory B cell population consists of large, dividing plasma cells. These cells are found in germinal centers, where their continued survival depends on exposure to small amounts of persistent antigen on dendritic cells. This long-lived memory population can survive for months or years. (In humans these plasma cells have a half-life of 8–15 years.) The antibodies they produce provide immediate immunity to microbial pathogens. These long-lived plasma cells probably develop in the bone marrow from a population of self-renewing, long-lived, slowly dividing memory B cells. These memory B cells require functional antigen receptors to survive, suggesting that constant antigen binding keeps them alive. For example, cats immunized with killed panleukopenia virus will continue to produce antibodies at low levels for many years. The source of these antibodies is believed to be the long-lived plasma cells stimulated to secrete antibodies by exposure to PAMPs and T cell help.

In general, only live attenuated viral vaccines (or virus-like particles, Chapter 3) can induce antibody responses that persist for many years in the absence of antigen re-exposure. If vaccines are administered too frequently, this will interfere with the generation of memory cells and thus reduce protection. Optimal boosting responses generally require long intervals between doses. In humans this is at least 3 to 4 months. A similar consideration applies to revaccination of animals. The longer the interval, the better the secondary response.

If a second dose of antigen is given to a primed animal, it will encounter large numbers of memory B cells, which respond in the manner described previously. As a result, a secondary immune response is much greater than a primary immune response. The lag period is shorter because more antibodies are produced, and they can be detected earlier. IgG is also produced in preference to the IgM characteristic of the primary response. In addition, memory B cells characteristically display and secrete antibodies with a much higher antigen affinity than primary plasma cells because of somatic mutation and affinity maturation.

Note that memory B cells do not produce antibodies and thus are not protective. If they are to be protective they must be reactivated by exposure to antigen. This may result from infection, or from cross-reaction with antigens produced by the normal microbiota. Once activated, they proliferate and differentiate rapidly into high-affinity antibody-producing plasma cells. This recall response requires less antigen and does not absolutely require CD4+ T cell help. As a result, the secondary response is much more rapidly established.

Memory T Cells

Naïve CD8$^+$T cells are long-lived cells that continuously recirculate between tissues, the blood-stream, and lymphoid organs. Once they encounter antigen, they multiply rapidly in an effort to keep pace with the growth of invading pathogens. The number of responding cells may increase more than 1000-fold within a few days. They reach a peak 5 to 7 days after infection when pathogen-specific, cytotoxic T cells can make up 50% to 70% of the total CD8$^+$ T cell population. In contrast to the prolonged B cell responses, however, the effector phase of T cell responses is relatively brief. Indeed, cytotoxicity is seen only in the presence of antigen. This is logical. Excessive sustained cytotoxic activities by T cells or overproduction of cytokines could cause severe tissue damage.

As with other lymphocytes, asymmetric division of an effector T cell generates two daughter cells with different fates. The T cell begins to divide even before it separates from the antigen-presenting cell. The dividing T cell is polarized because one pole of the cell contains the antigen-binding structures. The other pole contains molecules excluded from the contact site. Thus when the cell divides, it forms two distinctly different daughter cells. The daughter cell adjacent to the contact site is the precursor of the effector T cells. The daughter cell formed at the opposite pole is the precursor of the memory T cells. The proximal cell has increased expression of effector molecules. The distal cell has increased lipid metabolism, increased expression of antiapoptotic molecules and lives very much longer. Once the infection has been eliminated, up to 95% of effector T cells undergo apoptosis 1 to 2 weeks after infection.

Memory T cells persist for a very long time lurking in the tissues and lymphoid organs and remaining, in effect, functionally silent until they re-encounter antigen. When that happens they respond very rapidly indeed.

Because they quietly persist in the body, memory T cells are effectively turned off. Their DNA remains active, but they use epigenetic checkpoint mechanisms to block the transcription of cytokine genes. Thus memory T cells contain the RNA transcripts for cytokines such as IFN-γ, but these are not translated into proteins in the absence of antigen. Memory T cells accumulate over an animal's life and can be the most abundant T cell population in older animals. Compared with naïve T cells, memory T cells are easier to activate, live longer, and have enhanced effector activity. As a result, they mount a strong rapid cytokine response when they next encounter the antigen and can provide life-long protection against pathogens.

Three types of memory T cells have been identified. These are central memory cells (Tcm), effector memory T cells (Tem), and tissue-resident memory T cells.

Tcm cells circulate through secondary lymphoid tissues, such as lymph nodes, awaiting the arrival of invaders. They lack immediate effector function but have very rapid proliferative responses. Their role is to recognize antigens presented by DCs and undergo rapid proliferation and differentiation so generating a large wave of effector cells.

Tem cells, in contrast, circulate through nonlymphoid tissues and survey frontline barriers and diseased tissues for invading pathogens. They have receptors enabling them to converge on inflamed tissues, where they immediately recognize and attack invaders without the need to differentiate further. Antigen persistence regulates the relative proportions of Tcm and Tem cells. Tcm cells predominate when the antigen is effectively cleared from the body whereas Tem cells predominate in chronic infections where the antigen persists.

Tissue-resident memory T cells occupy organs such as the skin, lungs, and intestine. They provide a first response to pathogens invading through mucosal surfaces. They rapidly produce cytokines after infection. They do not circulate in peripheral blood.

All three memory T cell populations express either CD4 or CD8 and persist in the absence of antigen. CD8+ memory cells tend to accumulate under epithelial surfaces, whereas CD4+ memory cells are scattered through the tissues in memory lymphocyte clusters. These cells slowly divide and replenish their numbers. They can be thought of as adult stem cells. The size of the immune system is fixed somewhat, but the Tem cell pool can double without loss of preexisting memory cells.

The survival of memory T cells depends upon the presence of two cytokines, IL-7 and IL-15. These survival cytokines maintain the memory cells in a state of continuous slow proliferation. Bacterial PAMPs such as the lipopeptides may also promote the long-term survival of memory T cells even in the absence of persistent antigen.

Memory T cells can be distinguished from naïve T cells by their phenotype, by secreting a different mixture of cytokines, and by their behavior. For example, memory T cells express high levels of a receptor that binds both IL-2 and IL-15. They express increased amounts of adhesion molecules, so they can bind more efficiently to antigen-presenting cells. They produce more IL-4 and IFN-γ and respond more strongly to stimulation of their TCR. They continue to divide very slowly, in the absence of antigen.

Over an animal's lifetime, immunological memories accumulate. Older animals have more memory cells than young animals and are thus much better prepared to respond to antigens than younger animals. Repeated vaccination generates new memory cells. However, the size of the memory cell compartment expands to accommodate them. Previously generated memory cells are not removed to make space for the newcomers.

A Word of Caution

Immunologic memory is real in the sense that most animals or people only develop many infectious diseases once, perhaps when young, and their subsequent resistance may persist for the rest of their life. This has been attributed to long-lived memory cells. There is however a second reason for prolonged immunity—inadvertent boosting. Thus for many common infections an individual may indeed develop immunological memory but they may then be boosted by exposure to that agent in the course of daily life. A good example was measles where a single infection appeared to confer life-long immunity. When measles was a common infection, individuals would encounter the virus repeatedly and be boosted without realizing it. Now that measles is rare it is clear that human immunologic memory is by no means as prolonged as once thought. We no longer regularly encounter measles virus and repeated revaccination is now required to maintain immunity. A similar phenomenon may occur with common animal infections such as *Bordetella bronchiseptica,* one cause of kennel cough in dogs.

Sources of Additional Information

Barnett, B.E., Ciocca, M.L., Goenka, R., Barnett, L.G., Wu, J., Laufer, T.M., et al. (2012). Asymmetric B cell division in the germinal center reaction. *Science,* 335, 342–344.

Brodovitch, A., Bongrand, P., Pierres, A. (2013). T lymphocytes sense antigens within seconds and make a decision within one minute. *J Immunol,* 191, 2064–2071.

Ciocca, M.L., Barnett, B.E., Burkhardt, J.K., Chang, J.T., Reiner, S.L. (2012). Cutting edge: Asymmetric memory T cell division in response to rechallenge. *J Immunol,* 188, 4145–4148.

Cresswell, P., Lanzavecchia, A. (2001). Antigen processing and recognition. *Curr Opin Immunol,* 13, 11–12.

Iwasaki, A., Medzhitov, R. (2010). Regulation of adaptive immunity by the innate immune system. *Science,* 327, 291–295.

Jensen, P.E. (2007). Recent advances in antigen processing and presentation. *Nat Immunol,* 8, 1041–1048.

Pichichero, M.E. (2008). Vaccine-induced immunologic memory and pace of pathogenesis: predicting the need for boosters. *Expert Rev Vaccines,* 7, 1299–1303.

Summerfield, A., Auray, G., Ricklin, M. (2015). Comparative dendritic cell biology of veterinary mammals. *Ann Rev Anim Biosci*, 3, 533–557.

Schenkel, J.M., Masopust, D. (2014). Tissue-resident memory T cells. *Immunity,* 41, 886–897.

Sprent, J., Tough, D.F. (2001). T cell death and memory. *Science*, 293, 245–247.

Vezys, V., Yates, A., Casey, K.A., et al. (2009). Memory CD8 T-cell compartment grows in size with immunological experience. *Nature*, 457, 196–200.

Zimmermann, P., Curtis, N. (2018). The influence of the intestinal microbiome on vaccine responses. *Vaccine,* 36, 4433–4439.

Zinkernagel, R.M. (2018). What if protective immunity is antigen-driven and not due to so-called "memory" B and T cells? *Immunol Rev,* 283, 238–246.

Nonliving Vaccines

Soon after Louis Pasteur identified the basic principles of vaccinology, Salmon and Smith demonstrated that killed Salmonella bacteria could serve as an effective vaccine. This simple empirical approach was rapidly adopted, and many diverse killed bacterial vaccines were rapidly developed. For example, killed typhoid vaccines were administered to British soldiers by the end of the nineteenth century. They worked but were somewhat toxic and caused significant morbidity. Today whole-cell killed *Bordetella pertussis* vaccine is still given to children in many countries to protect against whooping cough because it is cheaper than the less toxic acellular vaccine.

This approach to developing vaccines can be summarized as "isolate, inactivate, and inject." This has worked well and is especially effective in the production of autogenous vaccines (Chapter 18). The great advantages of this type of vaccine are its safety and simplicity—and thus reduced cost.

Technically speaking the term "killed vaccines" applies to the death of living organisms such as bacteria. Likewise, the term "inactivated vaccines" applies to the treatment of molecular constructs such as viruses.

This type of vaccine may contain either a very complex antigenic mixture such as that found in killed whole organisms, or the vaccine components may be purified to various degrees. Unnecessary or toxic components may be removed, but the vaccine may be enriched with those antigens that are directly responsible for the protective immune response. The degree of purification demanded will depend upon the costs of the purification process and any adverse effects mediated by the unwanted/unnecessary components.

The major problem with these nonliving vaccines is that they cannot invade host cells. As a result, they act as exogenous antigens and stimulate type 2 immune responses and antibody formation rather than type 1 cell mediated responses. Therefore they may provide only weak or transient immunity against viruses or intracellular bacteria. In addition, killed vaccines, depending upon their purity and toxicity, may require administration of multiple doses to generate strong prolonged immunity. Each vaccine dose increases the chances of the recipient developing allergic or other adverse reactions. In many cases these killed/inactivated/subunit vaccines also require adjuvants that carry with them the potential to induce innate immune responses resulting in other problems.

Until the 1990s, most veterinary vaccines either contained inactivated/killed organisms that were adjuvanted with alum or oil, or they were modified live vaccines (Table 3.1). Increased knowledge of microbial genetics has revolutionized the way in which vaccine antigens can be generated. These vaccines may now contain cultures of organisms that have been killed by

TABLE 3.1 ■ The Advantages and Disadvantages of Living and Inactivated Vaccines

Advantages of Killed Vaccines	Advantages of Modified Live Vaccines
No reversion to virulence or toxicity	Stimulates CMI in addition to antibodies
No mutation or recombination	Cheap
Stable on storage	No need for adjuvants
No residual virulence	Fewer boosters required
Fewer regulatory constraints	Can be used on mucosal surfaces

CMI, Cell-mediated immunity.

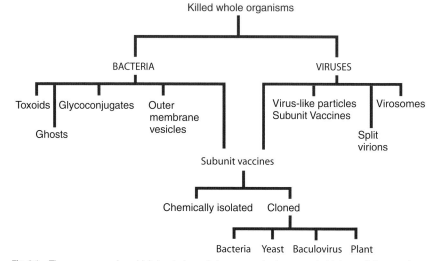

Fig. 3.1   The many ways by which bacteria and viruses can be incorporated into nonliving vaccines.

chemical or physical means; inactivated toxins (toxoids); or highly purified subunits, the antigenic components of microorganisms that have been purified from cultures by chemical or physical processes, or have been produced by recombinant DNA techniques (Fig. 3.1).

Bacterial Vaccines

Methods of Inactivation

Organisms killed for use in vaccines must remain as structurally similar to the living organisms as possible. Therefore crude methods of killing that cause major changes in antigen structure as a result of protein denaturation are usually unsatisfactory. Chemical inactivation must not alter the structure of the antigens responsible for stimulating protective immunity. One such chemical is formaldehyde, which cross-links multiple lysine residues on the toxin to form highly stable methylene bridges. These confer structural rigidity on these proteins and neutralize their toxicity. Proteins may also be mildly denatured by acetone or alcohol treatment. Alkylating agents that cross-link nucleic acid chains are also suitable for killing organisms because by leaving the surface proteins of organisms unchanged, they do not affect their antigenicity. Examples of alkylating agents include ethylene oxide, ethyleneimine, acetyl ethyleneimine, and β-propiolactone, all of which are used in veterinary vaccines (Fig. 3.2).

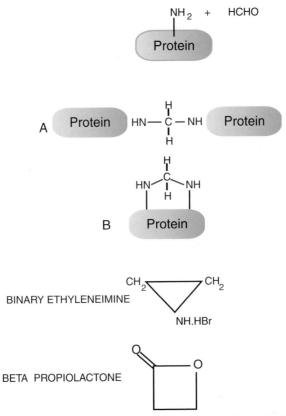

Fig. 3.2 The cross-linking effect of formaldehyde by generating methylene bridges. The figure also shows the structure of binary ethyleneimine and β-propiolactone, two major microbial inactivating agents used in veterinary vaccines.

BACTERINS

Vaccines containing whole, killed bacteria are called bacterins. The bacteria can be grown in large volumes in bioreactors. It is usual to then kill the bacteria with formaldehyde and add aluminum or oil-emulsion adjuvants. The formaldehyde can be neutralized with sodium thiosulfate or sodium bisulfite. The antibody responses to these vaccines are directed against many different bacterial antigens, both essential and unimportant. The immunity produced by these simple bacterins is relatively short-lived, usually lasting no longer than one year and sometimes considerably less. For instance, a formalized swine erysipelas (*Erysipelothrix rhusiopathiae*) bacterin protects pigs for only four to five months. *Streptococcus equi* bacterins protect horses for less than one year, even though recovery from a natural case of strangles may confer a lifelong immunity.

One important issue, especially when using coliform and *Campylobacter* bacterins, is that of strain specificity. Multiple strains of each organism occur in nature, and successful vaccination requires immunization with appropriately matched strains. This is sometimes not possible if a commercial vaccine is employed. One method of overcoming this difficulty is to use autogenous vaccines. These are vaccines that contain organisms obtained either from animals on the farm where the disease problem is occurring, or from the infected animal itself. These can be very successful if carefully prepared because the vaccine will contain all the antigens required for protection in that specific location. As an alternative to the use of autogenous vaccines, some manufacturers produce polyvalent vaccines containing a mixture of antigenic types. For example, leptospirosis vaccines commonly contain up to five different serovars. This practice, although effective, is inefficient because only a few of the antigenic components employed may be required in any given location.

Although simple to make and generally inexpensive, bacterins are not always effective. They also may contain unwanted toxic components such as endotoxins. For this reason, many companies purify bacterins at additional cost. Remember too that not all the antigens in a bacterium can trigger a protective immune response. Some antigens, such as those found on the bacterial surface, are of much greater importance than internal proteins. Thus to the extent afforded by economics, efficacy, and safety, inactivated vaccines may be purified. Killed bacterial vaccines are usually stable in storage so that maintenance of the cold chain is not a major issue. Once the antigens are purified, then the vaccine can be formulated by adding adjuvants to enhance its immunogenicity and stabilizers to increase its storage life. If it is to be used in multidose vials, then preservatives must also be added.

TOXOIDS

Many bacterial pathogens cause disease by producing potent exotoxins. The most important are toxins from the Clostridia: *Clostridium tetani*, *Clostridium perfringens*, and *Clostridium botulinum*. The immunoprophylaxis of tetanus is restricted to toxin neutralization. *Cl. tetani* produces a toxin called tetanospasmin. This acts on presynaptic motor nerve cells to cause excessive motor neuron activity leading to extreme muscle spasms, respiratory paralysis, and death. Growing *Cl. tetani* in a semisynthetic medium produces large quantities of toxin. The toxin is released into the supernatant and can be treated with formaldehyde to fix the protein and block the conformational changes that make it toxic. It is then called tetanus toxoid. Next, the supernatant is ultrafiltered to get rid of unwanted proteins. Toxoids are available for most clostridial diseases and for infections caused by *Mannheimia haemolytica*. A toxoid is also available for vaccination against bites from *Crotalus atrox,* the Western diamondback rattlesnake.

Tetanus toxoid with an aluminum hydroxide adjuvant is given by intramuscular injection for routine prophylaxis, and a single injection of this vaccine will induce protective immunity in 10 to 14 days. The antibodies directed against the toxin have a higher affinity for the toxin than does the toxin receptor. Thus in infected wounds the antibodies bind the toxin as it is produced. The toxin molecules cannot therefore bind their receptors on neurons and are effectively neutralized. Antitoxins to the other clostridial toxins such as *Cl. botulinum* or *Cl. perfringens* act in a similar matter.

Toxoids are safe and cannot revert to virulence. They cannot spread to other animals. They are very stable and resistant to damage by temperature and light. They generally induce good humoral immunity but not cell-mediated immunity. As with other nonliving vaccines, toxoids are not always highly immunogenic. As a result, multiple doses may be needed to assure immunity. Additionally, an adjuvant, usually an aluminum salt, must be incorporated into the vaccine. Local reactions such as redness, swelling, and induration at the injection site may develop within a few hours. These usually resolve within 72 hours.

Conventional immunological wisdom would suggest that the use of antibodies against tetanus toxin (tetanus immune globulin) should interfere with the immune response to toxoid and must therefore be avoided. This is not a problem in practice however, and both may be successfully administered simultaneously (at different sites) without problems. This may be because of the relatively small amount of immune globulin usually needed to protect animals.

BACTERIN-TOXOIDS

Some veterinary vaccines combine both toxoids and killed bacteria in a single dose by the simple expedient of adding formaldehyde to a whole culture. These products, sometimes called anacultures or bacterin-toxoids, are used to vaccinate against *Clostridium haemolyticum* and *Cl. perfringens*. Trypsinization of the mixture may make it more immunogenic. Other bacterin-toxoids may have improved efficacy by adding other purified immunogenic antigens. For example, *Escherichia coli* bacterins against enteric colibacillosis in calves and pigs may be made more effective by the addition of additional fimbrial adhesion proteins such as F4 (K88), F5 (K99), F6, F7, and F18. Antibodies to these antigens prevent *Escherichia coli* binding to the intestinal wall and thus contribute significantly to protection. Similarly, *Mannheimia* bacterins enriched with the white cell-killing leukotoxoid are more effective than conventional bacterins in preventing bovine respiratory disease.

Subunit Vaccines

One problem with the use of whole killed organisms in vaccines is that they contain many components that are either nonantigenic or induce nonprotective responses, or, most importantly, may be toxic or allergenic. Thus in the interests of safety and efficacy it is often desirable to isolate and purify individual microbial antigens or subunits. These subunit vaccines may be isolated by classical physicochemical fractionation techniques or by gene cloning. Subunit vaccines only contain a part of the target organism and as a result vaccinated animals only respond to those subunits. By definition they are noninfectious and nonreplicating. Their great advantages include not only increased safety and reduced toxicity, but also the potential to use antibody assays to distinguish vaccinated from infected animals.

An example of the importance of subunit vaccines is seen when vaccinating against either *Bordetella pertussis* in children or *Bordetella bronchiseptica* in dogs. Originally these infections were controlled by the use of whole heat-killed bacterial vaccines. Unfortunately they had significant toxicity and induced inflammation and "soreness" in vaccinated children. Because of these problems, there has been a transition to the use of "acellular" vaccines. These contain a mixture of purified bacterial subcomponents. There are several different vaccines of this type because there is no consensus on the ideal composition of an acellular vaccine. They differ in the number of subunits included such as pertussis toxin, filamentous hemagglutinin, outer membrane proteins, or fimbrial antigens. These acellular vaccines also contain much less endotoxin and are thus considerably less toxic than whole cell vaccines. Although widely accepted, they are somewhat less effective with a shorter duration of immunity besides being more expensive.

CORE ANTIGENS

Another approach to the development of subunit vaccines against gram-negative bacteria is the use of common core antigens. The outer layer of the gram-negative bacterial cell wall consists of lipopolysaccharide. This lipopolysaccharide is formed by a variable oligosaccharide (O antigen) bound to a highly conserved core polysaccharide and to lipid A. The O antigen varies greatly among gram-negative bacteria so that an immune response against one O antigen confers no immunity against bacteria expressing other O antigens. In contrast, the underlying core polysaccharide is conserved between gram-negative bacteria of different species and genera. Thus an immune response directed against this common core structure has the potential to protect against many different gram-negative bacteria. Mutant strains of *E. coli* (J5) and *Salmonella enterica* Minnesota and Typhimurium (Re) have been used as sources of core antigen. J5 is a rough mutant that is deficient in uridine diphosphate galactose 4-epimerase. As a result, the organism makes an

incomplete oligosaccharide side chain, and has lost most of the outer lipopolysaccharide structure. Immunization with a J5 bacterin thus provides protection against multiple gram-
negative bacteria such as *E. coli, Klebsiella pneumoniae, Actinobacillus pleuropneumoniae,* and
Haemophilus influenzae (type B). A J5 bacterin has also been reported to protect calves against
organisms such as *S. enterica* Typhimurium and *E. coli,* and pigs against *A. pleuropneumoniae.*
The most encouraging results have been obtained when vaccinating against coliform mastitis
(Chapter 16).

GLYCOCONJUGATE VACCINES

Many important bacterial antigens consist of capsular polysaccharides or glycoproteins whose
immunogenic structures are carbohydrate side-chains. Unlike protein antigens that trigger
T cell-dependent B cell responses, bacterial polysaccharides cannot bind to MHC molecules
and hence cannot trigger T cell help (They are "T-independent"), and they also cannot trigger
the reactions needed for survival, affinity, maturation and extensive B cell proliferation. As
a result, B cells can only produce low affinity immunoglobin (Ig)M antibodies against polysaccharides. They do not induce an IgM to IgG switch, they fail to induce a booster response,
and they do not induce T cell memory. Thus pure bacterial polysaccharides are very poor
vaccine antigens (Fig. 3.3).

However, if these same polysaccharides are chemically conjugated to a carrier protein, the
complex will elicit a T-dependent response and memory B cells that can be effectively boosted
by the same glycoconjugate. This method has therefore been used very successfully to develop
effective glycoconjugate vaccines.

Glycoconjugate vaccines against meningococcus, pneumococcus, and *H. influenzae* are available and highly efficacious in adult humans. (They are however poorly immunogenic in infants

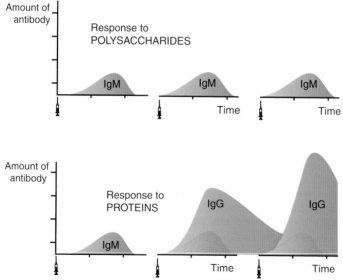

Fig. 3.3 Immune responses to carbohydrate antigens and to glycoconjugate vaccines. T-independent antigens such as polysaccharides do not stimulate a class switch, they do not increase in antibody affinity, and
they do not stimulate immunologic memory. They make very poor vaccines until chemically linked to a protein
carrier molecule. *Ig,* Immunoglobin.

and the elderly.) The Vi polysaccharide of *Salmonella typhi* is also rendered much more immunogenic by conjugation to several carrier proteins. Examples of carrier proteins include tetanus and diphtheria toxoids, in addition to bacterial proteins from *Neisseria meningitides* and *H. influenzae*. Thus Prevnar 13 is a pneumococcal vaccine for humans consisting of a mixture of pneumococcal polysaccharides from 13 pneumococcal serotypes chemically conjugated to a nontoxic variant of diphtheria toxin.

In attempting to vaccinate pigs against *A. pleuropneumoniae* a glycoconjugate vaccine has been prepared by coupling the serotype-1 capsular polysaccharide (CP) or the lipopolysaccharide (LPS) to the *A. pleuropneumoniae* hemolysin protein. Pigs receiving these experimental vaccines made antibodies against both the CP and the LPS. Similar successes have been obtained in mice by conjugating *M. haemolytica* O-specific polysaccharide to bovine serum albumin. It has even proved possible to engineer *E. coli* to produce and export glycoconjugates with the polysaccharides already linked to carrier proteins. These will greatly simplify production and reduce the cost of these vaccines.

OUTER MEMBRANE VESICLES

Outer membrane vesicles (OMVs) are spherical particles 20 to 300 nm in diameter released by gram-negative bacteria. They are generated by the budding out of the bacterial outer membrane and thus contain many bacterial membrane components. OMVs are highly immunogenic and can induce potent protective immune responses. An antiNeisseria OMV-based vaccine is available for humans. Bacteria can be engineered to increase vesicle production, reduce LPS toxicity, and increase expression of protective antigens. OMVs are readily phagocytosed by antigen processing cells and carry many pathogen-associated molecular patterns (PAMPs) including LPS, lipoproteins, and peptidoglycans. They induce a potent type 1 immune response. They can be readily obtained in large quantities from culture supernatants. Their main limitation is their strain specificity.

Other heterologous proteins may be incorporated into OMVs. For example, Leishmania antigens have been incorporated into *E. coli* OMVs. Very encouraging results have been obtained using OMVs derived from *B. bronchiseptica* to protect experimental animals.

CLONED ANTIGENS

Gene cloning is a technology that can be used to produce large very quantities of purified microbial antigen for use in vaccines (Fig. 3.4). In this process DNA encoding the antigen of interest is first isolated from the pathogen. This DNA is then inserted into a plasmid that is then transfected into a bacterium or yeast in such a way that it is functional. The recombinant protein is expressed in large amounts when the bacteria or yeast are grown.

E. coli has been widely used as the host organism that can be readily transfected with a plasmid containing the gene encoding the vaccine antigen of interest. The recombinant *E. coli* can then be induced to synthesize large amounts of this specific protein. There are however limitations to this process because the new protein may be incorrectly folded, and its posttranslational modifications, such as glycosylation, may also be wrong. Removing unwanted *E. coli* components may also be difficult or expensive.

As an alternative to *E. coli*, the methyltrophic yeast *Pichia pastoris* has been used as a source of recombinant antigens for vaccine use. This yeast secretes the expressed proteins, is high yielding, and generates appropriate posttranslational modifications. The cloned antigens are expressed in their native form so that protein folding is appropriate and conformational epitopes can be generated (Chapter 5). The other widely employed yeast expression system has been baker's yeast, *Saccharomyces cerevisiae*.

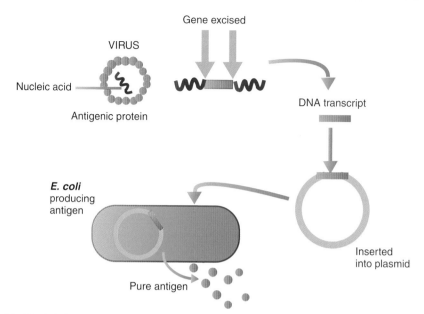

Fig. 3.4 The isolation and purification of microbial antigens through gene cloning. Thus the gene encoding the protective antigen from the organism of interest is incorporated into a plasmid. It is then inserted into a vector such as *Escherichia coli*. The gene product is thus expressed in the bacterium in large quantities.

A third possible source of recombinant antigens for vaccines is through the use of an insect baculovirus vector called nuclear polyhedrosis virus from the "alfalfa looper" moth (*Autographa californica*). Baculoviruses are insect viruses that have a promoter region that causes them to make enormous quantities of the viral polyhedron protein. Replacing the polyhedron gene with a gene encoding the antigen of interest thus generates large amounts of the new recombinant protein. Baculoviruses also grow in insect ovarian cells (from the Fall armyworm). This makes them inherently safe because they are unable to grow in mammalian cells. Additionally, there is no known adventitious agent that can grow in both insect and mammalian cells. This methodology has been developed for the production of vaccines against porcine circovirus type 2 and classical swine fever virus as well as influenza virus. Glycosylation and posttranslational folding may also differ from that in mammalian cells

An example of a recombinant antibacterial vaccine is that directed against the Lyme disease agent, *Borrelia burgdorferi*. Thus the gene for OspA, the immunodominant outer surface lipoprotein of *B. burgdorferi*, has been cloned into *E. coli*. The recombinant protein expressed by the *E. coli* is purified and used as a vaccine when combined with adjuvant. This vaccine is unique because ticks feeding on immunized animals ingest the antibodies made by the vaccinated animal. These antibodies then kill the bacteria within the tick midgut and so prevent their dissemination to the tick salivary glands. They thus prevent transmission by the tick vector.

Gene cloning techniques are useful in any situation where pure protein antigens need to be produced in large quantities. Unfortunately, as described earlier, very pure proteins are often poor antigens because they are not effectively delivered to antigen-sensitive cells and may not be correctly folded. They also lack the PAMPs released by intact organisms so they fail to generate innate immune responses. An alternative method of delivering a recombinant antigen in a vaccine is to clone the gene of interest into an attenuated living carrier organism (Chapter 4).

IRON TRANSPORT PROTEINS

Iron is an essential growth factor for many pathogenic bacteria. The bacteria take up iron from their environment by the use of iron-binding proteins called siderophores. These siderophores have such a high affinity for ferric iron that they can take it from the host's iron-binding proteins. Bacteria have a siderophore receptor on their outer membrane that facilitates the transfer of this iron into the cell. Antibodies directed specifically against these siderophores or their cell surface receptors (porins) will effectively block bacterial iron acquisition and thus inhibit bacterial growth. If bacteria are cultured in a low iron environment, they express increased quantities of their iron acquisition proteins. These can be harvested and their siderophore receptors and porins (SRP®) purified. These proteins can then be used in vaccines.

The SRP antigens of the major gram-negative enterobacteria are highly conserved. As a result, SRP-containing vaccines have been successfully used to control Klebsiella mastitis in dairy cattle and for reducing the burden of O157:H7 *E. coli* in feedlot cattle. An SRP vaccine directed against *S. enterica*, serotype Newport, increased milk production in uninfected dairy cattle.

BACTERIAL GHOSTS

Bacterial "ghosts" are the empty cell envelopes of gram-negative bacteria. They have no cytoplasm and no chromosomal or plasmid DNA, but have a conserved cellular morphology and all cell surface structures. They are constructed using the cloned bacteriophage lysis gene, E. This protein fuses the inner and outer membranes of gram-negative bacteria to form a transmembrane pore through which the bacterial cytoplasm escapes. For safety reasons, any remaining DNA is destroyed by nucleases during the production process. Thus these ghosts contain no genetic information. However, when used as vaccines they are highly immunogenic. Because of their structure they have intrinsic adjuvant activity and can induce both adaptive and innate immune responses. Once lyophilized they are very stable. These ghosts appear to be excellent alternatives to killed bacterial vaccines (especially because their antigenic components are not denatured). Bacterial ghost technology has been applied to the pig pathogen, *A. pleuropneumoniae*. When administered orally it generated sterile immunity and cross-protection between serotypes. When given intramuscularly it was protective but did not induce sterile immunity. Ghosts have also been generated against the bovine pathogens *Pasteurella multocida* and *M. haemolytica*. They appear to be very effective in many animal experimental systems. Ghosts have also been prepared against diverse veterinary gram-negative pathogens, especially Salmonellae and *E. coli*, with encouraging results.

VIRAL VACCINES
Whole Virus Vaccines

There are many different ways of making antiviral vaccines (Fig. 3.5). Vaccines may simply contain inactivated viruses. The classical example of this is Jonas Salk's poliomyelitis vaccine that consisted of formalized monkey cell tissue culture derived virus. Similar to killed bacterial vaccines these inactivated viral vaccines are cheap to produce and relatively safe. For example, influenza vaccines are made by first growing large quantities of the influenza virus in embryonated chicken eggs. The virus is isolated and then broken up with detergents. The important influenza virus antigen, the hemagglutinin, is then purified and is the major vaccine immunogen. However, immunity to killed viruses such as influenza may be short-lived. One additional problem with viral vaccines is that many of the important viruses such as influenza or bluetongue consist of multiple highly variable strains. Consequently, they may not be effective when strains change and new vaccines must be produced at regular intervals.

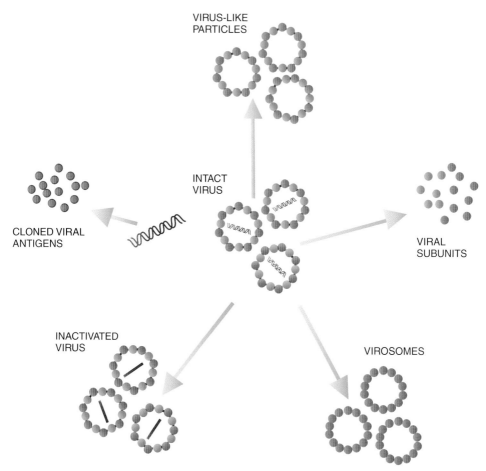

Fig. 3.5 The many ways by which viral antigens can be incorporated into vaccines.

VIRUS-LIKE PARTICLES

In general, resistance to virus infections depends on an immune response directed against antigens on the surface of the virus or on virus-infected cells. Subunit vaccines directed against isolated surface antigens tend to be poorly immunogenic. Virus-like particles (VLPs) are subunit vaccines that assemble into structures resembling the outer protein shell of viruses. They do not contain a viral genome and cannot spread the infection (Fig. 3.6). They have the same shape and size as native viruses such as icosahedrons or rods. VLPs are diverse nanoparticles 20 to 800 nm in size. They may be made using viral protein subunits to form, in effect, a natural viral capsid. Subunit vaccines, as described earlier, are often poor immunogens because of incorrect folding or poor presentation to antigen presenting cells. VLPs in contrast, are the optimal size and present dense repeating protein arrays and conformational epitopes similar to those of intact viruses. Thus VLPs can serve as modular vaccine platforms for a diverse range of viral diseases.

VLPs present the immune system with multiple viral epitopes in the correct conformation. Because they are composed of viral proteins, they can activate helper T cells, induce a strong

WHOLE VIRUS 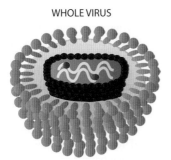 VIRUS-LIKE PARTICLE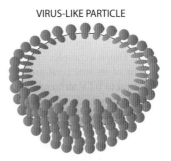

Fig. 3.6 The structure of virus-like particles. These are essentially virus particles that do not contain genetic material. These "empty shells" are fully immunogenic and trigger a protective response against the original virus.

antibody response with affinity maturation, and generate long-lived memory cells. They are efficiently taken up and processed by dendritic cells and presented by MHC class I molecules to cytotoxic T cells. This ability to target dendritic cells makes VLPs highly effective immunogens, and, as a result, adjuvants may not be required. Because of their immunogenicity, VLPs need lower doses as compared with conventional subunit vaccines, and this reduces vaccine costs.

Additional antigenic proteins can be incorporated into VLPs including TLR ligands, or other cell-targeting molecules such as CpG oligonucleotides. These can then activate memory cells and influence the Th1/Th2 polarity of the resulting immune response. In effect, VLPs are self-adjuvanting vaccines. If VLPs are sufficiently small (25–40 nm), they are not retained at the injection site but can penetrate tissue barriers, travel to draining lymph nodes, and are readily endocytosed by antigen-presenting cells. When coupled to specific-cell targeting molecules, these nanoparticles are much more effective than microparticles at being taken up by antigen-presenting cells. VLPs promote DC activation and presentation of antigens to both MHC class I and class II molecules so they can prime both $CD4^+$ and $CD8^+$ T cells.

Two VLP-based vaccines are currently used in humans, one against hepatitis B virus and the other against human papilloma virus. The hepatitis B vaccine uses monophosphoryl lipid A (MPL) added to alum as an adjuvant to induce a Th1 response and cytotoxic T cells. This human hepatitis B vaccine was the first to use VLPs and also the first anticancer vaccine because hepatitis B can cause liver cancer.

VLP-based vaccines have been generated for numerous veterinary pathogens ranging from small nonenveloped viruses such as parvoviruses and circoviruses to complex enveloped viruses such as Newcastle disease virus. Other veterinary vaccines that contain VLPs include those directed against foot-and-mouth disease and avian influenza. Encouraging results have also been obtained with caliciviruses, parvoviruses, birnaviruses, and nodaviruses, all of which can form VLPs with just a single capsid protein.

VLPs can be generated by several different expression systems involving yeasts, bacteria such as *E.coli*, mammalian cells, plants, or insect cells. They coexpress multiple viral proteins that are then allowed to self-assemble. The most promising production system involves the use of insect cells to grow baculoviruses. These baculovirus infected cells can be induced to produce large amounts of correctly folded viral proteins. They have much higher expression levels than mammalian cells and can produce multiple viral proteins at one time. These proteins also interact within the cell cytoplasm to generate a very much higher yield of VLPs. VLPs from viruses with multilayered capsids obviously present greater technical difficulties in the manufacturing process. Generally, expression of only one or two capsid proteins is sufficient to generate VLPs. On the other hand, more complex viruses may require expression of several viral capsid proteins. The purification process of VLPs is similar to the purification of virus vaccines except that the safety requirements are less stringent because VLPs are unable to replicate or cause disease.

Bluetongue (BTV), a significant disease of sheep and cattle is caused by insect-transmitted bluetongue virus. This is a complex virus, but it has proved possible to use the baculovirus system to express all four of its structural proteins and assemble these into VLPs. They appear to be structurally identical to BTV although lacking a viral genome. A vaccine consisting of these VLPs induced neutralizing antibodies and strong immunity in sheep against homologous virus. Interestingly, the VLPs induced a stronger and longer immune response than when the sheep were vaccinated with the same subunits not assembled into VLPs. One problem with vaccination against BTV is the existence of multiple, antigenically different serotypes. However, it may be possible to overcome this by the use of VLPs from different serotypes.

VLPs can be modified for vaccine use in several different ways. Therefore they can be altered to remove a specific antigen thus making them suitable for DIVA purposes. In addition to stimulating immune responses to viral pathogens, VLPs can be linked to heterologous antigens and used to deliver these antigens, such as proteins from bacteria or other viruses, to the immune system.

Isolated small peptides are often too small to be immunogenic. (They lack helper T cell epitopes in addition to their B cell epitopes). They must therefore be conjugated to carrier proteins to generate helper T cell responses. Self-assembling peptide nanoparticles (SAPNs) have also been used in efforts to optimize the immune response to viral antigens by assembling multiple copies of the peptide in the form of repetitive antigen arrays. They can form a repeating structure consisting of large numbers of identical peptide chains. These multicopy antigen structures can significantly increase the antibody responses to peptides. Two-copy arrays are good but four-copy arrays are much better.

VIROSOMES

Virosomes are liposomes expressing viral antigens. Liposomes are lipid-based vesicles with an aqueous core surrounded by a phospholipid bilayer. Cationic liposomes bind antigenic proteins as a result of their surface charge. Viral antigens may be enclosed in the aqueous core, absorbed into the phospholipid bilayer or adsorbed onto the liposome surface. Purified viral antigens can be used to make antigenic virosomes. Experimental vaccines incorporating Newcastle disease virosomes have worked well in chickens. As with VLPs, virosomes can deliver many other antigens such as oligonucleotides, peptides, antigenic fragments, and RNA, and can serve as modular vaccine platforms. Many different viral antigens can be incorporated into the lipid bilayer of the virosome. It is even possible to target the virosomes to specific cell types such as antigen presenting cells.

SUBUNIT VACCINES

The simplest method to produce a subunit vaccine is to break an organism into its component parts. For example, influenza vaccines are grown in eggs and the virus membrane disrupted by means of a surfactant. This releases the envelope and also the internal nuclear and matrix proteins. The vaccines are further purified by centrifugation to remove the internal viral core. Split virion vaccines do not undergo further purification so they usually contain more protein and thus are more likely to cause local reactions. However comparative efficacy studies suggest that split-virion flu vaccines are more effective than subunit vaccines. It appears that the internal viral core proteins stimulate greater cell-mediated responses. It is also possible to isolate and use the two major influenza antigens, hemagglutinin and neuraminidase, in a vaccine so as to minimize toxic effects.

CLONED ANTIGENS

The first successful use of gene cloning to prepare an antigen involved foot-and-mouth disease virus (FMDV). The protective antigen of FMDV (VP1) was well recognized, and the genes that coded for this protein had been mapped. The RNA genome of the FMDV was isolated and transcribed into DNA by reverse transcriptase. The resulting DNA was then carefully cut by restriction endonucleases so that it only contained the gene for VP1. This DNA was then inserted into a plasmid, the plasmid inserted into *E. coli*, and the bacteria grown. The bacteria synthesized large quantities of VP1, which was harvested, purified, and incorporated into a vaccine. The process was highly efficient because 4×10^7 doses of foot-and-mouth vaccine could be obtained from 10 L of *E. coli* grown to 10^{12} organisms per milliliter. Unfortunately, the immunity produced in response to vaccination with this highly purified antigen was inferior to that produced by whole killed virus vaccine and required a 1000-fold higher dose to induce comparable protection.

The first commercially available recombinant veterinary vaccine was made against feline leukemia virus (FeLV). The major envelope protein of FeLV, gp70, is the antigen largely responsible for inducing a protective immune response in cats. The gene for gp70 (a glycoprotein of 70 kDa) plus a small portion of a linked protein called p15e (a protein of 15 kDa from the envelope) was isolated and inserted into *E. coli*, which then synthesized large amounts of the combined proteins. The recombinant protein was harvested, purified, mixed with a saponin adjuvant, and used as a vaccine.

An alternative approach is to deliver vaccine antigens within yeast cells. Yeast-based vaccines also show high antigen expression levels, are considered very safe, may be "self-adjuvanting" (in other words, trigger innate immunity), and their antigens undergo appropriate posttranslational modification such as glycosylation. Many yeast-based vaccines are currently under development, especially for poultry and swine.

Oral vaccination has long been considered a desirable route of administration for animals but has been hindered by the ability of the gastrointestinal tract to digest and destroy oral antigens. Such vaccines have been delivered in the form of plant materials. Cloning of vaccine antigen genes into plants has been successfully achieved for viruses such as transmissible gastroenteritis, hepatitis B, Norwalk, and Newcastle disease. The plants employed include tobacco, potato, soybean, rice, and maize. A subunit Newcastle disease vaccine produced in suspension-cultured tobacco cells produced by Dow AgroSciences was licensed by US Department of Agriculture in 2006. The plant cells were grown in an indoor, biocontained production system thus minimizing consumer concerns about genetically modified organism (GMO) plants. The vaccine contains the viral hemagglutinin and neuraminidase generated in transformed plant cells grown in suspension culture. Given to 1-day-old chicks by subcutaneous injection and boosted two weeks later, it is safe and effective in protecting poultry against Newcastle Disease Virus. It has not been commercially marketed.

The DIVA Principle

Conventional vaccines, either live or inactivated, are designed to generate an immune response that is similar to that caused by natural infections. As a result, the antibody response to such a vaccine cannot usually be distinguished from that caused by a natural infection. This is a major impediment to their use, especially in situations where serology is used to identify infected animals as a preliminary to their selective removal. It is highly desirable that newer vaccines using recombinant technology are able to induce an antibody response that can be differentiated from that induced by natural infection. The acronym DIVA is used to describe such vaccines. It stands for DIFFERENTIATING INFECTED FROM VACCINATED ANIMALS.

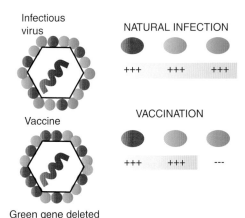

Infectious virus

NATURAL INFECTION

Vaccine

VACCINATION

Green gene deleted

Fig. 3.7 The DIVA principle. Removal of an antigen from a whole microbial vaccine ensures that antibodies against that antigen do not develop. If they are detected they imply that the animal has encountered the whole organism. Thus this methodology permits serologic differentiation between infected and vaccinated animals.

In general, DIVA technology involves either removing from the vaccine one or more of the antigens that are found in the circulating field strains of the agent (deletion mutants) (Fig. 3.7). Alternatively, one can use subunit vaccines that are also missing specific antigens. If antigens are absent from a vaccine, detection of antibodies to these antigens implies a natural infection. Conversely, it is possible to insert a new antigen into the vaccine so that detection of antibodies to this antigen identifies the animal as vaccinated. An appropriate screening test, such as an enzyme-linked immunosorbent assay, must be available to screen for the missing antigen. Ideally DIVA vaccines allow disease eradication to occur simultaneously with mass vaccination programs.

Sources of Additional Information

A complete web-based database of available veterinary vaccines is available at the Vaccine Investigation and Online Information Network (VIOLIN) at http://www.violinet.org/vevax/index.

Ada, G. (2001). Vaccines and vaccination. *N Engl J Med*, 345, 1042–1051.

Babiuk, L.A. (2002). Vaccination: a management tool in veterinary medicine, *Vet J*, 164, 188–201.

Crisci, E., Barcena, J., Montoya, M. (2012). Virus-like particles: The new frontier of vaccines for animal viral infections. *Vet Immunol Immunopathol*, 14, 211–225.

Francis, M.F. (2018). Recent advances in vaccine technologies. *Vet Clin Small Anim*, 48, 231–241.

Gerdts, V., Mutwiri, G, Richards, J., Van Drunen Littel-Van Den Hurk, S., Potter, A.A. (2013). Carrier molecules for use in veterinary vaccines. *Vaccine*, 31, 596–602.

Lee, D.H., Bae, S.W., Park, J.K., Kwon, J.H., Yuk, S.S., Song, J.M., et al. (2013). Virus-like particle vaccine protects against H3N2 canine influenza virus in dog. *Vaccine,* 31, 3268–3273.

Liu, F., Ge, S., Li, L., Wu, X., Wang, Z. (2012). Virus-like particles: potential veterinary vaccine immunogens. *Res Vet Sci*, 93, 553–559.

Norimatsu, M., Chance, V., Dougan, G., et al. (2004). Live *Salmonella enterica* serovar Typhimurium (*S. typhimurium*) elicit dendritic cell responses that differ from those induced by killed S. typhimurium. *Vet Immunol Immunopathol*, 98, 193–201.

Pabst, O., Hornef, M. (2014). Gut microbiota: a natural adjuvant for vaccination. *Immunity*, 41, 349–351.

Pennock, N.D., Kedl, J.D., Kedl, R.M. (2016). T Cell vaccinology: beyond the reflection of infectious responses. *Trends Immunol*, 37, 170–180.

Plotkin, S.A. (2010). Correlates of protection induced by vaccination. *Clin Vaccine Immunol*, 17, 1055–1065.

Shin, M.K., Yoo, H.S. (2013). Animal vaccines based on orally presented yeast recombinants, *Vaccine*, 31, 4287–4292.

Living Vaccines

When the first vaccines were developed by Louis Pasteur and his colleagues, there was a dispute between the proponents of killed/inactivated vaccines and those that believed that living organisms were required to induce protective immune responses. It did not take long to prove that killed organisms could also induce protective immunity. However, vaccines containing living organisms that can replicate in their host do have some advantages over inactivated products. Moreover, the advantages and disadvantages of each vaccine type tend to complement each other, and each has appropriate and inappropriate uses.

Unfortunately, two of the prerequisites of an ideal vaccine, high antigenicity and absence of adverse side effects, are sometimes incompatible. Vaccines containing replicating organisms may trigger innate immune responses as they infect host cells and tissues. As a result, vaccinated animals may develop a very mild, short lasting "sickness" such as fever, inappetence, or depression. Inactivated vaccines are generally less immunogenic than their modified live counterparts. Live vaccines are better able to stimulate cell-mediated immunity against the targeted pathogen because they replicate to a limited extent within the vaccinated animal. The live organisms may enter cells and be processed as endogenous antigens. As a result, they can trigger a type 1 immune response dominated by $CD8^+$ cytotoxic T cells. This may result in a mild infection, but it generates long-lasting protection similar to that in animals that recover from the actual disease. The organisms used in these live vaccines may, however, also have the potential to gain virulence and thus cause disease. Vaccines containing killed organisms, in contrast, act as exogenous antigens. They tend to stimulate type 2 responses dominated by $CD4^+$ T cells and antibodies. This may not generate a very strong protective response to some organisms, but they may provide adequate protection and are often safer.

Note that by triggering innate immunity, live viral vaccines can retain their ability to induce interferon production. This can occur within a few hours of administration. As a result they may confer very rapid protection (Fig. 4.1). This may be important if these vaccines are used to stop an epidemic that has already started.

ANTIGEN PROCESSING

As described in Chapter 2, cell-mediated immune responses are primarily directed against abnormal cells such as those infected with viruses. Cytotoxic T cells recognize antigen fragments bound to MHC class I molecules expressed on infected cells. To stimulate these cytotoxic responses, the foreign invader must grow inside the cells. These endogenous antigens are therefore the key to stimulating cell-mediated responses. Killed antigens or their subunits cannot do this and

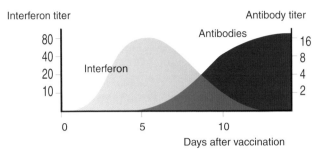

Fig. 4.1 The sequential production of interferon and antibodies induced in calves following intranasal live vaccine against bovine herpesvirus. Modified live vaccines have the potential to confer very rapid immunity in a vaccinated animal, long before antibodies are produced.

therefore stimulate predominantly type 2, antibody-mediated responses. Only live organisms capable of inducing intracellular protein synthesis can trigger cell-mediated responses. Thus live vaccines have an immunogenic ability lacking in inactivated vaccines.

Attenuation

Virulent living organisms cannot normally be used in vaccines otherwise they will cause disease. As described in Chapter 1, some early vaccination attempts included administering infectious material by unusual routes. This was a hazardous procedure and only one such procedure is in use today—vaccination against contagious ecthyma of sheep. Contagious ecthyma (also called *soremouth* or *orf*) is a viral skin disease of lambs that causes massive scab formation around the mouth, prevents feeding, and results in a failure to thrive. The disease has little systemic effect. Lambs recover completely within a few weeks and are then solidly immune. It is usual therefore to vaccinate lambs by rubbing infected scab material into scratches made in the inner aspect of the lamb's thigh or other hairless area. The development of lesions at this site has no untoward effect on the lambs, and they become solidly immune. Because vaccinated animals may spread the disease, however, they must be separated from unvaccinated animals for a few weeks.

The soremouth example notwithstanding, this is not a common procedure. Under normal circumstances microbial virulence must be reduced so that, although still living, the organisms in vaccines may replicate to a limited extent but can no longer cause disease. This process is called attenuation. The level of attenuation is critical to vaccine success. Attenuation must be a key property of the organism and not dependent on fully functional host defenses. It should not lead to the development of a persistent carrier state. However, the attenuated organisms need to be sufficiently invasive and persistent to stimulate a protective immune response. Underattenuation will result in residual virulence and disease; overattenuation may result in an ineffective vaccine. Once organisms are attenuated sufficiently to be used safely, these vaccines are classified as *modified live vaccines* (MLV).

Bacterial Attenuation

The traditional method of attenuating bacteria or viruses was to grow them for a long period of time in culture. It was hoped that over time, random mutations would accumulate and effectively reduce microbial virulence. This often worked, especially with agents with a small genome such as viruses. It occasionally worked with bacteria as well, but this was uncommon and unpredictable. It is difficult to attenuate bacteria. They have a large genome and, unless the genes that control virulence are specifically targeted, they will not reliably lose virulence. It is exceedingly difficult to attenuate bacteria simply by passaging them many times in vitro.

RANDOM MUTAGENESIS

The traditional methods of attenuation were empirical at a time when there was little understanding of the changes induced by the attenuation process. They usually involved adapting organisms to growth in unusual conditions so that as they mutated, they lost their adaptation to their usual host. For example, Albert Calmette and Camille Guérin passaged *Mycobacterium bovis* in an alkaline medium containing sterile bovine bile 230 times every 21 days from 1908 to 1921. This led to several genetic changes in the organism that resulted in its gradual attenuation for humans. This is the Bacille Calmette-Guérin (BCG) strain of *M. bovis*. It is widely used as a vaccine against tuberculosis, but its effectiveness varies between countries. It is widely used in Europe but not in North America. (Interestingly, Calmette also developed the first antivenom for snakebite.)

The vaccine strain of *Bacillus anthracis* was developed by Max Sterne in 1935. He grew anthrax in 50% serum agar under an atmosphere rich in CO_2 so that it lost its virulence. *B. anthracis* has virulence factors encoded on two plasmids, pXO1 and pXO2. The Sterne strain has lost its pXO2 plasmid. This encodes the bacterial capsule, a thick layer of polysaccharide that protects the bacteria against phagocytosis. Thus it cannot form a capsule, and as a result is susceptible to phagocytosis and is relatively avirulent. The anthrax vaccine is prepared as a spore suspension. It is administered to livestock in a dose containing up to 10 million spores with a saponin adjuvant, and it has an excellent safety record.

A group of brucellosis cultures were maintained by John Buck of the US Department of Agriculture's Bureau of Animal Industry on his desk at room temperature for "well over a year." They were then evaluated for immunogenicity and stability. The nineteenth culture was significantly less pathogenic than the others and remained stable while passaged and transmitted. This was licensed as the Brucella vaccine strain 19 in 1941. *Brucella abortus* strain 19 vaccine formed the basis of Brucella eradication in many countries. Its lack of virulence is the result of a deletion of 702 base pairs that encode the erythritol catabolic genes. As a result, strain 19 is unable to use erythritol, a sugar found in abundance in the bovine placenta.

Other examples of attenuated bacterial strains used in vaccines include an attenuated strain of *Brucella suis* (Strain 2), used in China for the prevention of brucellosis in goats, sheep, cattle, and pigs. Streptomycin was used to derive the attenuated Rev.1 strain from a virulent culture of *Brucella melitensis*. A rough strain of *Salmonella enterica* Dublin (strain 51) is used as a vaccine in Europe to protect calves at two to four weeks of age. Immunity to salmonellosis involves macrophage activation and is thus relatively nonspecific.

Unfortunately, genetic stability cannot always be guaranteed in these attenuated strains. This is of special concern in bacterial vaccine strains that were generated as a result of random mutagenesis. Multiple passages of the organism in the laboratory on growth media, cell cultures, or in eggs resulted in random mutations of unknown genes. This attenuation may simply be caused by the loss of a single gene that could equally well mutate back again. Back-mutation or genome reassortment, using genes from related bacteria, may occur and thus the attenuated organisms may suddenly regain their virulence.

GENE DELETION

A much more reliable method of making bacteria avirulent is by deliberate genetic manipulation. Gambling with random mutagenesis is no longer acceptable. Molecular/genetic techniques now enable us to generate gene-deleted attenuated bacteria with defined properties (Fig. 4.2).

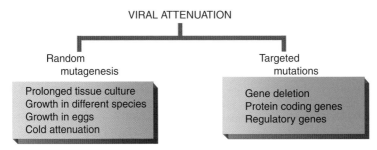

Fig. 4.2 The ways by which viruses may be rendered avirulent for use in vaccines. These can be broadly divided into two methods, either random mutagenesis or much more targeted genetic techniques.

Attenuating mutations can be targeted to specific genes and designed to eliminate any signs of disease or undesirable adverse reactions. The mutations generated in this way can be made irreversible. When selecting these genes however, it is important that the mutated organism be capable of replicating for a sufficient length of time in the vaccinated animal to induce strong primary and memory responses.

Bacterial attenuating mutations are generally made in two types of genes—housekeeping genes and virulence genes. Housekeeping genes are directly involved in the bacterial central metabolic pathway. Examples of such genes include *aro*A that encodes a protein controlling aromatic amino acid biosynthesis, *crp* the gene encoding the cAMP receptor protein, and *cya* the adenylate cyclase gene.

Deletion of the *aro*A gene blocks synthesis of aromatic amino acids. As a result the bacteria can only grow in a medium where these amino acids are provided. Within an animal their growth is restricted and they cannot persist. However, they live long enough to induce an immune response. These deletions are made in genes located on the bacterial chromosome, not on plasmids, and as a result they are very stable. They involve deletion of very large pieces of genes so that reversions are highly improbable. Because they have evolved within a specific bacterial species, these genes are unlikely to be replaced by corresponding gene segments from nearby unrelated bacteria. Because of the short survival time of these bacteria *in vivo*, they have insufficient time to regain gene segments.

Bacteria attenuated by deletion of the aromatic pathway genes have been used in many different vaccines. For example, an *aro*A-deleted strain of *Streptococcus equi* has been used as a vaccine against equine strangles. It was attenuated by deletion of a 1 kb segment of the *aro*A gene. The vaccine is applied to the inner side of the upper lips. It produces high antibody titers in vaccinated horses and provides protection against experimental challenge with virulent *S. equi*. Thus it does not propagate in horses and because it is not shed it cannot spread to in contact animals. It is currently licensed under the name *Equilis Strep*E by Intervet in the European Union.

A modified live vaccine is available that contains streptomycin-dependent Mannheimia haemolytica and *Pasteurella multocida*. These mutant bacteria depend on the presence of high levels streptomycin for protein synthesis. When these organisms are administered to an animal, residual streptomycin permits limited growth. Once the streptomycin has gone, the organisms will die, but not before they have stimulated a protective immune response.

Other examples of bacterial virulence genes that may be deleted include the genes directly involved in toxin synthesis and genes involved in the regulation of the virulence genes. As a result an organism is rendered nonpathogenic. It should be pointed out, however, that toxins are often the prime targets of the protective immune response so that the complete deletion of their genes would remove the toxin and make the vaccine nonimmunogenic. Therefore we generally seek to eliminate or inactivate the genes encoding the toxic parts of the molecule while retaining the immunogenic parts. This works well for tetanus and diphtheria vaccines in addition to cholera.

Viral Attenuation

Like bacteria, attenuation of viruses is a key step in making safe, effective, modified live vaccines. Unlike bacteria with their large complex genomes, viruses have a very much smaller genome. This may be readily manipulated to generate potential viral vaccines. Viral virulence is influenced by the ability of the virus to bind to their target cell receptors, the size of the infecting dose, its genetics, and its ability to stimulate and resist innate immune defenses such as inhibition by interferon.

Adaptation to Unusual Species

Viruses have traditionally been attenuated by prolonged growth in cells or species to which they are not naturally adapted. For example, rinderpest virus, which was normally a pathogen of cattle, was first attenuated by growth in goats, then in rabbits. Eventually, a vaccine devoid of residual virulence was developed by passaging it 90 times in tissue culture. On investigation, this attenuated virus was found to contain a combination of many less-attenuating mutations distributed throughout its genome. Similar examples include the adaptation of African horse sickness virus to mice and of canine distemper virus to ferrets.

Growth in Tissue Culture

The traditional method of virus attenuation has been prolonged tissue culture. This was the method used by Albert Sabin when he developed the first human oral polio vaccine. In these cases virus attenuation was accomplished by culturing the organism in cells to which they are not adapted. Sabin grew human poliovirus in monkey cells. Mutants developing during this cell-culture passage lost the ability to cause paralysis in humans. These were then selected for lack of virulence in monkeys. In another example, virulent canine distemper virus preferentially attacks lymphoid cells. For vaccine purposes therefore, this virus was cultured in canine kidney cells. In adapting to these culture conditions, it lost its ability to cause severe disease in dogs.

Attenuation in Eggs

Chicken eggs are cheap and available in large quantities. Some mammalian viruses may therefore be attenuated by prolonged growth in eggs. For example, the Flury strain of rabies vaccine was attenuated by passage in eggs and lost its virulence for normal dogs and cats.

Cold Attenuation

Viral growth is influenced by the temperature within the host animal. Thus while the deep body is at a constant temperature, the temperature on body surfaces where viruses first invade may be significantly lower. Viruses may therefore be attenuated by adapting them to grow at lower temperatures. For example, a virus such as influenza is grown in embryonated eggs. Then incubation temperatures are gradually reduced from 34°C to 25°C. The virus is passaged multiple times at each temperature step. Viral survival at this low temperature depends on the development of mutations in multiple genes. At the same time, the virus loses its ability to grow at normal body temperature, 39°C.

Once cold adaptation is successfully achieved, a stable clone can be evaluated for use as an intranasal spray vaccine. The attenuated virus will grow in the nasal cavity but not farther down the respiratory tract, thus minimizing adverse reactions caused by residual virulence.

Chemical Mutagenesis

Instead of simply relying on random mutagenesis to generate attenuated strains of viruses, it is possible to add mutagenic chemicals to cultures to enhance the process. These chemicals generally act by inserting incorrect nucleotides into nucleic acids during replication. For DNA viruses, 5-bromodeoxyuridine is commonly used whereas 5-fluorouracil is used for RNA viruses. For example, 5-fluorouracil has been used to attenuate respiratory syncytial virus. Other mutagens include hydroxylamine that has been used on foot and mouth disease virus, and nitrous acid and 5-azacytidine that have been used on Eastern equine encephalitis virus. The viruses can be cloned after exposure to the mutagens and clones screened for small plaque size or temperature sensitivity. (The smaller-than-usual plaques that form in a cell monolayer suggest that the virus has a reduced ability to spread, replicate, and kill cells, and implies lower virulence.) If an attenuating mutation has been identified in an isolate, then the mutated gene sequence can be excised and inserted into another strain of the agent. This is called site-directed mutagenesis. This has worked well for negative-stranded RNA viruses such as rabies.

Targeted Attenuation

Our ability to manipulate viral genomes enables us to use several other strategies to engineer irreversibly attenuated viruses for use in vaccines. These strategies can include replacement of viral genes with genes from related viruses, thus effectively inserting new mutations. Another possible strategy is simply to alter the order of genes in the attenuated virus. It is also possible to combine mutations from several partially attenuated strains. The simplest process, however, is simply to delete selected genes.

GENE-DELETED VACCINES

Deletion or mutation of certain critical genes can generate defective viruses that cannot replicate in their hosts. These defective viruses can however be grown in helper cells that provide the missing genes. Although the virus cannot complete its life cycle, its genes are still expressed and thus generate endogenous antigens. Single cycle viruses that are defective in a single protein required for assembly or viral spread represent variations on this method. An example of a successful gene-deleted vaccine is that against the herpesvirus that causes pseudorabies in swine (Fig. 4.3). The enzyme, thymidine kinase (TK), is required by herpesviruses to replicate in nondividing cells such as epidermal and neuronal cells, which themselves have low levels of thymidylate metabolism. Viruses lacking the *TK* gene can therefore infect these cells but cannot replicate and cannot cause disease. Vaccines containing these TK-minus mutants not only confer effective protection, but also block cell invasion by virulent pseudorabies viruses, and prevent the development of a persistent carrier state.

Leaderless Vaccines

Another way of attenuating a virus is to eliminate the sequence for a critical leader gene. For example, it is possible to develop a foot-and-mouth disease virus in which the gene for the leader protease is deleted (Fig. 4.4). In this virus the viral RNA encodes all the virus genes at one time. A result it is translated as a large "polyprotein." This polyprotein is then posttranslationally cleaved by a protease into four structural proteins and 10 nonstructural proteins. The protease autocatalytically cleaves itself off the polyprotein and then initiates gene translation of the 5' end of host RNA. As a result, deleting the protease gene ensures that the leaderless virus cannot replicate and can be used in a vaccine.

Marker Vaccines

Genetic manipulation can also be used to make viruses that trigger a characteristic and diagnostic immune response. These are used in "marker vaccines." For example, pseudorabies virus

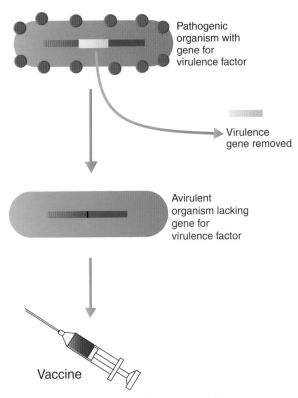

Fig. 4.3 The attenuation of a virulent organism by the targeted deletion of virulence genes ensures that a virus such as pseudorabies becomes irreversibly attenuated. In addition, if the gene also encodes a major antigen that can be detected by serologic assays, then its removal permits vaccinated animals to be distinguished from infected ones.

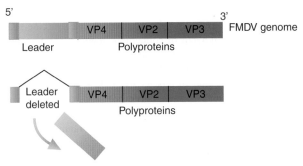

Fig. 4.4. The generation of a leaderless attenuated vaccine virus. This technique has been used for the attenuation of foot and mouth disease virus. *FMVD*, Foot-and-mouth disease virus.

expresses two glycoprotein antigens called gX and gI. These are potent antigens, yet neither is essential for viral growth or virulence. They are expressed by all field isolates of this virus and so naturally infected animals will make antibodies to both gX and gI. An attenuated pseudorabies vaccine has therefore been produced using a virus that lacks these proteins. As a result, vaccinated pigs will not make antibodies to gX or gI, but naturally infected pigs will. The vaccine will not cause positive serological reactions in assays for anti-gX or -gI, and the presence of antibodies to gX and gI in a pig is evidence that the animal has been exposed to field strains of pseudorabies virus. This is an example of how a vaccine may be made that eliminates the confusion caused when seeking to differentiate infected from vaccinated animals (DIVA). This permits eradication of specific infectious diseases much more economically and rapidly than conventional methods because an animal will not make antibodies against antigens that are not present in the vaccine.

Gene-deleted vaccines have been developed in a similar manner for bovine herpesvirus-1 (BHV-1). Thus a TK-minus strain is safe and effective in a vaccine. Likewise, a DIVA vaccine for BHV-1 has been made by deleting glycoprotein E, another viral protein not required for viral invasion. Specific diagnostic tests based on detection of gE have been developed. Another example of a DIVA vaccine is the insertion of an influenza B gene into an avian influenza A vaccine. Because influenza B does not infect birds, the presence of antiinfluenza B antibodies confirms vaccination.

DISA Vaccines

Ideally it should be possible to generate a safe and effective vaccine by deleting a single critical component required for the spread of a highly pathogenic virus. These DISA vaccines (Disabled Inactivated Single Antigen) contain attenuated viruses that cannot spread between cells or animals. These virus vaccines induce a fully competent immune response except against the missing protein. This also includes effective cytotoxic T cell responses. These have been developed against bluetongue virus and African horse sickness virus.

Safety Issues

The disadvantage of attenuated live vaccines produced by traditional methods is their potential for reversion to virulence. Genes may mutate again. Viruses may recombine with other viruses. Viruses may simply readapt back to their original host and disease reoccur.

Genetically modified organisms such as those described above must be stable over multiple generations. This includes not only reversion while they are within the vaccinated animal but also if they escape into the environment. Most importantly, mutation leading to a gain of virulence must not occur. Deletion mutations must therefore be made in genes that are known to be stable and not flanked by mobile elements. Likewise any gene duplications or inactive duplicates of the target gene must be identified. For example, the most widely used vaccine strain of *Mycoplasma mycoides* (Strain T1/44), the causal agent of contagious bovine pleuropneumonia, is known to revert to pathogenicity. This strain was developed from a Tanzanian isolate by 44 passages in embryonated eggs. Analysis has shown that the deletion mutants that cause its attenuation are located in a region with multiple tandem repeats and that active copies of the virulence gene persist on other repeats. As a result recombination events and reversion to virulence are highly possible.

Gene transfer from a vaccine strain of bacteria to other organisms can occur via bacteriophages or mobile genetic elements such as plasmids and transposons. Important examples include antibiotic resistance and toxin genes. Although not usually found in mobile elements, the location of the virulence genes must be assessed. For example, cholera toxin genes are located on prophages and can be actively transmitted between bacteria by bacteriophages. Conversely, gene transfer to the attenuated vaccine strain must also be considered. These are all a potential cause of concern when using modified live vaccines.

Sources of Additional Information

A complete web-based database of available veterinary vaccines is available at the Vaccine Investigation and Online Information Network (VIOLIN) at http://www.violinet.org/vevax/index.

Crowe, J.E., Bui, P.T., London, W.T., Davis, A.R., Hung, P.P., Chanock, R.M., Murphy, B.R. (1994). Satisfactorily attenuated and protective mutants derived from a partially attenuated cold-passaged respiratory syncytial virus mutant by introduction of additional attenuating mutations during chemical mutagenesis. *Vaccine,* 12, 691–699.

Chitlaru, T., Israeli, M., Rotem, S., Elia, U., Bar-haim, E., et al. (2017). A novel live attenuated anthrax spore vaccine based on an acapsular *Bacillus anthracis* Sterne strain with mutations in the *htrA*, *lef* and *cya* genes. *Vaccine,* 35, 6030–6040.

Curtiss, R. (2002). Bacterial infectious disease control by vaccine development. *J Clin Invest,* 110, 1061–1066.

Field, H.J., Wildy, P. (1978). The pathogenicity of thymidine kinase-deficient mutants of herpes simplex virus in mice. *J Hyg (Lond),* 81, 267–277.

Lauring, A.S., Jones, J.O., Andino, R. (2010). Rationalizing the development of live attenuated virus vaccines. *Nat Biotechnol,* 28, 573-579.

Maassab, H.F., Bryant, M.L. (1999). The development of live attenuated cold-adapted influenza virus vaccine for humans. *Rev Med Virol,* 9, 237–244.

Minor, P.D. (2015). Live attenuated vaccines: Historical successes and current challenges. *Virology,* 479, 379–392.

Sah, P., Medlock, J., Fitzpatrick, M.C., Singer, B.H., Galvani, A.P. (2018). Optimizing the impact of low-efficacy influenza vaccines. *Proc Natl Acad Sci U S A,* 115, 5151–5156.

Smith, G.A., Young, P.L., Rodwell, B.J., Kelly, M.A., Storie, G.J., Farrah, C.A., Mattick, J.S. (1994). Development and trial of a bovine herpesvirus 1-thymidine kinase deletion virus as a vaccine. *Aust Vet J,* 71, 65–70.

Recombinant Vectored Vaccines

As noted in Chapter 4, empirical microbial attenuation by traditional processes is an unpredictable and somewhat hazardous way of making a live vaccine. Targeted attenuation by gene deletion or deliberate mutation of an organism generates a significantly safer product. But an even better solution is available—the use of recombinant vectored viruses in vaccines. Avirulent viruses may be genetically modified to express antigens from the organism of interest. When used in vaccines they can safely combine optimal antigenicity against the selected pathogen with the minimal virulence of the vector virus. These recombinant vectored vaccines have many advantages. They allow the simultaneous expression of multiple antigenic determinants and also avoid the hazards of whole pathogenic viruses, maximizing their safety. The recombinant organisms are much easier to grow than the original pathogen, and this results in a more consistent product along with a much shorter production and development time. More importantly, the ability of vectored vaccines to infect cells and so express endogenous antigens ensures that they are very efficient at inducing both antibody- and strong T cell–mediated responses against intracellular pathogens.

Vectors

Agents that carry selected genes encoding foreign antigens are known as vectors. Genetically engineered vectors can either be used as vaccines themselves or used to produce large amounts of antigens *in vitro* that can then be incorporated into vaccines. Vectors include bacteria, DNA viruses, yeasts, plasmids, and even plants (Fig. 5.1). Some microbial vectors may also replicate within an animal and as a result stimulate protective immune responses, provided they only cause abortive infections.

Genes encoding protein antigens can be cloned directly into viruses. Instead of isolating and purifying the antigens, the recombinant virus vector itself may simply be used as a vaccine. Experimental recombinant vaccines used as vaccine platforms have usually used large DNA viruses such as poxviruses, adenoviruses, and herpesviruses, or bacteria such as *Mycobacterium bovis*, BCG, lactobacillus, or salmonella as vectors. The organisms that have been most widely employed for this purpose in veterinary medicine are poxviruses such as vaccinia, fowlpox, and canarypox.

Viral vectored vaccines have the advantage of being able to induce both antibody- and cell-mediated immune responses without the need for an adjuvant. They do not require complex purification. They can generate antigens in the correct conformation and they can deliver more than one antigen at a time. As a result, these vaccines are safe, they cannot be transmitted by arthropods, and they are not excreted in body fluids. Their major advantage is that the antigens are synthesized within infected cells and thus act as endogenous antigens. They produce a

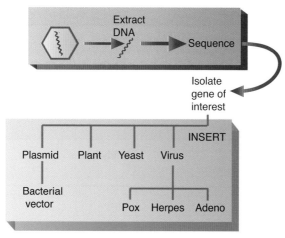

Fig. 5.1 The various methods of generating live recombinant vaccines. The gene encoding the antigen of interest is isolated, inserted into a plasmid. This plasmid can then be inserted into many different potential vectors.

"balanced" immune response compared to inactivated viral vaccines. In selecting viral vectors for vaccine use, safety is of paramount importance, whereas other considerations include vector stability and the ability to scale-up production.

POXVIRUS VECTORS

Poxviruses are the most widely used vectors in vaccines because they have a very large genome that can accommodate large inserts. For example, mammalian poxviruses such as vaccinia have a 190 kb genome, whereas fowlpox and canarypox have genomes of more than 300 kb. As a result, a 10 kb base-pair segment of the vaccinia genome can be removed and up to 30,000 base-pairs of foreign DNA can be inserted without affecting virus infectivity. Multiple foreign genes can therefore be inserted into a single vector. By splicing genes from selected pathogens into a poxvirus vector and using this as a vaccine, we can immunize recipients against all these pathogens. Unlike other DNA viruses, poxviruses have their own transcription machinery, RNA polymerase, and posttranscriptional modifying enzymes so this permits self-sufficient replication in the cytoplasm of infected cells. They can express high levels of the new antigen. Moreover, these recombinant proteins undergo appropriate processing steps, including glycosylation and membrane transport within the poxvirus. The poxviruses are also easy to administer by dermal scratching or by ingestion.

The first widely employed vaccine vector was vaccinia virus, the "cowpox" vaccine used to protect humans against smallpox. There were some safety concerns regarding the use of vaccinia because it is not completely innocuous, especially in immunosuppressed recipients. This problem was solved by using highly attenuated, replication-deficient strains of the virus. For example, modified vaccinia virus ankara (MVA) was grown for 570 serial passages in chick embryo fibroblasts and lost about 10% of its genome. It can no longer replicate in mammalian cells. As a vector it is highly efficient and it stimulates powerful cell-mediated immune responses in children and the elderly.

The earliest of such vaccines used the avirulent Copenhagen strain of vaccinia virus to express rabies virus glycoprotein. This virus strain has had 19 genes encoding virulence genes deleted, resulting in a highly attenuated organism. The cDNA for the rabies virus glycoprotein G was

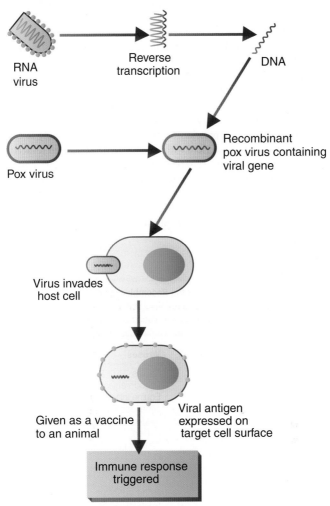

Fig. 5.2 The production of an oral vaccinia rabies recombinant vaccine. Vaccinia has been selected because its genome can accommodate a very large gene insert. In addition, the recombinant vaccinia readily induces protective immunity following oral vaccination.

then inserted into the thymidine kinase (TK) gene of vaccinia. As a result, the vaccinia expressed the rabies glycoprotein and at the same time attenuated the vaccinia virus (Fig. 5.2). This glycoprotein can induce virus-neutralizing antibodies and so confer protection against rabies. Vaccination with this rabies-vaccinia recombinant (RABORAL V-RG) results in the production of antibodies to the glycoprotein and the development of immunity. This vaccine has been successfully used as an oral bait vaccine administered to raccoons, coyotes, arctic and gray foxes. This form of the vaccine can be distributed by dropping from aircraft (Chapter 20).

The Copenhagen strain of vaccinia has been further attenuated by elimination of unwanted genes to produce the NYVAC strain. This strain has also been used in several animal vaccines including those directed against wildlife rabies, pseudorabies in pigs, equine influenza, Japanese encephalitis in pigs, and rabies in cats and dogs. Other mammalian poxviruses that have been investigated for their functionality as vaccine vectors include capripox, swinepox, parapox, and the myxoma virus.

Highly effective recombinant vaccines were also developed for rinderpest; these consisted of a vaccinia or capripox vector containing the hemagglutinin *(HA)* or fusion *(F)* genes of the rinderpest virus. This recombinant capripox vaccine can also protect cattle against lumpy skin disease (Chapter 16).

The most widely employed and successful poxvirus vector is the host-range restricted strain of canarypox virus (ALVAC). This virus grows only in birds but it is capable of entering mammalian cells, generating antigens, and so immunizing mammals. It does not replicate after entering a mammalian cell, and expression of the inserted antigens only lasts about six hours. Immunity to canarypox does not interfere with a recipient's response to revaccination. Nor does it appear to induce the formation of canarypox neutralizing antibodies. The canarypox vector system has been used as a platform for many different vaccines including canine distemper, equine influenza, West Nile virus, feline leukemia, and rabies viruses (Table 5.1). The currently used vector was originally isolated from an infected canary, but was then passaged 200 times in chick embryo fibroblasts before being plaque purified four times.

TABLE 5.1 ■ Some of the Recombinant Viral Vectored Vaccines That Are Commercially Available or Under Development. A Recombinant: Vaccine Vector Database, Vaxvec, is Available at http://violinet.org.vaxvec.

Vector	Viruses
Vaccinia	Rabies
	Pseudorabies
	Equine influenza
	Japanese encephalitis
Capripox	Rinderpest/PPR
Canarypox	Rabies
	Distemper
	FPV
	Equine influenza
	West Nile
	Feline leukemia
Fowlpox	Avian influenza
	Laryngotracheitis
	Newcastle disease
Marek's/HVT	Newcastle disease
	Infectious bronchitis
	Avian influenza
	Infectious bursal disease
Adenoviruses	FMDV
	Rift Valley Fever
	Rabies
	Distemper
	Pseudorabies
	PPR
Newcastle Disease	Avian influenza
	Infectious bursal disease

FPV, Feline panleukopenia virus; *FMDV*, foot-and-mouth disease virus; *PPR*, *peste des petites* ruminants.

Canarypox recombinant vaccines expressing measles virus fusion proteins and hemagglutinins have also been used to vaccinate dogs against distemper. Likewise, recombinant vaccines expressing the F and HA proteins of distemper are protective in dogs and ferrets. Canarypox recombinant vaccines expressing the feline leukemia virus capsid (*gag*) gene, parts of the subgroup A envelope (*env*) gene, and the polymerase gene (*pol*) are protective in kittens. Vaccines containing canarypox recombinants expressing the hemagglutinin from two strains of equine influenza H3N8 are immunogenic in horses and protect against naturally acquired disease. The canarypox recombinant West Nile virus vaccine available in Europe expresses the prM-E polyprotein gene. Both equine vaccines are adjuvanted with carbopol, a complex organic polymer (Chapter 15).

A recombinant rabies G-protein, canarypox vectored vaccine was 100 times more effective than an equivalent fowlpox vectored vaccine and of similar efficacy to a vaccinia vectored recombinant. Canarypox recombinant vaccines expressing the rabies G-protein work well in dogs and cats, protecting them for at least three years. More importantly these vaccines work in puppies in the presence of maternal antirabies antibodies.

The first commercially available vectored vaccine used a fowlpox vector. Fowlpox is a common pathogen of chickens and there are numerous avirulent vaccine strains available. It has also been possible to engineer species-specific avian poxviruses such as fowlpox strain 9 (FP9) to generate recombinant viral vaccines for poultry (Chapter 19). Deletion of its thymidine kinase gene does not affect its replication. Therefore new genes can be readily inserted into that region of its genome. Fowlpox-based recombinants expressing Newcastle disease hemagglutinin (HA) and fusion (F) proteins have been widely used as vaccines to protect one-day-old chicks and provide lifetime immunity to Newcastle disease virus (NDV) even in the presence of maternal antibodies. The HA and F proteins of NDV are potent antigens that induce neutralizing antibodies. This vaccine has the additional benefit of conferring immunity against fowlpox. Another reason for its good safety profile is that NDV replicates in the upper respiratory tract, whereas fowlpox virus replicates in the skin. Other fowlpox recombinant poultry vaccines may incorporate genes from infectious laryngotracheitis virus or from *Mycoplasma gallisepticum*.

Avipox viruses such as fowlpox and canarypox are naturally restricted to birds in which they can replicate. They have an abortive replication cycle in mammals and as a result they are very safe. Because the vector does not replicate within the recipient it cannot spread to others.

ADENOVIRUS VECTORS

Adenoviruses are a large family of double stranded DNA viruses that cause respiratory and gastrointestinal disease in humans and animals. They elicit strong cell-mediated and antibody-mediated immune responses. They have a wide host range and infect multiple cell types. They can be delivered by injection and orally. The most commonly used vector is human adenovirus-5. The adenovirus genome is a linear chain consisting of 36 kb of DNA. Recombinant adenovirus vaccines usually have two envelope genes deleted, E1 and E3. Loss of E1 renders the virus unable to replicate whereas E3 is involved in evading host immunity and is not required for viral replication. Deletion of both these genes makes space available for an inserted transgene. Replication competent adenoviral vectors can also be produced by simply removing the E3 gene. There is less vacant space, but they are much more immunogenic.

Adenoviruses work well as vaccine vectors because they can deliver antigens very efficiently to dendritic cells and upregulate their production of costimulatory cytokines and chemokines. They may be either replication-competent or replication-deficient but still achieve gene expression. Replication competent adenoviruses can contain a 3 to 4 kilobase (kb) insert whereas the replication deficient adenoviruses can contain a 7 to 8 kb insert. They can thus express large quantities of foreign antigen. Replication competent adenovirus vectors will grow for a short period but not cause disease. They also target epithelial cells so they can stimulate both systemic and mucosal immunity. These adenovirus vectors are unlikely to cause tumors because they do not integrate their DNA into the genome of the host cell. They can also be made thermostable, a factor that greatly simplifies their storage. Unfortunately, adenovirus capsids stimulate toll-like receptors and other pattern recognition receptors and thus trigger inflammation. This is a significant disadvantage because the inflammatory response results in the loss of a large quantity of vectors and transgenes. Another problem encountered in humans is preexisting immunity to adenovirus-5, a rather common mild respiratory pathogen. This can significantly inhibit the effectiveness of adenovirus-vectored vaccines. Prime-boost protocols using different vectors may be needed to overcome this problem.

A Rift valley fever–adenovirus recombinant vaccine is effective in sheep and goats. A canine distemper-adenovirus recombinant vaccine appears to be effective in puppies born to distemper-immune mothers, and an adenovirus recombinant vaccine is protective against swine pseudorabies. A foot-and-mouth disease (FMD)–adenovirus recombinant vaccine has received conditional approval in the United States. It contains the nucleotide sequence encoding the FMD virus (FMDV) polyprotein P1-2A structural proteins and the 3C protease genes inserted into the E1 region of a replication incompetent adenovirus-5 vector. A human cytomegalovirus promoter was inserted to control expression of the FMDV genes. When combined with a lipid/polymer adjuvant, this vaccine protected against clinical FMD and prevented viral shedding. Vaccinated animals can be differentiated from naturally infected animals by their lack of antibodies to the FMDV nonstructural proteins.

A *peste des petites* ruminants (PPR)-adenovirus recombinant vaccine has been developed that expresses the surface glycoproteins of PPR virus (PPRV). Vaccinated animals therefore make high levels of antibodies against the surface glycoprotein but totally lack antibodies against the nucleocapsid core protein. This is an inexpensive vaccine that can be used in low value small ruminants.

A rabies-adenovirus recombinant vaccine incorporating a glycoprotein gene from the attenuated ERA strain has been developed and widely employed in Canada as an oral bait vaccine in skunks and raccoons (ONRAB, Artemis Technologies).

HERPESVIRUS VECTORS

Herpesvirus genomes contain several nonessential regions that can be removed to accommodate large segments of foreign DNA without preventing their replication. Although many viruses have been tested in poultry for use as vectors, one virus, herpesvirus of turkeys (HVT), appears to be optimal. HVT is currently employed as a vaccine against Marek's disease. Its genome is well defined and it can cause persistent infection in the presence of maternal antibodies. A single dose of HVT can result in life-long immunity when delivered *in ovo* to an 18-day-old embryo. As a result, several different HVT-recombinant vaccines have been developed. These may contain the fusion protein of Newcastle disease virus, the VP2 protein of infectious bursal disease virus, the glycoprotein G gene of laryngotracheitis, or the hemagglutinin of H5 avian influenza.

OTHER VIRAL VECTORS

Avirulent strains of NDV, notably B1 and LaSota, are widely used as vaccines in poultry. Both strains have a good safety record. As a result, bivalent NDV-vectored vaccines have been developed that express a single foreign gene. Examples include the insertion of a hemagglutinin gene from avian influenza virus and the insertion of the VP2 gene from infectious bursal disease virus. Other studies have targeted infectious bronchitis and infectious laryngotracheitis. They are not yet commercially available.

PLANT-BASED VACCINES

Oral vaccination has long been considered a desirable route of administration for animals but has been hindered by the ability of the gastrointestinal tract to digest and destroy ingested antigens. Although highly desirable from the point of view of the user, it often requires a large dose of antigen to elicit a protective response. Such vaccines can, however, be economically delivered in the form of recombinant plant material. Various plants such as tobacco, rice, maize, potato, alfalfa, and soybean have been used as vectors for introduced viral genes.

Plant production systems may include the use of entire plants grown in the field or greenhouses, or plant cell cultures grown in bulk. The manufacturing process is simple; many such as corn or alfalfa are natural feeds, and the fact that the antigens are enclosed within cellular plant cell walls means that they survive the digestive process.

To be used as bioreactors, plants can be transformed in many different ways. For example, genes can be introduced into plants using the gram-negative bacterium *Agrobacterium tumefaciens*. This organism contains a natural plasmid that is introduced into a plant genome and transcribed within plant cells. Insertion of this plasmid results in abnormal plant hormone production that causes crown gall disease. Most of the plasmid DNA can however be replaced with the gene encoding an antigen of interest. Once the gene is stably integrated into a plant, a master seed bank can be established that serves as a permanent source of vaccine antigen.

An alternative technique is to target the chloroplast genome rather than the nuclear genome. Chloroplasts, like mitochondria, originate from cyanobacteria that were initially incorporated into an early eukaryotic cell. Now they are present in all green plant cells. They have a small genome that can incorporate and express introduced antigen genes. As a result, all the green parts of the plant may express large amounts of vaccine antigen. These genes are not transmitted in pollen so there is less chance of out-crossing to other nearby plants.

One other way to incorporate antigen genes into plants is through transient expression by plant viruses. Thus engineered tobacco mosaic virus grows well in tobacco plants and can trigger production of very large amounts of the introduced protein. Unfortunately, these recombinant viruses retain their infectivity and may spread to other plants prompting environmental safety concerns. New time-saving technologies to introduce vaccine genes into plants include infiltration processes where the Agrobacterium or viral vectors are simply injected into leaves. Given the problem of vaccine costs in livestock, it is clear that plant-based vaccines have great potential in the veterinary marketplace.

A Newcastle disease vaccine produced in suspension-cultured tobacco cells has been licensed in the United States. The NDV glycoprotein has also been expressed in potato, maize, and rice. The spike protein gene of infectious bronchitis has also been introduced into potato. The VP2 protective antigen from infectious bursal disease virus has been expressed in rice and tobacco. Plant-based pig vaccines that are being studied include those against the fimbriae of enterotoxic *Escherichia coli* that have been produced in alfalfa chloroplasts as well as rice, barley, and tobacco; transmissible gastroenteritis S protein has been produced in corn. The FMD antigen VP1 has been produced in tobacco (using bamboo mosaic virus) in addition to potato, alfalfa, and tomato. Bovine virus diarrhea E2 protein has also been expressed in alfalfa. Rabies G protein has been expressed in many plants including maize. When fed to sheep, it protected them from rabies virus challenge.

It is clear that plant-based vaccines expressed in normal animal food plants, such as alfalfa or corn, without the need for any purification process have the greatest potential to provide very cheap and highly effective vaccines to livestock. When they become available, they will transform the vaccine industry. The main impediments to their use are regulatory and environmental concerns centered on the use of genetically modified plants in human food.

Chimeric Virus Vaccines

It is possible to insert proteins from one virus into another carrier virus to produce a chimeric viral vaccine (Fig. 5.3). The antigens on these chimeric viruses are arranged in the same configuration as in the original virus and are present at high density. One example of a chimeric vaccine involves the use of a yellow fever viral chimera to protect against West Nile virus infection in horses. This technology inserts the envelope genes of West Nile virus into the capsid and accompanying nonstructural genes of the attenuated yellow fever vaccine strain YF-17D. The result is a yellow fever–West Nile virus chimera that is much less neuroinvasive and hence much safer as a vaccine than either of the parent viruses. This has been licensed by US Department of Agriculture.

Another example of a licensed chimeric vaccine is that against porcine circovirus (PCV). In this case, the capsid gene of virulent PCV2 (ORF2) is inserted into nonpathogenic PCV1 to produce a nonpathogenic chimera that can then be administered as a vaccine.

Safety Issues

Before recombinant bacterial vaccines are released, certain safety issues must be resolved. Thus the precise functions, locations, and stability of the genes to be mutated, any possible reversion mechanisms, any possible recombinant effects with other inactive genes, the potential for gene transfer both from and to other organisms by phage transduction, transposon or plasmid transfer, and complementation must all be addressed.

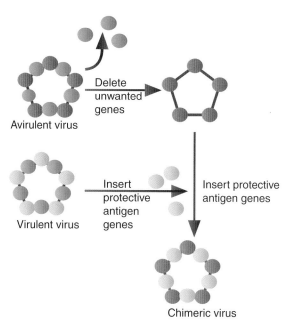

Fig. 5.3 The construction of a chimeric vaccine. Selected protein antigens from an avirulent virus are replaced by similar antigens from a related pathogen. These chimeras thus combine the avirulence of one virus with the immunogenicity of another.

Sources of Additional Information

A recombinant vaccine vector database, Vaxvec, is available at http://violinet.org.vaxvec.

Baron, M.D., Iqbal, M., Nair, V. (2018). Recent advances in viral vectors in veterinary vaccinology. *Curr Opin Virology, 29*, 1–7.

Choi, K.S. (2017). Newcastle disease virus vectored vaccines as bivalent or antigen delivery vaccines. *Clin Exp Vaccine Res, 6*, 72–82.

Choi, Y., Chang, J. (2013). Viral vectors for vaccine applications. *Clin Exp Vaccine Res, 2*, 97–105.

Deng, S., Martin, C., Patil, R., Zhu, F., et al. (2015). Vaxvec. The first web-based recombinant vector database and its data analysis. *Vaccine, 33*, 6938–6946.

Draper, S.J., Heeney, J.L. (2010). Viruses as vaccine vectors for infectious diseases and cancer. *Nature Reviews, 8*, 62–73.

Ewer, K.J., Lambe, T., Rollier, C.S., Spencer, A.J., Hill, A.V., Dorrell, L. (2016). Viral vectors as vaccine platforms: from immunogenicity to impact. *Curr Opin Immunol, 41*, 47–54.

Frey, J. (2007). Biological safety concepts of genetically modified live bacterial vaccines. *Vaccine, 25*, 5598–5605.

Medina, E., Guzman, C.A. (2001). Use of live bacterial vaccine vectors for antigen delivery: Potential and limitations. *Vaccine, 19*, 1573–1580.

Poulet, H., Minke, J., Pardo, M.C., Juillard, V., Nordgren, R., Audonnet, J.C. (2007). Development and registration of recombinant veterinary vaccines. The example of the canarypox vector platform. *Vaccine, 25*, 5606–5612.

Ramezanpour, B., Haan, I., Osterhaus, A., Claassen, E. (2016). Vector-based genetically modified vaccines: Exploiting Jenner's legacy. *Vaccine, 34*, 6436–6448.

Shahid, N., Daniell, (2016). H. Plant-based oral vaccines against zoonotic and non-zoonotic diseases. *Plant Biotechnol J, 14*, 2079–2099.

Takeyama, N., Kiyono, H., Yuki, Y. (2015). Plant-based vaccines for animals and humans: Recent advances in technology and clinical trials. *Ther Adv Vaccines, 3*, 139–154.

Takeyama, N., Yuki, Y., Tokuhara, D., Oruku, K., Mejima, M., Kurokawa, S., Kuroda, M., Kodama, T., et al. (2015). Oral rice-based vaccine induces passive and active immunity against enterotoxigenic *E. coli*-mediated diarrhea in pigs. *Vaccine, 33*, 5204–5211.

Weli, S.C., Tryland, M. (2011). Avipoxviruses: Infection biology and their use as vaccine vectors. *Virology J, 8*, 49. Retrieved from http://www.virologyj.com/content/8/1/49.

Zanotto, C., Pozzi, E., Pacchioni, S., Volonte, L., Morghen, C.D.G., Radaelli, A. (2010). Canarypox and fowlpox viruses as recombinant vaccine vectors: A biological and immunological comparison. *Antiviral Res, 88*, 53–63.

CHAPTER 6

Nucleic Acid Vaccines and Reverse Vaccinology

Many current vaccines were developed years ago using what are now considered outdated technologies. In spite of being phenomenally successful, these technologies have proved unable to make progress against some major human diseases such as tuberculosis, malaria, or human immunodeficiency virus/acquired immunodeficiency syndrome (HIV/AIDS). In addition, they cannot be developed rapidly enough to control explosive outbreaks of diseases such as Ebola or Zika, or even new strains of influenza. Over the past few decades, however, the development of vaccines has been transformed by the introduction of innovative technologies. As a result, the possibilities of developing new effective vaccines against these diseases are increasingly plausible. It is important to point out, however, that veterinary vaccine production is governed by the marketplace. An innovative and effective technology that works in humans and appeals to scientists may not be sufficiently economical to produce nor to satisfy animal vaccine needs. Nevertheless, two new technologies are in the process of transforming veterinary vaccinology. These are the development of DNA-plasmid vaccines and of reverse vaccinology.

DNA-Plasmid Vaccines

In conventional vaccines, a modified live virus is injected into an animal. The virus infects cells and then uses its genome to encode viral antigens. These antigens are processed and fragments expressed on the cell surface. The expressed viral proteins are recognized as foreign by B and T cells, and the animal responds by mounting antibody or cell-mediated immune responses. An alternative way to trigger these responses is to inject a DNA plasmid (a piece of circular DNA, usually from *Escherichia coli* that acts as a vector) containing the genes encoding the specific protein antigen of interest (Fig. 6.1). When this DNA plasmid enters a cell nucleus in a recipient animal, it will be transcribed into mRNA. The mRNA is transported to the cell cytoplasm and translated into protein. The recipient cells will therefore synthesize and express the foreign antigen. As with virus-encoded proteins, this endogenous antigen will be processed, bound to MHC class I molecules, and expressed on the cell surface. It will then prime both B and T cell responses and trigger cytotoxic T cell responses and antibody production. The plasmid, however, unlike viral vectors, cannot replicate in mammalian cells and it encodes only the target antigen.

There are several DNA-plasmid vaccines approved for use in animals and numerous others are in various stages of development for humans. Although yet to reach significant commercial production, DNA vaccines appear to be ideal for organisms that are difficult or dangerous to grow in the laboratory. They are very stable at room temperature and relatively easy to manufacture to

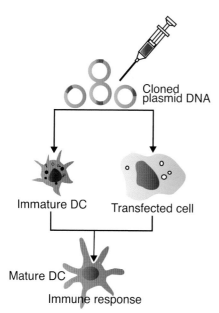

Cloned plasmid DNA

Immature DC   Transfected cell

Mature DC

Immune response

Fig. 6.1 The principle of DNA vaccination. The gene encoding the antigen of interest is first incorporated into a plasmid. The plasmid is then inserted into the cells of the host animal. The antigen gene is functional and can thus be transcribed and translated into the antigenic protein that acts as an endogenous antigen. *DC,* Dendritic cells.

consistent specifications. DNA vaccines are often more effective than recombinant proteins and avoid the need for complex vectors. The DNA sequence of a plasmid can be easily modified to manipulate the type 1 T helper to type 2 T helper (Th1/Th2) ratio in the induced response. Likewise the DNA can be combined with genes for cytokines, and also adjuvants, polymeric carriers, or viral vectors (Table 6.1).

VACCINE PRODUCTION

The selected DNA sequence from the organism of interest is isolated and inserted into a bacterial plasmid usually obtained from *E. coli*. In addition to the genes encoding the vaccine antigen or antigens of interest, the plasmid must also contain a strong promoter sequence upstream (usually from another virus like Rous sarcoma virus or cytomegalovirus), in addition to a transcriptional termination/polyadenylation sequence downstream. When the plasmid enters the cell nucleus,

TABLE 6.1 ■ **A Comparison of the Advantages of Conventional and DNA-Plasmid Based Vaccines**

Conventional Vaccines	DNA-Plasmid Vaccines
Not limited to protein antigens	Very safe
No risk of inducing anti-DNA antibodies	Presented by both MHC class I and II molecules
Less risk of tolerance induction	Can be polarized to Th1 or Th2 responses
No risk of affecting the genes controlling cell growth	Relatively easy and cheap to produce
Difficult to polarize responses to Th1 or Th2	No need for adjuvants
More strongly immunogenic	Correct antigen folding
Low doses required	Persistent response
Immunity develops rapidly	Very specific for an antigen

MHC, Major histocompatibility complex; *Th1,* type 1 helper T cell.

the promoter causes transcription of the mRNA of the antigen gene. The polyadenylation sequence is required for the mRNA to leave the nucleus and enter the cytoplasm. Plasmids may be modified in many ways to improve antigen yield and immunogenicity. Some plasmids may be engineered to express more than one antigen or perhaps an antigen plus an immunostimulatory protein separated by a spacer. Alternatively, a mixture of two plasmids, one expressing the antigen gene and one expressing a cytokine gene, may be administered at the same time. Protein expression may also be optimized by changing the plasmid codon usage. (Pathogens often have a somewhat different codon usage than do eukaryotic cells, so this can be modified to match the target species and so increase transcription efficiency.)

VACCINE ADMINISTRATION

Genetically engineered plasmids are usually suspended in saline and injected intramuscularly into an animal where they are taken up by the skeletal muscle cells. This is the limiting step for these vaccines because the physical barriers of the cell wall and the nuclear membrane interfere with plasmid uptake while DNA in the extracellular space is rapidly degraded. Several approaches have been taken to overcome this problem. For example, if the muscle cells are first damaged by mycotoxins or by the use of hypertonic saline solution, this may assist penetration into cells. Plasmid penetration is also enhanced by the use of "adjuvants" such as lipid complexes, microcapsules, or nonionic copolymers. Aluminum phosphate seems especially effective in improving DNA vaccine efficiency.

DNA vaccines may also be injected subcutaneously where the plasmids are deposited in extracellular spaces. They can then be carried to draining lymph nodes where they are probably taken up by antigen presenting cells.

Once it enters a cell, like a virus, the DNA plasmid is transcribed into messenger RNA and translated into the endogenous target protein. The newly generated protein then undergoes appropriate processing, is bound to MHC class I molecules, and presented to the antigen-presenting cells. These carry the peptide to the draining lymph node where it is presented to T and B cells. This leads to the production not only of neutralizing antibodies but also of cytotoxic T cells because the antigen is endogenous. These expressed peptides have an authentic tertiary structure and posttranslational modifications such as glycosylation. The immune response to these peptides is also enhanced because the bacterial DNA in the plasmid itself contains unmethylated CpG motifs that are recognized by toll-like receptor 9 (TLR9). As a result, they initiate innate immune responses, activate dendritic cells, and eventually promote a strong Th1 response.

This type of DNA-plasmid has been used to protect horses against West Nile virus infection (West-Nile Innovator, Ft Dodge). The commercial vaccine consists of a plasmid engineered to express high levels of the virus envelope (E) and premembrane (prM) proteins. In addition, the plasmid contains gene promoters and marker genes (Fig. 6.2). Upon injection with a biodegradable oil adjuvant, this plasmid enters cells and causes them to express the West Nile virus proteins. Other DNA vaccines have been licensed to prevent infectious hematopoietic necrosis and salmonid pancreas diseases in farmed Atlantic salmon (Chapter 21), and also melanomas in dogs (Chapter 23). This approach has also been applied experimentally to produce DNA vaccines against avian influenza, lymphocytic choriomeningitis, canine and feline rabies, canine parvovirus, bovine viral diarrhea, feline immunodeficiency virus, feline leukemia virus, pseudorabies, foot-and-mouth disease virus, bovine herpesvirus-1, and Newcastle disease. Although theoretically producing a response similar to that induced by attenuated live viral vaccines, these nucleic acid vaccines are ideally suited to protect against organisms that are difficult or dangerous to grow in the laboratory. Some DNA vaccines can also induce immunity even in the presence of very high titers of maternal antibodies. Although the maternal antibodies can block serological responses, the development of memory responses is not impaired.

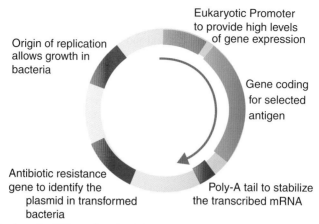

Fig. 6.2 The structure of a DNA vaccine plasmid. In this case it encodes the protective antigens from the West Nile virus. The plasmid also incorporates an antibiotic resistance gene so that it can be readily detected in tissues. This plasmid is used as a DNA vaccine in horses.

DNA-plasmid vaccination is well tolerated and after intramuscular injection most of the plasmids remain at the injection site for several weeks. Some may be transiently detected in the blood and other organs. Antibody responses after DNA vaccination increase slowly but are unusually prolonged when compared with a single protein injection. It may take as long as 12 weeks to reach peak antibody titers in mice.

CELL ENTRY

DNA plasmid vaccines must get inside target cells. This can be achieved by intramuscular injection of saline solutions although they require quite a lot of DNA (10 μg–1 mg). Much of the DNA in saline goes into the intracellular spaces and is therefore "wasted." Muscle cells may also take up the plasmids by phagocytosis or perhaps through specific receptors. Although intramuscular injection is very inefficient because the transfection rate is low (about 1%–5% of myofibrils in the vicinity of an intramuscular injection site), the expression of the transfected gene can persist for at least two months. Its encoded peptides are either treated as endogenous antigens and displayed on the cell surface or secreted and presented to antigen-processing cells. It may be that the skeletal muscle cells are not the most important pathways for antigen processing. The injected plasmid may simply be carried into the draining lymph node where it is taken up by dendritic cells. This processed antigen preferentially stimulates a Th1 response associated with IFN-γ production. It is possible to modify the DNA to bias the T cell response toward type 1 or type 2 responses simply by inserting appropriate cytokine genes.

Gene Guns

Plasmid entry into cells can also be achieved by "shooting" the DNA plasmids directly through the skin adsorbed onto microscopic gold or tungsten nanoparticles. These are fired by a "gene gun" using compressed helium (Fig. 6.3). The "gene gun" delivers the plasmid-coated particles directly to the cell cytoplasm. Saline injections promote a Th1 response. By bypassing TLR9, the gene gun technique preferentially stimulates Th2 responses. The use of a gene gun is more efficient than injection because some of this DNA is taken up by dendritic cells bypassing more conventional endocytosis mechanisms, and it therefore minimizes degradation.

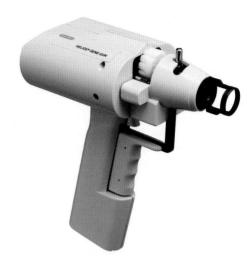

Fig. 6.3 A Helios gene gun. It uses a low-pressure pulse of helium to sweep DNA, RNA, or protein-coated gold particles from the inner wall of a small plastic cartridge directly into target cells. (From Bio-Rad Inc. With permission.)

Electroporation

Another way to overcome the problems associated with getting DNA plasmids inside cells is electroporation. This combines an intramuscular injection with the local application of a pulsed electric field of 50 to 1000 v through needle electrodes for a few micro- or milliseconds. After this electrical pulse the muscle cell membranes become temporarily permeable and open pores that allow the plasmids to enter the cell. For intradermal electroporation, the electrodes are placed on the skin and the pulses stimulate the skin dendritic cells to take up the plasmids. These very short pulses are well tolerated (by humans) and cause minimal erythema and irritation. It is difficult to see how this method could be applied in a practical manner to many domestic animal species. Most dendritic cells only express the plasmids for a few days whereas the muscle cells do so for several months. Thus the intramuscular route is preferred.

PROBLEMS

The major impediment to the development of DNA vaccines is their low immunogenicity because of the relatively low transfection efficiency of the plasmid. In other words, large amounts of DNA are injected and very little antigen is expressed. Up to several milligrams of DNA must be injected to induce a strong immune response. They also only work for protein antigens. The purification required to separate the plasmid from contaminating cellular DNA and RNA is expensive. One way to solve the efficacy problem is to enhance plasmid uptake by using different routes and methods of administration such as gene guns or electroporation. Alternatively, the plasmids may be delivered in association with regulatory cytokine genes, such as those for GM-CSF, IFN-γ, IL-2, and IL-12. The plasmids may also be adsorbed onto cationic microparticles that are then phagocytosed by antigen presenting cells.

PRIME-BOOST STRATEGIES

It has long been normal practice to use exactly the same vaccine for boosting an immune response as was employed when priming an animal. This approach has many advantages, not the least of which is simplicity in manufacturing and regulating vaccine production. There is, however, no reason why different forms of a vaccine should not be used for priming and for boosting if this will induce an optimal response. This approach is known as a heterologous prime-boost strategy. Under some circumstances this may result in significantly improved vaccine effectiveness. The heterologous prime-boost approach is somewhat empirical, and researchers may simply test numerous vaccine combinations to determine which combination yields the best results. Prime-boosting has been investigated in efforts to improve the effectiveness of DNA plasmid vaccines, because it is clear that DNA-plasmid vaccines alone may not be sufficient to trigger a protective immune response. However greatly improved results may be obtained by boosting with a conventional or virus vectored vaccine. Combinations may involve priming with one DNA plasmid, but boosting with either another plasmid, perhaps in another vector, or with recombinant protein antigens. These strategies may increase the avidity and persistence of antibody responses and also increase cytotoxic T cell responses.

It should be noted that no DNA-plasmid vaccines for human use have yet been approved. They have not been as immunogenic in humans as in laboratory animals. Primates need ten times as much DNA as rodents do because a human serum protein, amyloid P, binds plasmids and inhibits their transfection. Although DNA-plasmid vaccines do not currently have great advantages over conventional protein vaccines, they may provide the solution to diseases not currently well controlled by conventional antigens such as malaria and tuberculosis.

RNA Vaccines

Messenger RNA is produced by transcription of DNA and translated into proteins. Thus when it enters cells it triggers protein expression. This mRNA is only transiently expressed, and as a result is potentially safer than persistent DNA. RNA can be synthesized so that it incorporates open reading frames that encode proteins combined with sequences at both termini that regulate translation and protein expression. Whereas conventional vaccines require large and expensive production facilities, RNA synthesis is relatively simple. It can be readily produced by a standardized process reducing both cost and time. Only information about the RNA sequence is required and there is no need to handle dangerous pathogens. RNA is relatively stable as long as it is not exposed to RNase. RNA is also self-adjuvanting in that it is a potent stimulator of interferon production. It should also be pointed out that RNA, unlike DNA, does not need to get into the cell nucleus. It is sufficient for it to cross the cell membrane into the cytoplasm. In fact, naked mRNA is spontaneously taken up by many cell types and expressed within minutes. Its stability can be further enhanced by chemical changes or incorporation into nanoparticles such as dendrimers (highly branched proteins).

RNA can be delivered to cells in two forms, conventional mRNA or self-amplifying mRNAs also called replicons. Both types of RNA are safe and well tolerated and induce antigen-specific immune responses. Conventional mRNA vaccines have largely been developed for use in human cancers. They encode tumor specific antigens that can trigger a protective immune response.

Most of the infectious disease focus has however been on self-amplifying vectors—replicons, derived from alphaviruses because these are highly effective and require a much lower dose of RNA to induce a protective immune response. Replicons are defined as nucleic acids that contain the instructions for their own replication.

ALPHAVIRUS REPLICONS

Alphaviruses are positive-sense, single-stranded RNA viruses. Examples of alphaviruses include Eastern, Western, and Venezuelan encephalitis viruses, Sindbis virus, and Semliki Forest virus. All can be used as vaccine vectors because their genome is relatively simple, and they generate large quantities of RNA in the cytoplasm of infected cells. Their 5' end encodes nonstructural proteins that are responsible for this cytoplasmic RNA replication. Their 3' end encodes structural proteins plus a

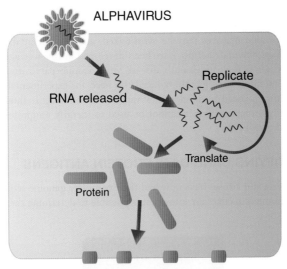

Fig. 6.4 The principle of Alphavirus replicon RNA vaccines. The RNA replicon consists of two components, a component encoding the genes for the transcriptase and a component encoding the antigen genes to be expressed. Once within a cell, the replicon copies itself and generates large quantities of the encoded antigenic protein.

promoter region (Fig. 6.4). If foreign genes of interest are inserted in place of the alphavirus structural genes, the viral RNA will continue to replicate and translate large amounts of the foreign proteins. Because of their very efficient promoters, the newly synthesized proteins may account for 10% to 20% of the total cell protein. It is also possible to incorporate genes for viral capsids or glycoproteins into the replicon so that virus-like particles form and effectively package and protect the RNA. They are not, however, able to replicate or produce progeny virus. If more promoter sites are inserted downstream, several different genes can be expressed and are able to generate multivalent vaccines.

The most commonly used alphavirus vector has been Venezuelan equine encephalitis virus. RNA replicon vaccines that have been investigated with encouraging results include those directed against swine influenza, avian influenza, foot-and-mouth disease, equine arteritis, porcine respiratory and reproductive syndrome, and Nipah virus. Three RNA replicon vaccines have been licensed by US Department of Agriculture. These are directed against porcine epidemic diarrhea, swine influenza H3N2, and highly pathogenic avian influenza H5N2.

Reverse Vaccinology

The first complete bacterial genome was sequenced in 1995. That opened the possibility of using this information to identify all the antigenic proteins of a pathogen. This data can then be used to select potential protective epitopes from these proteins without the need to grow the specific microorganisms and it permits the rational design of vaccines based solely on genomic data.

Epitopes, otherwise called antigenic determinants, are the short peptides from protein antigens that are recognized by antibodies or bind to MHC molecules on the cells of the immune system. These epitopes are the essential structures that must be present in vaccines to trigger protective immune responses. Thus "vaccinomics" can be used to accurately identify protective epitopes that may then be experimentally tested in animals, a process called reverse vaccinology. The procedures require identification of the cell surface proteins of interest. Once identified their structure can be predicted. Then their important epitopes, especially those that bind to common MHC molecules and are likely recognized by CD4$^+$ and CD8$^+$ T cells, can be identified (Fig. 6.5).

The protective protein epitopes may be synthesized, and experimental vaccines made and tested in animals. Experimental vaccines have been developed in this way against several veterinary pathogens including foot-and-mouth disease virus, canine parvovirus, and influenza A. *In silico* prediction methods have greatly reduced the need for experimental testing in animals in addition to the time needed to develop new vaccines (Table 6.2). It should be noted that a major defect in this approach is that it cannot be used to identify nonprotein epitopes such as polysaccharides and glycolipids.

STEP 1. IDENTIFYING CANDIDATE PROTEIN ANTIGENS

Thousands of bacteria and viruses have now had their complete genome sequences determined. Now that these genome sequences are known, it is possible to determine the precise amino acid

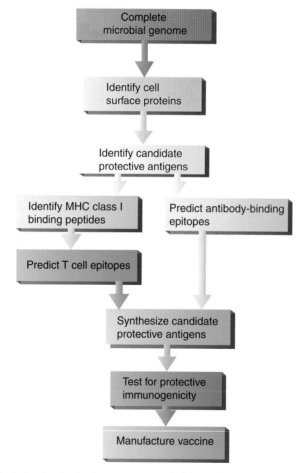

Fig. 6.5 A flowchart showing the basic processes required to produce a new vaccine through reverse vaccinology. In effect the protective antigens are first identified by computational methods before they are tested in animals. *MHC*, Major histocompatibility complex.

TABLE 6.2 ■ Conventional and Reverse Vaccinology—A Comparison

	Conventional	Reverse
Antigens to be identified	10–20 identified biochemically	All the protein antigens encoded in the genome
Antigenic properties	The most abundant or antigenic.	All possible antigens irrespective of antigenicity or amount. The most conserved antigens can be identified
Polysaccharide antigens	Significant antigens in conventional vaccines	Cannot be identified
T cell and B cell epitopes	Limited to well characterized antigens	Almost all T cell epitopes can be identified. Less so for B cell epitopes
Efficacy	Determined by extensive animal testing.	Predicted first and then confirmed by animal testing

sequence of the proteins encoded by their genes. One can then compute and characterize these sequences and the structure of all potential surface and secreted proteins of an organism, including those that are present in very small quantities or were previously unknown. The next step is to use bioinformatics algorithms to identify those proteins that are most conserved across multiple strains and predict their most important antigenic epitopes—their "antigenome." Not all epitopes identified in a pathogen are equal in their ability to induce neutralizing antibodies or trigger T cell responses, but it is possible to select those most likely to stimulate antibody- or cell-mediated responses. These are called the immunodominant epitopes. Normally about 40 to 50 immunogenic proteins are selected for screening. Some of these, especially those found on the surface of the organisms, are likely to have immunodominant epitopes that can be incorporated into vaccines. Genomics analysis software enables not only the sequences of these proteins to be determined but also their three-dimensional structure. Another approach is to assume that all protective antigens have a characteristic epitope structure (or protective signature). Computer analysis of all known protective antigens has identified many possible such signatures. These can then be used to predict potential candidate vaccine epitopes.

This computational approach has been supplemented by other techniques such as directly isolating all the surface peptides from a bacterium. The isolated peptides can then be loaded into a mass spectrometer that can identify and quantitate all the antigens on the microbial surface. This approach has also identified many previously unknown antigens. One interesting example is the discovery of pili on the surface of gram-positive bacteria. Pili were not previously known to be present on gram-positive bacteria, although known for years to be present on gram-negative bacteria. Antigens from the pili of streptococci and pneumococci have been found to determine their host species specificity.

Thus reverse vaccinology techniques need no more than the genome sequence of the organism to derive the entire antigenome of each pathogen and so identify the best possible vaccine candidate antigens. They can identify unique antigens that may improve existing vaccines in addition to identifying protective epitopes on organisms that have not been controlled by conventional vaccination techniques (Box 6.1).

Immunoinformatics can be used to convert this large-scale immunologic data using computational approaches to obtain practical results. Once these protective epitopes have been identified it may be possible to combine them in a single molecule and discard nonprotective epitopes. Such a vaccine has been developed for the prevention of canine leishmaniasis (Chapter 13).

BOX 6.1 ■ A Flea Vaccine From Reverse Vaccinology?

The transcriptome of the cat flea *Ctenocephalides felis* has been used to identify candidate protective antigens based on analysis of its secreted proteins. (The transcriptome is derived from the flea's RNA. This is reversely transcribed into DNA and the DNA sequenced.) This DNA sequence can then be analyzed and its protein amino acid sequences determined. T and B cell epitopes can then be predicted from these protein sequences. A candidate vaccine derived in this manner has reduced the hatchability of eggs from fleas that fed on immunized cats. It is an encouraging start.

Contreras, M., et al. (2018). A reverse vaccinology approach to the identification of Ctenocephalides felis candidate protective antigens for the control of cat flea infestations. *Parasites and Vectors,* 11(1), 43.

STEP 2. IDENTIFYING T CELL EPITOPES

Epitopes that will activate helper T cells must be identified to determine their ability to bind to the antigen-binding sites on major histocompatibility complex (MHC) class I and II molecules. Remember T cells will only recognize epitopes if they are first bound to an MHC molecule. To do this, the typical target protein sequence is broken down into overlapping nine amino acid frames and these are screened for their ability to bind the MHC antigen-binding groove. Sequences can be identified that bind strongly to the antigen-binding groove of MHC molecules and are potential vaccine candidates. Many MHC-binding algorithms have been published that help identify these peptides.

MHC class I binding predictors have proven to be very efficient and accurate. It is also possible to analyze each step in the antigen-processing pathway. The sites where proteasomes will cleave the antigen can be predicted. It is possible to predict which of these peptide fragments will bind to transporter proteins and also those that will bind to the MHC class I antigen–binding groove. There is now an integrated whole antigen processing pathway software available that combines all these processes. Prediction of MHC class II binding epitopes is currently much less accurate because MHC class II binding is much less stringent than class I.

All these analyses aim to identify the shortest peptides within an antigen that can stimulate CD4 or CD8 T cells, differentiate those that can bind to MHC class I and class II and determine their binding affinity. Epitope screening can be optimized for a specific viral population or used to generate a "universal" vaccine. In humans this approach may lead to personal immunotherapy. All of these can be assessed through multiple sophisticated software programs.

This approach has been successfully employed to predicting those foot-and-mouth disease virus (FMDV) peptides that will bind to bovine leukocyte antigen (BoLA) class I, the bovine MHC. The ability of these antigenic peptides each containing 8 to 11 amino acids from the P1 structural polyprotein of FMDV to bind BoLA has been determined.

STEP 3. IDENTIFYING B CELL EPITOPES

Predicting the epitopes that will stimulate B cells and hence antibody formation is much more difficult than predicting T cell epitopes. T cells can only recognize short antigenic peptides bound to MHC molecules. B cell receptors, in contrast, can potentially recognize any exposed surface region of an antigen and this may not be a protein. Thus B cell epitope prediction remains imperfect and hence unsatisfactory. Identifying B cell epitopes therefore requires solving the three-dimensional (3D) structure of antigen-antibody complexes, identifying epitopes on the exterior of the molecule, and evaluating the antigen-antibody interaction. For example, hydrophobic amino acids will likely be found in the interior of a protein whereas hydrophilic ones are more likely to be on its surface. B cell epitope prediction is therefore based on amino acid properties such as hydrophobicity, charge, exposed surface area, and structure. These surface epitopes may be linear and determined by the amino acid sequence of the antigen. Alternatively, the epitopes may be conformational and based on the way the peptide chain folds. If the epitope is conformational then the complete 3D structure of the antigen must be generated to predict its immunogenicity. Conformational epitopes may also cause difficulties when making a synthetic vaccine because they must retain their conformation to be functional. It is also possible to obtain more predictive information about the B cell epitopes of a pathogen by analyzing the antibodies produced by recovering convalescent animals. These antibodies can be examined for their ability to react with selected viral epitopes in an effort to determine which are immunogenic. This was the method employed to develop the first Ebola virus vaccines.

STEP 4. SYNTHESIZING AND TESTING THE VACCINE

Once the candidate T and B cell epitopes have been identified, the most promising ones can be synthesized and tested in animals. The candidate epitopes can be narrowed to those that make the most potent immune response, generate broadly neutralizing antibodies, and confer protective immunity. Multiple protective antigens can then be pooled in the vaccine or attached to nanoparticles. Reverse vaccinology has an additional benefit. It enables epitopes to be selected that can bind successfully to MHC class I binding sites and so preferentially stimulate cell-mediated immunity. Molecular modeling is able to predict such peptides. It is indeed possible to prepare a collection of peptides that can bind to the predominant MHC molecules in a population and then combine them in a cocktail designed to immunize the greatest proportion of the susceptible population. Multimerization of these peptides may increase their antigenicity. Synthetic peptides are easy to store and transport. Synthetic antigenic peptides have been developed for use in vaccines directed against canine parvovirus and foot-and-mouth disease virus.

OTHER APPROACHES

In addition to the "classical" approach described, two variant approaches may also be made. One is to compare the potential epitopes on several closely related strains of the agent. Although these differ between strains, there will be a core antigenome shared by all the members of the same species. These core genes can then be analyzed to identify shared epitopes and used to make a vaccine that is be effective against all members of the species irrespective of their strain diversity.

Another approach is to compare the genomes of virulent and avirulent strains of the same species. In this way the genes encoding pathogenicity determinants can be identified and vaccines developed that will only inhibit pathogenic strains while leaving avirulent commensals unaffected.

NEW VACCINES

Reverse vaccinology has been applied to many bacterial pathogens, For example, it was used to identify all the surface antigens on Group B *Neisseria meningitidis*. The process identified 91 previously unknown surface antigens. Of these, 28 induced bactericidal antibodies. The four major antigens inducing the best and broadest bactericidal activity were then expressed in *E. coli* vectors, purified and incorporated into a successful multicomponent vaccine. This led eventually to a commercially successful human vaccine.

An example of the use of reverse vaccinology to generate new veterinary vaccines is the case of *Histophilus somni*. This bacterium is associated with the bovine respiratory disease complex and there are some moderately successful vaccines available against it. Whole genome sequencing was performed on six field isolates of *H. somni*. The genomes were assembled and then their protein-coding regions were ranked on the basis of their predicted surface expression and their conservation between all the strains. A vaccine containing a pool of six selected recombinant proteins has been tested in cattle with encouraging results.

It has also been possible to make a pairwise comparison of the predicted T cell epitope content between many different strains of swine influenza virus. The T cell epitopes of the influenza virus were selected based on their predicted binding by SLA class I and II as well as assessing their T cell-facing epitopes and epitope similarities. The SLA data was predicted based on human models and the published pig genome. When compared with an existing inactivated swine flu vaccine, a higher T cell epitope relatedness score was associated with greater protection by a vaccine. When the epitopes on the hemagglutinin of 23 different viral strains were compared with the vaccine, it was possible to show how protection occurred in the absence of cross-reactive hemagglutination inhibiting antibodies. Protection in that case was the result of cross-conserved T cell epitopes. Thus it is possible to predict whether a new or existing vaccine will be protective against newly emerging influenza strains. A similar epitope comparison study has been used to predict the relative protection afforded by different commercial vaccines against different strains of porcine circovirus (Fig. 6.6).

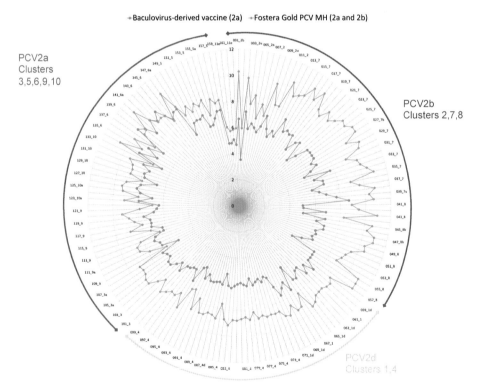

Fig. 6.6 An epitope comparison study on two swine Circovirus vaccines. One, in orange, is baculovirus-derived. The other in black, is a conventional circovirus vaccine. Around the outside are 161 different field strains of porcine circovirus. Two different PCV2 vaccines were analyzed for their ability to stimulate a T cell response against each strain. The closer the jagged line is to the outside, the greater its immunogenicity. (Courtesy of Zoetis and Dr. Meggan Bandrick)

MOSAIC VACCINES

Once all the naturally occurring T cell epitopes of an organism have been identified, it is possible to combine the best and most diverse of these epitopes into a single protein. The resulting "mosaic" protein resembles a microbial protein, but is assembled from the set of natural epitopes based on computer optimization. Generally they are assembled from peptides 9 to 12 amino acids in length because this is the size of an epitope recognized by cytotoxic T cells. Once their optimal sequence is determined, the protein can be generated in an appropriate vector and used as a vaccine. Mosaic vaccines designed to prevent HIV/AIDS are currently undergoing trials. It is hoped that by increasing the diversity of T cell epitopes in the vaccine that there will be greater "coverage" of the viral antigens and hence a reduction in the virus's ability to "escape." An experimental mosaic vaccine has been developed against porcine respiratory and reproductive syndrome virus (PRRSV). Two T cell epitope sequences were selected using bioinformatic techniques from the viral envelope glycoprotein GP5 and combined to generate a DNA vaccine. This was administered to young piglets by gene gun or electroporation. The vaccine proved to be immunogenic and induced partial protection as reflected by a decreased viral load and lung lesion scores.

With appropriate epitope selection, it is also possible to make a mosaic vaccine that affords protection against multiple viruses. Optimal epitope coverage probably only requires two to three carefully selected epitopes. Adding additional epitopes increases coverage but with diminishing returns if rare epitopes are incorporated into the mosaic vaccine. Adding additional epitopes also increases the vaccine cost and complexity.

Systems Immunology

In some respects, we are remarkably ignorant about the reasons why some vaccines are very effective while others fail. Understanding the immunologic mechanisms of action of successful vaccines is essential to the rational design of future vaccines. Systems immunology is an interdisciplinary approach that integrates all of the multiple areas of immunology together with transcriptomics, metabolomics, and proteomics. Once these are integrated and the networks identified, and their structure and dynamics elucidated, it is then possible to clarify the precise rules that regulate how the body responds to specific antigens. Sometimes these factors have been underappreciated. For example, Fc receptor activity is important in protection against HIV. As a result, it is possible to design rational vaccines that can induce optimally protective immune responses.

Another area that would benefit from a systems vaccinology approach is identification of the mechanisms by which adjuvants work. Recombinant vaccines depend upon adjuvants to stimulate a protective response and their mechanisms of activity are unclear. An example of such an approach is the systematic analysis of changes in transcriptomes in sheep blood following vaccination against foot-and-mouth disease using several different adjuvants.

The emergence of new diseases and the need for diverse anticancer vaccines has provided a sense of urgency in the rapid production of new vaccines. They can no longer be produced at the leisurely pace of past products. The need for new influenza viruses on an annual basis to keep pace with emerging strains is but one example of this process. Vaccine manufacturers are seeking to build simpler vaccines, developing new, diverse vector systems that will be highly productive expression systems, and using virus-like particles to support a "plug and play" approach. New antigens may simply be inserted into existing virus-like particles or bacterial ghosts (Chapter 3). Modern modular vaccine production facilities should ideally permit the very rapid establishment of a new product line.

The repertoires of B and T cells in response to infection or vaccination can provide insights to strategies for improving vaccines. It is important to examine functional specialization of lymphocytes. Understanding immune cell repertoires is central to generating monoclonal antibodies or cancer-specific T cells. High throughput single cell genomic analyses have revolutionized the study of B and T cell repertoires. For example, it can sequence both the light and heavy chains expressed by a B cell, and so determine its true genotype. Using this approach might make it possible to determine an individual's history of infections and predict their response to vaccines. Studies have, for example, shown that after immunizing mice against influenza, half of the B cells produced did not appear to target known flu antigens. They only appeared after vaccination with antigen, not the adjuvant. Perhaps the B cells are responding to new antigens (neo-epitopes)—otherwise called "dark antigens."

Sources of Additional Information

A web-based database on DNA vaccines is available at http://www.violinet.org/dnavaxdb.

Babiuk, L.A., Pontarollo, R., Babiuk, S., et al. (2003). Induction of immune responses by DNA vaccines in large animals. *Vaccine*, 21, 649–658.

Backert, L., Kohlbacher, O. (2015). Immunoinformatics and epitope prediction in the age of genomic medicine. *Genome Med,* 7, 119.

Bosworth, B., Erdman, M.M., Stine, D.L., Harris, I., Irwin, C., Jens, M., et al. (2010). Replicon particle vaccine protects swine against influenza. *Comp Immunol Microbiol Infect Dis,* 33, e99–e103.

Brun, A., Barcena, J., Blanco, E., Borrego, B., Dory, D., et al. (2011). Current strategies for subunit and genetic viral veterinary vaccine development. *Virus Res,* 15, 1–12.

Dunham, S.P. (2002). The application of nucleic acid vaccines in veterinary medicine, *Res Vet Sci,* 73, 9–16.

Francis, M.J. (2018). Recent advances in vaccine technologies. *Vet Clin Small Anim,* 48, 231–241.

Kramps, T., Elbers, K. (Eds), (2017). Introduction to RNA vaccines. *In RNA vaccines: Methods and Protocols, Methods in Molecular Biology.* New York: Springer Science.

Lundstrom, K. (2016). Replicon RNA viral vectors as vaccines. *Vaccines,* 7, 4(4). doi: 10.3390/vaccines 4040039.

Moss, R.B. (2009). Prospects for control of emerging infectious diseases with plasmid DNA vaccines, *J Immune Based Ther Vacc,* 7, 3. doi: 10.1186/1476-8518-7-3.

Nabel, G.J. (2013). Designing tomorrow's vaccines. *N Engl J Med,* 368, 551–560.

Pandya, M., Rasmussen, M., Hansen, A., Nielsen, M., Buus, S., Golde, W., Barlow, J. (2015). A modern approach for epitope prediction: Identification of foot-and-mouth disease virus peptides binding bovine leukocyte antigen (BoLA) class I molecules. *Immunogenetics,* 67, 691–703.

Pulendran, B., Li, S., Nakaya, H.I. (2010). Systems vaccinology. *Immunity* 33, 516–529.

Rappuoli, R., Bottomly, M.J., D'Oro, U., Finco, O., De Gregorio, E. (2016). Reverse vaccinology 2.0: Human immunology instructs vaccine antigen design. *J Exp Med,* 213, 469–481.

Russell, P.H., Mackie, A. (2001). Eye-drop DNA can induce IgA in the tears and bile of chickens, *Vet Immunol Immunopathol,* 10, 327–332.

Sanchez-Trincado, J.L., Gomez-Perosanz, M., Reche, P.A. (2017). Fundamentals and methods for T- and B-cell epitope prediction. *J Immunol Res.* 2680160.

Sette, A., Rappuoli, R. (2010). Reverse vaccinology: developing vaccines in the era of genomics. *Immunity,* 33, 530–541.

Soria-Guerra, R.E., Nieto-Gomez, R., Govea-Alonso, D.O., Rosales-Mendoza, S. (2015). An overview of bioinformatics tools for epitope prediction: Implications on vaccine development *J Biomed Inform,* 53, 405–414.

Ulmer, J.B., Geall, A.J. (2016). Recent innovations in RNA vaccines. *Curr Opin Immunol,* 41, 18–22.

Vander Veen, R.L., Harris, D.L., Kamrud, K.I. (2012). Alphavirus replicon vaccines. *Anim Health Res Rev,* 1, 1–9.

Williams, J.A. (2013). Vector design for improved DNA vaccine efficacy, safety and production. *Vaccines,* 1, 225–249.

Yamanouchi, K., Barrett, T., Kai, C. (1998). New approaches to the development of virus vaccines for veterinary use. *Rev Sci Tech,* 17, 641–653.

CHAPTER 7

Adjuvants and Adjuvanticity

OUTLINE

How Adjuvants Work

Types of Adjuvants

Damage-Associated Molecular
Patterns-Type Adjuvants

Pathogen-Associated Molecular
Patterns-Type Adjuvants

Particulate Adjuvants

Attenuated live vaccines are not always practical or available for many infectious diseases. This is especially the case when natural infections do not confer adequate protective immunity. If these infections are to be prevented, then killed, inactivated or subunit vaccines must be used, and in many case these vaccines are poorly immunogenic. They therefore require additional components called adjuvants to enhance their immunogenicity, prolong their effect, and provide adequate protection. Adjuvants are also essential for the effectiveness of many recombinant vaccines (Table 7.1)

In 1924, Gaston Ramon, a French veterinarian working at the Pasteur Institute, observed that the antibody levels in horses immunized with tetanus or diphtheria toxoids were higher in animals that developed injection site abscesses. Ramon then induced sterile abscesses by injecting starch, breadcrumbs, or tapioca together with the toxoids and was able to enhance antibody production still further. Thus substances that induced inflammation at the injection site promoted antibody formation. In 1926, Alexander Glenny did essentially the same thing by injecting a foreign antigen together with alum (aluminum potassium sulfate). As a result, the addition of aluminum salts to enhance vaccine efficacy became a standard procedure. To maximize the effectiveness of vaccines, especially those containing killed organisms or highly purified antigens, it is now common practice to add substances, called adjuvants, to a vaccine (*adjuvare* is the Latin verb for "to help"). These adjuvants trigger innate responses that in turn promote the adaptive responses and so provide long-term protection. Adjuvants can increase the speed or the magnitude of the adaptive response to vaccines. They may permit a reduction in the dose of antigen injected or in the numbers of doses needed to induce satisfactory immunity. Adjuvants have also been used to induce appropriate bias in the adaptive response (toward a type 1 or type 2 response), and they are essential if long-term memory is to be established to soluble antigens. On the other hand, it is sometimes difficult to find the correct balance between adjuvant toxicity and immune stimulation to optimize safety and efficacy.

Until recently little attention has been paid to how adjuvants work and their mechanisms of action were speculative. Vaccine adjuvants were defined by what they do and the "science" of adjuvants has been empirical. In other words, stuff was added to vaccines to see if it improved either the strength or duration of the immune response. As a result, adjuvants appear, at first sight, to be an eclectic mixture of natural extracts and inorganic salts, and also particles such as emulsions, nanoparticles, and liposomes.

75

TABLE 7.1 ■ Some Commonly Used Adjuvants in Veterinary Vaccines

Adjuvant Name	Type	Contents
Emulsigen-D MVP Laboratories	Oil in water emulsion	Mineral oil plus dimethyldioctadecyl ammonium bromide
MF59 (Novartis)	Oil in water emulsion	Squalene, Tween 80, Span 85, citrate buffer
ISCOMs	Nanoparticles	Cholesterol, phospholipids, saponins
ISCOMATRIX	Combination	Saponin, Cholesterol, dipalmitoyl phosphatidyl-choline
MetaStim Fort Dodge	Oil emulsion	Oil with emulsifier
Havlogen Merck Animal Health	Polymer	Carbopol
AS04 Glaxo Smith Kline	Alum adsorbed TLR agonist	Alum, Monophosphoryl Lipid A (MPLA)
AS03 Glaxo Smith Kline	Oil in water emulsion	Squalene, Polysorbate 80, α-tocopherol
TS6, Boehringer Ingelheim	Oil in water emulsion	Light mineral oil plus multiple lipophilic and hydrophilic surfactants

TLR, Toll-like receptor.

How Adjuvants Work

Innate immune responses are needed to initiate protective adaptive immunity. The early innate immune response plays a key role in determining the magnitude, quality, and duration of the adaptive immune responses. Very highly purified antigens make poor vaccines because they lack the signals that trigger innate immune responses and as a result cannot generate the downstream signaling required to enhance adaptive responses. Conversely, modified live vaccines, when mimicking natural infections, cause cell damage, trigger the release of pathogen-associated molecular patterns (PAMPs) and damage-associated molecular patterns (DAMPs), and promote strong innate and adaptive responses. In effect therefore, adjuvants trigger the mandatory innate response needed to optimize the adaptive responses and promote the uptake of vaccine antigens by antigen-presenting cells—essentially dendritic cells (Fig. 7.1). They do this in two ways. First, they trigger innate immune responses that provide a stimulus for dendritic cell function and antigen presentation. Alternatively (or additionally) they deliver the antigen in a form optimized for dendritic cell processing and antigen presentation.

Innate immune responses are triggered when pattern-recognition receptors detect microbial invasion and tissue damage. Molecules released by tissue damage (DAMPs) or molecules from foreign microbes (PAMPs) trigger innate responses through pattern-recognition receptors (PRRs) (Fig. 7.2). The activation of PRRs and other cellular receptors on dendritic cells triggers cytokine release. These cytokines promote helper T cell responses, while these in turn activate B and T cells and so promote adaptive immunity.

Some adjuvants cause cell and tissue damage and so provide the body with DAMPs. These DAMP-type adjuvants act by chemical irritation or have direct toxic effects. Thus adjuvants such as the saponins and some emulsions cause cell lysis at the injection site. Saponins are amphipathic soap-like glycosides that can form complexes with cell membrane cholesterol resulting in membrane destruction. The toxicity of emulsions is caused by the presence of short-chain detergent-like molecules that lyse cell membranes. Longer chains are less toxic but poorer adjuvants. The emulsifiers used in water/oil emulsions may have similar toxic effects. Aluminum salts are also cytotoxic and cause the release of DNA, uric acid, and adenosine from dying cells. All these adjuvants release DAMPs that bind to receptors on antigen presenting cells and activate their

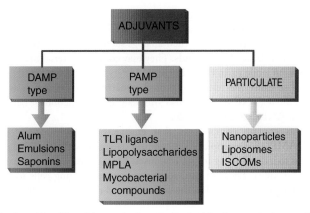

Fig. 7.1 A classification of the different types of adjuvants. Each of the three major types relies on stimulation of innate immunity and the resulting enhancement of the antigen-processing step in adaptive immunity. *ISCOMs, Immune stimulating complexes.*

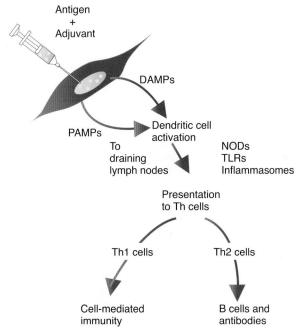

Fig. 7.2 The basic mechanisms by which adjuvants work. *DAMPS, damage-associated molecular complexes; NODs, nucleotide oligomerization domains; PAMPs, Pathogen-associated molecular patterns; TLRs, Toll-like receptors.*

inflammasome pathway. This generates cytokines leading to helper T cell activation. (Inflammasomes are multiprotein complexes whose activation stimulates the production of cytokines such as interleukin (IL)-1 and IL-18 and so promote both innate and adaptive immunity.)

A second type of adjuvant contains microbial products, PAMPs, the essential "danger" signals that also trigger innate immune processes. These PAMP-type adjuvants also provide signals through pattern recognition receptors such as the toll-like receptors (TLRs) and so activate dendritic cells. PAMP-type adjuvants contain killed bacteria, or microbial molecules such as flagellin (a TLR5 ligand), lipopolysaccharide (LPS) (a TLR 4/2 ligand), DNA containing CpG oligodeoxynucleotides (a TLR 9 ligand), their analogs such as monophosphoryl lipid A (MPLA, a TLR4/2 ligand), or synthetic TLR ligands. They may contain bacterial toxins like cholera toxin (CT) or *Escherichia coli* labile toxin (LT). These PAMP-type adjuvants directly activate PRRs on dendritic cells and so cause the release of proinflammatory cytokines such as IL-1, IL-6, and tumor necrosis factor-α (TNF-α). They also stimulate the production of neutrophil-attracting chemokines such as CCL-3, -4, -8, and -20.

Many adjuvants contain components that engage both pathways by using a mixture of PAMPs and DAMPs. For example, TLR agonists synergize with cell-damaging squalene oil-in-water emulsions to induce strong innate responses. This increases the release of the stimulatory cytokines and chemokines. These in turn recruit antigen-presenting cells to the injection site. They enhance antigen uptake as well as the activation and maturation of the antigen-presenting cells (Fig. 7.3).

Note, however, that because they stimulate innate immunity, adjuvants also promote inflammation. This occurs immediately after vaccination and accounts for the commonly observed transient local inflammatory reactions at the injection site. Depression, fever, and malaise, occasionally encountered after animals are vaccinated, result from cytokines at the injection site overflowing into the circulation and acting on the brain. Thus one of the challenges in developing new adjuvanted vaccines is to generate the most potent ones and minimizing their adverse effects, especially inflammation.

Antigen-processing cells are the key to effective adjuvant action. Once activated, these cells take up antigen based on its size, its charge, and its hydrophobicity. They then mature, express high levels of major histocompatibility complex (MHC) molecules, and effectively present the antigen to helper T cells. These cells are critical in determining the nature of the immune

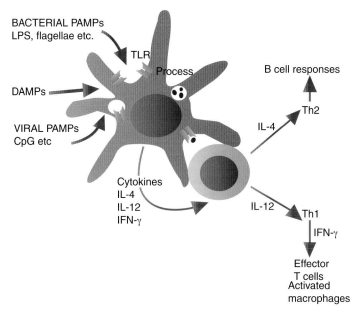

Fig. 7.3 The central role of adjuvants in stimulating antigen-presenting dendritic cells and so triggering a strong adaptive immune response. *CpGs, DAMPS, NODs, PAMPs, TLRs.*

response and can be directly influenced by adjuvants. Therefore a third type of adjuvant consists of particles optimized for ingestion and processing by antigen-presenting cells. The use of particles coated with antigen, cytokines, and costimulatory molecules as adjuvants has led to encouraging improvements in vaccine efficacy and provides a framework for future advances.

The Depot Effect

It was long believed that adjuvants, such as the aluminum salts, acted as antigen depots, slowly releasing the antigen into the body to trigger a prolonged immune response. This effect has probably been exaggerated. Surgical removal of the antigen-alum depot at two hours after injection has no influence on its adjuvanticity. Similar studies have shown a similar lack of depot effect for the oil-based adjuvant MF59 and for ISCOMS (immune stimulating complexes).

Types of Adjuvants

To mount an effective immune response, B cells need to generate at least 20,000 plasma cells, and many more T cells are needed to mount a cell-mediated response. Most modern adjuvants can generate sufficient B cells but not enough CD8 T cells. The few adjuvants that can stimulate adequate T cell responses rely on signaling through antigen processing cells.

Damage-Associated Molecular Patterns-Type Adjuvants

ALUMINUM ADJUVANTS

Aluminum adjuvants have been used since the 1920s and they are by far the most widely employed DAMP-type adjuvants. They are administered to millions of people annually and are both safe and cost-effective. Until recently alum (aluminum potassium sulfate $AlK(SO_4)_2$, was the only adjuvant globally licensed for human use. This has now generally been replaced by aluminum oxyhydroxide ($AlO[OH]$, aluminum hydroxyphosphate ($HAlO_5P$), or aluminum phosphate ($Al[PO_4]_3$). At a neutral pH the hydroxide binds to negatively charged proteins, whereas the phosphate binds positively charged proteins. These aluminum adjuvants either adsorb antigen to the salt nanoparticles or they can be coprecipitated with the antigen. Either method ensures that the antigen is tightly bound to the mineral matrix. It thus makes soluble antigens particulate so that they can be endocytosed and effectively processed. Calcium phosphate is also used as an adjuvant. It is less irritating than the aluminum salts and has been used in experimental vaccines.

Aluminum-adjuvanted vaccines induce tissue damage and cell death at the injection site. This releases DAMPs including DNA, uric acid, ATP, heat shock protein 70, and interleukins 1 and 33. These DAMPs then attract neutrophils with some eosinophils and lymphocytes. Alum causes dying neutrophils to release DNA to form extracellular traps and enhance dendritic cell T cell interactions. Recruitment of mature dendritic cells to the sites of injection is also enhanced. Subsequently macrophages are also attracted to these sites and these macrophages may then develop into dendritic cells. Alum appears to affect lipids in the plasma membrane and promotes dendritic cell homing to lymph nodes. Alum also stimulates the production of chemokines that attract neutrophils and eosinophils. Thus alum has multiple effects largely based on its tissue damaging properties. DNA is known to accumulate at sites of alum deposition and is apparently important because local DNase treatment blocks this adjuvant activity. It has been suggested that alum kills cells at the injection site, releasing DAMPs, which in turn activate host DCs. Recently it has also been demonstrated that alum signals through inflammasomes. DCs or macrophages stimulated with alum plus lipopolysaccharide induced IL-1β and IL-18 release. Alum however, is not good at generating Th1 CD8$^+$ cells and does not induce strong cytotoxic T cell responses.

Alum promotes the production of IL-4 enhancing Th2 responses to protein antigens and generates large numbers of B cells. As a result, while promoting antibody responses, these adjuvants have little effect on cell-mediated responses. Aluminum adjuvants greatly influence the primary immune response but have much less effect on secondary immune responses.

SAPONIN-BASED ADJUVANTS

Saponins are natural triterpene glycosides derived from plants. Their glycosides are hydrophilic whereas the triterpenes are lipophilic, and so saponins act like soap or detergents. The most important of the adjuvant saponins is Quil-A, a mixture of 23 different saponins derived from the inner bark of the South American soapbark tree (*Quillaja saponaria).* It is a potent DAMP-type adjuvant, but crude Quil-A is too toxic for use in humans. As a result, Quil-A has been fractionated and its active fractions identified. The most abundant of these fractions is QS-21. QS-21 combines the most potent adjuvant activity with minimal toxicity. Saponin-based adjuvants selectively stimulate Th1 and cytotoxic T cell responses because they direct antigens into endogenous processing pathways and enhance IFN-γ release by dendritic cells. The saponins cause tissue damage and so activate inflammasomes.

Saponins are employed as adjuvants for foot-and-mouth disease vaccines and recombinant feline leukemia vaccines in addition to experimental porcine respiratory and reproductive system virus (PRRSV) vaccines for pigs. Toxic saponin mixtures are used in anthrax vaccines, where they lyse tissue at the site of injection so that the anthrax vaccine spores may germinate.

Immune stimulating complexes (ISCOMs) are stable matrixes containing cholesterol, phospholipids, and a mixture of Quil-A saponins, and antigen. They assemble into very stable, spherical 40 nm cage-like structures with multiple copies of the antigen exposed on their surface. ISCOMs act as both DAMP-type and particulate adjuvants combined within the same particle. In general, the antibody response to an antigen incorporated in an ISCOM is about tenfold that of the same antigen in saline. They are highly effective in targeting antigens to dendritic cells. The sugar groups on the saponin bind to cell surface lectins on DCs and activate them. Saponins deliver proteins, not only to endosomes, but also to the cytosol of DCs so that they can be presented on MHC class I molecules. In addition, the saponins promote cytokine production and the expression of costimulatory molecules. Depending on the antigen employed, ISCOMs can stimulate either Th1 or Th2 responses. ISCOMATRIX is a particulate adjuvant consisting of cholesterol, phospholipid, and saponin without incorporated antigen. MATRIX-M also consists of nanoparticles made from purified saponins, cholesterol, and phospholipid.

EMULSION ADJUVANTS

Emulsions are generated when two immiscible liquids are mixed together. They occur in several different forms (Fig. 7.4). For example, a water-in-oil (W/O) emulsion consists of aqueous droplets suspended in a continuous oil phase. The best example of this is Freund's adjuvant. Because antigens are water soluble, the droplets are slowly released as the oil breaks down and this slows the degradation of the antigen. An alternative is to use an oil-in-water (O/W) emulsion, where oil droplets are suspended in a continuous aqueous phase. The best example of this is MF59, a commercial adjuvant used in human vaccines.

Mineral oil W/O emulsions tend to be more effective adjuvants but O/W emulsions have a better safety profile. They are less irritating and toxic than water in oil emulsions. In general, both types of emulsion cause cell damage and can be considered to be DAMP-type adjuvants.

One method of forming a slow-release antigen depot is to incorporate the antigen in a water-in-oil emulsion (droplets of the aqueous phase plus a surfactant such as Tween, Span, or lecithin emulsified in an oil phase). A light mineral oil stimulates a local, chronic inflammatory response,

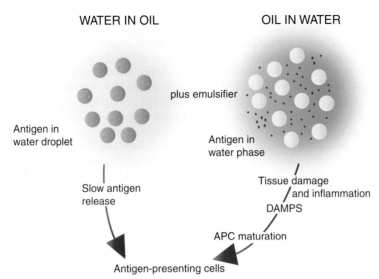

Fig. 7.4 Emulsion adjuvants may be prepared in several ways. The main division is between water in oil and oil in water adjuvants. They each act in a different fashion. A water in oil in water adjuvant may combine the best aspects of both, but may be difficult to manufacture consistently. *APCs, DAMPs.*

and as a result, a granuloma or abscess forms around the site of the inoculum. The antigen is slowly leached from the aqueous phase of the emulsion. These emulsion adjuvants may cause significant tissue irritation and destruction. Mineral oils are especially irritating. Nonmineral oils, although less irritating, are also less-effective adjuvants. The tissue damage generates DAMPs that stimulate both dendritic cells and macrophages.

Nanoemulsions are DAMP-type adjuvants consisting of oil-in-water emulsions containing both solvents and surfactants. An example of a nanoemulsion is MF59; an adjuvant used in human influenza vaccines. MF59 contains squalene combined with polysorbate 80 (Tween 80—an emulsifier) and sorbitan trioleate (Span 85). Squalene is a linear hydrocarbon found in many animal tissues, most notably the liver of sharks. It is a free-flowing oil that can be readily metabolized and is nontoxic. These nanoemulsions do not form a depot at the injection site, but the oil droplets stimulate immune cell recruitment and the emulsifiers cause cell damage. It is more potent and consistent than aluminum-based vaccines and induces Th1 type cell-mediated responses. MF59 also induces a mild local inflammatory reaction. The slow release of antigen from the emulsion may promote macrophage differentiation into dendritic cells. Antigen bound to the oil droplets promotes enhanced uptake by dendritic cells at the injection site, possibly by stimulating local chemokine production. They may also trigger local release of TNFα and IL-1β. MF59 recruits neutrophils, monocytes, eosinophils, and B cells to injection sites. This results in the increased transport of the antigen to draining lymph nodes. Interestingly none of the components of MF59 are adjuvants by themselves. By combining microarray and immunofluorescence assays it has been possible to compare the effects of MF59, and alum adjuvants. For example, MF59 induced the increased expression of 891 genes, whereas alum induced 312 genes. MF 59 was the most potent inducer of genes encoding cytokines, cytokine receptors, and adhesion molecules. MF59 has been used successfully to adjuvant a canine coronavirus vaccine.

Nanoemulsions using soybean oils have also shown encouraging results as adjuvants. These nanoemulsions may induce apoptosis in epithelial cells but then facilitate the uptake and processing of these cells by dendritic and other phagocytic cells. Because they have some antimicrobial activity they can also be used both to inactivate and adjuvant some vaccine preparations.

A diverse range of stable fluid oil-based microemulsion adjuvants are sold under the name of Montanide by SEPPIC (Société d'Exploitation de Produits Pour les Industries Chimiques, Paris). They may contain either a mineral oil or metabolizable oils such as squalene. Droplet size can range from 10 to 500 nm and they contain an emulsifier, mannide monooleate. They have been widely used in veterinary vaccines including those against Newcastle disease, *Mycoplasma hyopneumoniae*, foot-and-mouth disease in pigs and cattle, and in some fish vaccines. Other O/W emulsions used in veterinary vaccines include Emulsigen, from MVP laboratories, TS6, from Merial, and MetaStim, from Fort Dodge.

Multiphasic water-in-oil-in-water (W/O/W) emulsions have also been extensively studied, although few have been produced commercially. They may produce less severe reactions such as granulomas at the injection site, but because they tend to be unstable, are not widely used. They are employed in some Newcastle disease and bovine ephemeral fever vaccines.

Pathogen-Associated Molecular Patterns-Type Adjuvants

Many adjuvants consist simply of microbial products—PAMPS. They are designed to target specific PRRs such as the toll-like receptors (TLRs). As a result, they activate dendritic cells and macrophages and stimulate the production of key cytokines such as IL-1 and IL-12. Depending on the specific microbial product, they may enhance either Th1 or Th2 responses.

TLR4 ligands such as bacterial lipopolysaccharides (or their derivatives) have long been recognized as having adjuvant activity. Their toxicity, however, has limited their use. Lipopolysaccharides enhance antibody formation if given at about the same time as the antigen. They have no effect on cell-mediated responses, but they can break T cell tolerance, and they have a general immunostimulatory activity. Monophosphoryl lipid A (MPLA) is a detoxified bacterial lipopolysaccharide. The lipopolysaccharide is obtained from Salmonella, hydrolyzed, and converted to a mixture of acetylated di-glucosamines. MPLA has less than 1% of the toxicity of the parent endotoxin. Nevertheless, it still binds to TLR 4. This results in the production of interleukin 1 and stimulates the clonal expansion of CD4+T cells. MPLA therefore retains the ability to stimulate T cells without the proinflammatory activity of endotoxin. (It activates a subset of the genes activated by endotoxin). It may also stimulate higher levels of IL-10, an antiinflammatory cytokine. When MPLA from *Salmonella minnesota* lipopolysaccharide is combined with aluminum hydroxide it is called adjuvant system 4 (AS04) (GSK Biologicals). It is used in the highly successful hepatitis B and human papillomavirus vaccines.

Killed anaerobic corynebacteria, especially *Propionibacterium acnes*, have a similar effect. When used as adjuvants these bacteria enhance antibacterial and antitumor activity. The TLR5 ligand, bacterial flagellin acts as an adjuvant that promotes mixed Th1 and Th2 responses. Double-stranded RNA (dsRNA) is the ligand for TLR3, and synthetic dsRNA (for example, polyinosinic:polycytidylic acid [poly I:C]) is an effective adjuvant. The ligand for TLR7 and TLR8 is single-stranded RNA. It is rapidly degraded and therefore an impractical adjuvant. Unmethylated CpG oligodinucleotides that bind TLR9 are potent immunostimulatory adjuvants for Th1 responses. Synthetic TLR ligands, such as the imidazoquinolines, and some guanosine and adenosine analogs. may also be effective adjuvants.

In practice it has been found that multiple innate stimuli may be more effective than a single stimulus and that PAMP combination adjuvants that have multiple mechanisms of action appear to be most effective. They are especially effective when combined with emulsion adjuvants.

SYNTHETIC POLYMER ADJUVANTS

Large biocompatible polymers may also be effective adjuvants. This is probably because they physically restrict the antigen to the injection site and reduce systemic toxicity, and also prolong the local innate reaction. In polymer adjuvanted vaccines, the antigens and adjuvants are either covalently attached to the polymer or encapsulated within polymer particles.

Among the most important of these polymers are polylactic acid (PLA) and poly(lactic-coglycolic acid) (PLGA). These polymeric microparticles can simply be mixed with an antigen such as tetanus toxoid that then binds to the particles. The adsorbed toxoid is then gradually released into the tissues.

Chitosan is a linear polymer formed by the deacetylation of chitin. It consists of randomly arranged chains of β-(1-4)-linked-D-glucosamine and N-acetyl-D-glucosamine monomers. Chitosan binds to mannose receptors on macrophages, activates inflammasomes and complement, and stimulates cytokine production. It and its derivatives may be used as mucosal adjuvants. Chitosan nanoparticles can protect antigens or DNA from degradation and are effective adjuvants when given orally or intranasally. They have been used in bovine herpesvirus, Newcastle disease, and foot and mouth disease vaccines. Other complex carbohydrates that are potentially useful adjuvants include mannans, glucans, and inulin.

High molecular weight, cross-linked, polyacrylic acid polymers termed carbomers have been used as adjuvants in many veterinary vaccines. Many different derivatives have been synthesized. The original synthetic carbomer was trademarked as carbopol (Lubrizol Advanced Materials, Inc.). Carbopol is a synthetic anionic polymer of acrylic acid cross-linked with polyalkenyl ethers or divinyl alcohol. It thus forms a network structure stabilized by cross-linking. It has significant adjuvant properties. It does not have obvious toxicity and antigen can be mixed directly with the carbopol gel. It does not bind to, or modify, the antigen. When incorporated into a live PRRS vaccine in pigs, it appears to enhance cellular immunity by inducing IFN-γ producing cells and driving a strong Th1 polarization. Carbopol promotes the capture of antigen by inflammatory macrophages. It may be combined with other DAMP-type adjuvants such as MF59 or a lipid/polymer/saponin adjuvant to generate additive effects. Carbopol has also been used in equine influenza, porcine circovirus, and *M. hyopneumoniae* vaccines.

Another surface-active polymer that enhances adjuvant activity when added to a squalene emulsion is Pluronic block polymer. This consists of alternating hydrophilic blocks of polyoxyethylene and hydrophobic blocks of polyoxypropylene. These bind to the surface of the oil droplets and increase their protein binding ability. It is used in some commercial veterinary vaccines.

Particulate Adjuvants

The immune system can trap and process particles such as bacteria or other microorganisms much more efficiently than soluble antigens. As a result, many successful adjuvants incorporate vaccine antigens into readily phagocytosable particles (Fig. 7.5). These adjuvants include emulsions, microparticles, ISCOMs, and liposomes, and all are designed to deliver antigen efficiently to antigen-presenting cells. Liposomes are lipid-based synthetic nano- or microparticles 200–1000 nm in size constructed of amphipathic lipid molecules surrounding an inner aqueous core. They are biodegradable and nontoxic. Hydrophilic antigens are enclosed in the aqueous core whereas hydrophobic antigens are inserted in the lipid bilayer. The antigens are effectively trapped and processed, yet are also protected from rapid degradation. They have been used as adjuvants and delivery systems to encapsulate, protect, and enhance antigen uptake by antigen-presenting cells and have been used in influenza and hepatitis A vaccines. The cationic charge is essential for efficient antigen adsorption to the nanoparticle, for retention at the injection site, for activation of the dendritic cells, and for vaccine immunogenicity including the induction of Th1

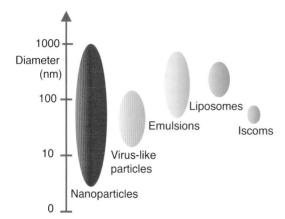

Fig. 7.5 Nanoparticle adjuvants come in many different sizes and this profoundly influences the nature of the immune response they induce. *ISCOMs*

type responses. These cationic liposomes can incorporate PAMPs such as trehalose trimycolate and MPLA. As described earlier, ISCOMS are complex lipid-based microparticles about 40 nm in size. All of these particulate adjuvants may be made more potent by incorporating PAMPs.

Nanotechnology uses particles with an overall size range of 1 to 1000 nanometers. These nanoparticles, nanoemulsions, or nanofibers can be used as adjuvants to promote responses to vaccines. They mimic viruses and bacteria in terms of size and structure. They can also encapsulate and so protect antigens from premature degradation. Because of their very small size, they effectively deliver peptides or proteins to antigen processing cells. Particles less than 1μm in diameter are ingested by pinocytosis; particles less than 120 nm are ingested by endocytosis. Particles smaller than 500 nm can freely enter the lymphatic system and travel to draining lymph nodes, where they are taken up by the antigen processing cells, but not by other cell types. They can activate dendritic cells and stimulate antigen processing. Nanoparticles are also biocompatible, biodegradable, and easy to produce. It is important to remember that biological molecules involved in immunity, especially antigens, allergens, and PAMPS, are also nanometers in size so particle size is critical. Conventional aluminum adjuvants employ microparticles (2–8 μm) and promote Th2 responses. However, if they are reduced to nanoparticle size (200–1500 nm) they favor Th1 responses.

Nanoparticle adjuvants show considerable promise in new vaccines. They can be made from many different compounds such as poly amino acids, polysaccharides, polystyrene, biodegradable polymers in addition to nondegradable elements such as gold, silver, iron, and silica. Polymers, lipids, scaffolds, microneedles, and other biomaterials can be used to improve vaccine efficacy. Some of these biomaterials include nanoparticles and microparticles formed from polymers or lipids that can be conjugated or targeted to immune cells. They offer significant benefits by being able to control the loading and unloading of immune cargoes. Nanoparticles have unique immunological properties that can be manipulated by altering their size, shape, charge, and hydrophobicity. They can be engineered to display a mixture of antigens and costimulating molecules on their surface so that the immune response is optimized. They can be coated with unique combinations of antigens, cytokines, adhesion molecules, immunomodulators, and costimulatory ligands, and in effect may be specifically tailored to generate key protective processes. By associating antigens with PRRs, nanoparticles can trigger cytotoxic lymphocyte responses to antigens that normally won't do this.

Nanoparticles have been used as vaccine carriers containing entrapped antigens or with antibodies or immunomodulators so that they are targeted directly at antigen-presenting cells. These nanoparticles are constructed from degradable synthetic polymers such as poly (lactide-co-glycolide)

(PLGA), copolymer hydrogels or nanogels, and cationic liposomes. PLGA nanocapsules have been used to deliver hepatitis virus B surface antigen in such a way that is rapidly taken up and transported to the endosomes of dendritic cells. PLGA may also directly activate immune pathways. Elipsoidal PLGA particles with a MHC-antigen complex and antiCD28 on its surface can mimic antigen presentation to stimulate T cells more effectively than spherical particles. Star-shaped gold nanoparticles attached to foot and mouth disease virus-like particles have demonstrated very effective adjuvant effects.

Nanoparticles under 500 nm in size traffic rapidly to draining lymph nodes whereas larger particles are retained at the injection site and are phagocytosed and carried to lymph nodes by antigen-presenting cells (APCs). Pulmonary macrophages and DCs take up 50 nm particles more efficiently than 500 nm particles. The chemistry and surface charge of the particles also affect responses. The correct biomaterials can increase antigen persistence. Porosity can increase the diffusion of intracellular proteases resulting in faster antigen processing and presentation.

COMBINED ADJUVANTS

Very powerful adjuvants can be constructed by combining PAMP and DAMP-type adjuvants in a single vaccine formulation. Typically, these combinations combine a DAMP adjuvant such as alum and the saponins, or a particulate carrier such as liposomes together with a PAMP such as MPLA, or CpG DNA. For example, an oil-based depot adjuvant can be mixed with killed *Mycobacterium tuberculosis* or *M. butyricum* incorporated into the water-in-oil emulsion using Arlacel A as an emulsifier. The mixture is called Freund's complete adjuvant (FCA). Not only does FCA form a depot, but the mycobacteria also contain muramyl dipeptide (*N*-acetylmuramyl-L-alanyl-D-isoglutamine), a PAMP that activates macrophages and dendritic cells. FCA works best when given subcutaneously or intradermally and when the antigen dose is relatively low. FCA promotes immunoglobulin (Ig)G production over IgM. It inhibits tolerance induction, favors delayed hypersensitivity reactions, accelerates graft rejection, and promotes resistance to tumors. FCA can be used to induce experimental autoimmune diseases, such as experimental allergic encephalitis and thyroiditis. It also stimulates macrophage activation, thus promoting their phagocytic and cytotoxic activities.

Use of oil-based adjuvants in animals intended for human consumption is problematic because the oil may cause significant injection site damage. Use of FCA is unacceptable in cattle, not only because of the mineral oil but also because its mycobacteria induce a positive tuberculin skin test in vaccinated animals. FCA is highly toxic in dogs and cats.

CYTOKINES

Cytokines can act as adjuvants. One possible strategy to improve responses to vaccinal antigens is to incorporate a cytokine into the vaccine. For example, interleukin-12 (IL-12) has been investigated in this matter. The intensity of the Th1 response to an inactivated pseudorabies vaccine, as measured by the numbers of IFN-γ-producing T cells is significantly increased in the presence of added IL-12. IL-18 has been incorporated into a Newcastle disease vaccine and in a bovine foot and mouth disease vaccine; and IL-7 has been added to a DNA vaccine against bursal disease. They are not yet commercially available and will likely add considerably to the cost of the product.

MUCOSAL ADJUVANTS

With the increased interest in intranasal or oral vaccines, there is a need to identify adjuvants that will enhance their effectiveness on mucosal surfaces. Mucosal surfaces act as physical barriers to prevent invasion, and as a result also exclude vaccine antigens and adjuvants. However, there are specialized antigen-sampling cells on these surfaces including M cells and intraepithelial dendritic cells. M cells can take up antigen and then transfer it to antigen presenting cells. Some antigens may also be taken up by goblet cells. The mucosal epithelium expresses many innate immune receptors including TLRs. Thus PAMPs such as muramyl dipeptide, poly I:C, flagellin, and CpG oligonucleotides work on mucosal sites. Some bacterial PAMPs such cholera toxin and the heat labile enterotoxin of *E. coli* can also act as mucosal adjuvants by stimulating dendritic cells. Cyclic dimeric guanosine monophosphate induces both Th1 and Th17 responses on mucosal surfaces. DAMP adjuvants can also act on mucosa to induce cell stress or damage. These include cyclodextrin and some oleic acid derivatives. They may simply work by inducing sufficient inflammation and mild damage to permit antigen entry. Some compounds added to intranasal adjuvants may prolong their half-lives on mucosal surfaces. A pectin that forms a gel on mucosal surfaces will increase the antigenicity of intranasal influenza vaccine by increasing the time it remains in contact with the mucosa. Other complex carbohydrates such as pullulans and mannans may have a similar effect.

Sources of Additional Information

Aoshi, T. (2017). Modes of action for mucosal vaccine adjuvants. *Viral Immunol, 30*, 463–470.

Aucouturier, J., Dupuis, L., Ganne, V. (2001). Adjuvants designed for veterinary and human vaccines. *Vaccine, 19*, 2666–2672.

Awate, S., Babiuk, L.A., Mutwiri, G. (2013). Mechanisms of action of adjuvants. *Front Immunol, 4*, 114.

Batista-Duharte, A., Martinez, D.T., Carlos, I.Z. (2018) Efficacy and safety of immunological adjuvants. Where is the cut-off? *Biomed Pharmacother, 105*, 616–624.

Bookstaver, M.L., Tsai, S.J., Bromberg, J.S., Jewell, C.M. (2018). Improving vaccine and immunotherapy design using biomaterials. *Trends Immunol, 39*, 135–150.

Brunner, R., Jensen-Jarolim, E., Pali-Scholl, I. (2010). The ABC of clinical and experimental adjuvants: A brief overview. *Immunol Lett, 128*, 29–35.

Burakova, Y., Madera, R., McVey, S., Schlup, J.R., Shi, J. (2018). Adjuvants for animal vaccines. *Viral Immunol, 31*, 11–22.

Coffman, R.L., Sher, A., Seder, R.A. (2010). Vaccine adjuvants: Putting innate immunity to work. *Immunity, 33*, 492–503.

Di Pasquale, A., Preiss, S., Tavares da Silva, F., Garcon, N. (2015). Vaccine adjuvants: From 1920 to 2015 and beyond. *Vaccines (Basel), 3*, 320–343.

Getts, D.R., Shea, L.D., Miller, S.D., King, N.J. (2015). Harnessing nanoparticles for immune modulation. *Trends Immunol, 36*, 419–427.

HogenEsch, H., O'Hagan, D.T., Fox, C.B. (2018). Optimizing the utilization of aluminum adjuvants in vaccines: You might just get what you want. *NPJ Vaccines, 3*, 51.

Horohov, D.W., Dunham, J., Liu, C., Betancourt, A., Stewart, J.C., et al. (2015). Characterization of the in situ immunological responses to vaccine adjuvants. *Vet Immunol Immunopathol, 164*, 24-29.

McKee, A.S., Munks, M.W., Marrack, P. (2007). How do adjuvants work? Important considerations for new generation adjuvants. *Immunity, 27*, 687–690.

MuZikova, G., Laga, R. (2016). Macromolecular systems for vaccine delivery. *Physiol Res, 65*, S203–S216.

O'Hagan, D.T., Friedland, L.R., Hanon, E., Didierlaurent, A.M. (2017). Towards an evidence based approach for the development of adjuvanted vaccines. *Curr Opin Immunol, 47*, 93–102.

Steinhagen, F., Kinjo, T., Bode, C., Klinman, D.M. (2011). TLR-based adjuvants. *Vaccine, 29*, 3341–3355.

Sulczewski, F.B., Liszbinski, R.B., Romao, P.R.T., Rodrigues Junior, L.C. (2018). Nanoparticle vaccines against viral infections. *Arch Virol, 163*(9), 2313–2325.

Sun, B., Yu, S., Zhao, D., Guo, S., Wang, X., Zhao, K. (2018). Polysaccharides as vaccine adjuvants. *Vaccine, 36*, 5226–5234.

The Administration of Vaccines

Although vaccine manufacturers produce high quality products, these will not be effective if administered by the wrong route, in the wrong dose, or at the wrong time. Thus careful and appropriate administration is required if maximum benefit is to be afforded by vaccination.

One must not lose sight of the objectives of vaccination. Vaccines are given to protect animals against significant infectious diseases to which they have a risk of exposure. Vaccines should therefore only be given when these benefits are obvious and outweigh any possible adverse effects. Potential risks include adverse reactions, the likelihood of acquiring the disease, and the severity of the disease. On the other hand, benefits include protection from infection and death, reduction in disease severity, and any contribution to herd immunity. Vaccines should be administered no more frequently than necessary to confer protection. It is of course equally inappropriate to vaccinate animals in such a way that any immunity conferred is insufficient to protect them. Veterinarians assessing vaccine risk must also consider any benefits to human health that might result from protection against zoonotic infections.

Since the 1990s, there has been a concerted effort to classify vaccines into those essential for animal health and thus mandatory (CORE vaccines) and those whose use depends upon specific risk assessment (nonCORE vaccines). That terminology is used here although it may be considered a false dichotomy. The use of every vaccine should be based on an objective and thorough risk assessment. The veterinarian must make their own professional judgment and an informed decision regarding vaccine use. Designation of core vaccines does not absolve them from their professional responsibilities in this respect.

Veterinarians should only use effective vaccines licensed by their national authorities and the vaccines must be used in accordance with the label directions. They should not be used unless the veterinarian has either diagnosed a specific disease or is aware of its presence in an area, because otherwise it is not possible to determine the benefits and risks of vaccination.

Vaccination Principles

VACCINATION SCHEDULES

Certain principles are common to all methods of active immunization. Most vaccines require an initial series in which the immune system is primed and protective immunity initiated, followed by revaccination (booster shots) at intervals to ensure that this protective immunity remains at an adequate level.

Initial Series

Because maternal antibodies passively protect newborn animals, it is not usually possible to vaccinate very young animals successfully. If protection is deemed necessary at this stage, the mother may be vaccinated during pregnancy. Maternal vaccinations should be timed so that peak antibody levels are achieved at the time of colostrum formation. Once an animal is born, successful active immunization is effective only after maternal antibodies have waned. Animals should be revaccinated 12 months later or at 1 year of age. It is unclear whether maternal antibodies can always block antibody responses to intranasal vaccines. Despite high levels of circulating maternal antibodies, maternal interference does not always occur and nasal antibody production is often unimpaired.

The timing of initial vaccinations may also be determined by disease epidemiology. Some diseases are seasonal, and vaccines may be given before outbreaks are anticipated. Examples of these include the vaccine against the lungworm, *Dictyocaulus viviparus,* given in early summer just before the anticipated lungworm season; the vaccine against anthrax given in spring; and the vaccine against *Clostridium chauvoei* given to sheep before turning them out to pasture. Bluetongue of lambs is spread by midges and is thus a disease of midsummer and early fall. Vaccination in spring will therefore protect lambs during the susceptible period. Similar considerations apply to mosquito-borne/wet season diseases.

Vaccination Intervals

When deciding on the optimal interval between the first immunization and the booster shot it is important to consider how B cells and T cells differentiate. These cells respond rapidly to antigen and generate effector cells or plasma cells. Once this phase is over, most effector cells die while the survivors differentiate into memory cells. Memory T cells may take several weeks after the primary immune response to reach maximal numbers. Only when this memory phase develops can a significant secondary response be induced. As a general rule it is better to wait for as long as possible between prime and boost. Boosting too soon may well result in suboptimal secondary responses. (But boosting too late may open a window of vulnerability). Excessive boosting of mice appears to drive T cells toward terminal differentiation and deplete the population of central memory cells. Similar considerations apply to B cell responses. They need time to develop memory cells and premature boosting runs the risk of generating suboptimal memory. Computer modeling suggests that an interval of several weeks is necessary to obtain optimal secondary responses. In children, 4 to 8 weeks is considered to be the minimal interval between the first two doses by the Centers for Disease Control and Prevention (CDC), whereas six months is the recommended interval between the second and third vaccine doses. Studies on revaccination with Clostridial vaccines in sheep also suggest that an interval of 8 weeks between vaccine doses is optimal. A study on boosting cattle with rabies vaccine suggested that the optimal response was obtained with a 180-day interval between vaccine doses.

Although experimental data suggest that vaccination intervals be somewhat longer than currently recommended, one must also remember that it is essential not to leave a window of susceptibility between vaccine doses. For practical purposes, it is generally recommended that in dogs and cats the minimal interval should be 2 to 3 weeks. For larger animals such as horses it is generally a minimum of 3 to 4 weeks. In general, the longer the interval between booster shots, the better it is for the induction of a maximal protective response. Decisions on vaccination frequency however must be at the discretion of the vaccinating veterinarian.

Revaccination

It is the persistence of memory cells after vaccination that provides an animal with long-term protection. The presence of long-lived plasma cells is associated with persistent antibody production so that a vaccinated animal may have antibodies in its bloodstream for many years after exposure to a vaccine.

Revaccination schedules depend on the duration of effective protection. This in turn depends on specific antigen content, whether the vaccine consists of living or dead organisms, and its route of administration. In the past, relatively poor vaccines may have required frequent administration, perhaps as often as every six months, to maintain an acceptable level of immunity. Modern vaccines usually produce a long-lasting protection, especially in companion animals. Many require revaccination only every three or four years, whereas for others, immunity may persist for an animal's lifetime. Even inactivated viral vaccines may protect individual animals against disease for many years. Unfortunately, the minimal duration of immunity has rarely been measured, until recently, and reliable figures are not available for many vaccines. Although serum antibodies can be monitored in vaccinated animals, tests have not been standardized, and there is no consensus regarding the interpretation of these antibody titers. Even animals that lack detectable antibodies may have significant cell-mediated resistance to disease. Nor is there much detailed information available regarding long-term immunity on mucosal surfaces. In general, immunity against feline panleukopenia, canine distemper, canine parvovirus, and canine adenovirus is considered to be relatively long lasting (>5 years). On the other hand, immunity to feline herpesvirus, feline calicivirus, and *Chlamydia* is believed to be relatively short. One problem in making these statements is the variability among individual animals and among different types and brands of vaccine. Thus recombinant canine distemper vaccines may induce shorter duration immunity than conventional, modified live vaccines. There may be a great difference between the shortest and longest duration of immunological memory within a group of animals. Duration of immunity studies are confounded by the fact that many older animals have increased innate resistance. Different vaccines within a category may differ significantly in their performance, and although all vaccines may induce immunity in the short term, it cannot be assumed that all confer long-term immunity. Manufacturers use different master seeds and different methods of antigen preparation. A significant difference exists between the minimal level of immunity required to protect most animals and the level of immunity required to ensure protection of all animals.

Annual revaccination was once the rule for most animal vaccines because this approach was administratively simple and had the advantage of ensuring that an animal was seen regularly by a veterinarian. It is clear, however, that modern vaccines such as those against canine distemper or feline herpesvirus induce protective immunity that can last for many years and that annual revaccination using these vaccines is excessive. A growing body of evidence now indicates that most modified live viral vaccines induce lifelong sterile immunity in dogs and cats. In contrast, immunity to bacteria is of much shorter duration and often may prevent disease but not infection. Old dogs and cats rarely die from vaccine-preventable disease, especially if they have been vaccinated as adults. In contrast, young animals die from such diseases, especially if not vaccinated or vaccinated prematurely.

A veterinarian should always assess the relative risks and benefits to an animal in determining the timing of any vaccination. It is therefore be good practice to use serum antibody assays such as rapid test ELISAs (enzyme-linked immunosorbent assays) or lateral flow assays, if available, to provide guidance on revaccination intervals. Persistent antibody titers determine whether an animal requires additional protection. These tests not only identify those animals that have responded to vaccination, they can determine if an animal is a nonresponder. They can determine if an animal that previously suffered from an adverse event really requires revaccination. They can determine whether an animal with an undocumented vaccine history needs to be vaccinated and with which vaccines. They can determine which animals in a shelter undergoing a disease outbreak are susceptible and so require vaccination. They can also determine whether revaccination is really necessary at three years. It should be pointed out, however, that animals with low or undetectable serum antibody levels may still be protected as a result of persistence of memory B and T cells capable of responding rapidly to reinfection. "Blind" revaccination should be avoided if appropriate serum antibody assays are available.

Notwithstanding this discussion, animal owners should be made aware that protection against an infectious disease can only be maintained reliably when vaccines are used in accordance with the protocol approved by the vaccine-licensing authorities. The duration of immunity claimed by a vaccine manufacturer is the minimum duration of immunity that is supported by the data available at the time the vaccine license is approved. This must always be taken into account when discussing revaccination protocols with an owner.

MATERNAL IMMUNITY

Mothers transfer antibodies to their offspring through feeding colostrum in most domestic mammals (Fig. 8.1). Once absorbed from the intestine, these maternal antibodies inhibit neonatal antibody synthesis by acting through regulatory pathways that ensure that the body does not make more antibodies than it needs. They inhibit B cells, not T cells. As a result, they prevent the successful vaccination of very young animals. This inhibition may persist for many months. Its duration depends primarily on the amount (titer) of antibodies transferred and the half-life of the immunoglobulins involved. This problem can be illustrated using the example of vaccination of puppies against canine distemper.

Maternal antibodies, absorbed from the puppy's intestine, reach maximal levels in serum by 12 to 24 hours after birth. These levels then decline slowly through normal protein catabolism. The catabolic rate of proteins is exponential and is expressed as a half-life. The half-life of specific antibodies against distemper and canine infectious hepatitis is 8.4 days. Experience has shown that, *on average*, the level of maternal antibodies to distemper in puppies declines to insignificant levels by about 10 to 12 weeks, but this may range from 6 to 16 weeks. (The titer of maternal antibodies, not the animal's age is the determining factor.) In a population of puppies, the proportion of susceptible animals therefore increases gradually from a very few or none at birth, to most puppies at 10 to 12 weeks. Consequently, very few newborn puppies can be successfully vaccinated, but most can be protected by 10 to 12 weeks. Rarely, a puppy may reach 15 or 16 weeks before it can be successfully vaccinated. If virus diseases were not so common, it would

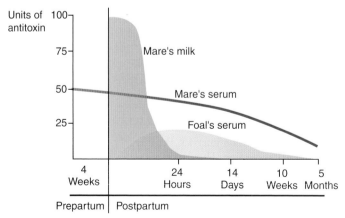

Fig. 8.1 The transfer of maternal antibodies from mares to foals. In this case antibodies to *Cl. perfringens* were measured in mare's serum, colostrum, and milk, and also in their foal's serum from birth to five months. (From Jeffcott, L.B. [1974]. Studies on passive immunity in the foal. I. γ-globulin and antibody variations associated with the maternal transfer of immunity and the onset of active immunity. *J. Comp. Pathol,* 84, 93–101.).

be sufficient to delay vaccination until all puppies were about 12 weeks old, when success could be almost guaranteed. In practice however, a delay of this type means that an increasing proportion of puppies, fully susceptible to disease, would be without immune protection—an unacceptable situation. Nor is it feasible to vaccinate all puppies repeatedly at short intervals from birth to 12 weeks, a procedure that would also ensure almost complete protection. Therefore a compromise must be reached.

The earliest recommended age to begin vaccinating a puppy or kitten with a reasonable expectation of success is at six weeks. Colostrum-deprived orphan pups lacking maternal antibodies, may be vaccinated at two weeks of age. Because it is impossible to predict the exact time of loss of specific maternal antibodies, any initial vaccination series will generally require administration of at least three doses. Current guidelines for essential canine and feline vaccines, for example, indicate that the first dose of vaccine should be administered as early as 6 to 8 weeks of age, and revaccinated at 2 to 4 week intervals until they are about 16 weeks of age. Strictly speaking these are not booster doses. They are simply designed to trigger a primary response as soon as possible after maternal antibodies have declined. Rabies is a core vaccine that should be given at 14 to 16 weeks. In kittens the half-life of maternal antibodies to feline panleukopenia is 9.5 days. The appropriate protocol would be to use three doses of the core vaccines (herpesvirus, calicivirus, and panleukopenia) at 8 to 9 weeks, 3 to 4 weeks later, and at 14 to 16 weeks; feline leukemia vaccine can be given at 8 weeks and 3 to 4 weeks later; and rabies vaccine can be given at 8 to 12 weeks, depending on the type of vaccine used (Fig. 8.2).

Similar considerations apply when vaccinating large farm animals (Fig. 8.3). The prime factor influencing the duration of maternal immunity is the level of antibodies in the mother's colostrum. In foals, maternal antibodies to tetanus toxin can persist for six months and antibodies to equine arteritis virus for as long as eight months. Antibodies to bovine viral diarrhea virus may persist for up to nine months in calves. The half-lives of maternal antibodies against equine influenza and equine arteritis virus antigens in the foal are 32 to 39 days respectively. As in puppies, a young foal may have nonprotective levels of maternal antibodies long before it can be vaccinated. Maternal antibodies, even at low titers, effectively block immune responses in young foals and calves, so premature vaccination may also be ineffective. The effective response to vaccines increases progressively after the first six months of life. A safe rule is that calves and foals should be vaccinated no earlier than three to four months of age, followed by one or two revaccinations at four-week intervals. The precise schedule will depend on the vaccine used and the species to

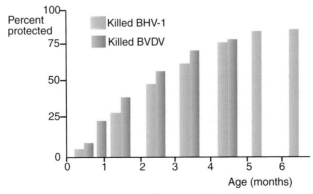

Fig. 8.2 The response of vaccinated calves to two different inactivated viral vaccines on calves between birth and six months of age. It is clear that vaccination before four to five months results in significantly reduced protection. *BHV*, bovine herpesvirus-1; *BVDV*, bovine virus diarrhea virus. (From data kindly provided by Dr. R.J. Schultz)

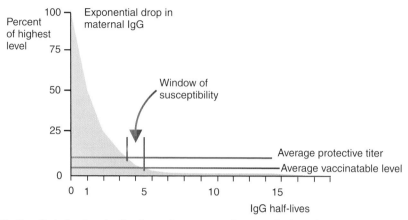

Fig. 8.3 The effect of maternal antibodies on the response of young animals such as puppies. Although immunoglobulins decline exponentially based on their half-life, the precise time at which they lose immunity and the time when they can be vaccinated depend upon the antibody titer. This protective titer varies between infectious agents and thus the time when the animal becomes susceptible will also vary. The presence of maternal antibodies also suppresses the puppy immune response to vaccination. The higher the maternal antibody titer, the greater the suppression. The time when a puppy can respond to a vaccine may not be the same as the time when it becomes disease susceptible. *Ig,* Immunoglobulin.

be vaccinated. Animals vaccinated before six months of age should always be revaccinated at six months or after weaning, to ensure protection.

Some live recombinant vaccines such as canarypox-vectored distemper in dogs or influenza in horses appear to be able to prime young animals in the presence of significant maternal antibodies. DNA vaccines against pseudorabies also appear to be effective in priming cell-mediated responses in piglets in the face of maternal immunity, whereas a DNA plasmid vaccine against bovine respiratory syncytial virus vaccine is not. Thus the ability of DNA vaccines to overcome maternal antibodies varies among species and agents.

Vaccination Strategies

Although the principles of vaccination have been known for many years, vaccines and vaccination procedures are continuing to improve in efficacy and safety. The earliest veterinary vaccines were often of limited efficacy and some had significant adverse effects, although these were considered acceptable when measured against the risks of acquiring disease. The vaccination protocols developed at that time reflected the inadequacies of these vaccines. Ongoing developments in vaccine design and production have resulted in great improvements in both safety and effectiveness. These improvements permit a reassessment of the relative risks and benefits of vaccination. Vaccination is not always a totally innocuous procedure. For this reason, the use of any vaccine should be accompanied by a risk/benefit analysis conducted by the veterinarian in consultation with the animal's owner. Vaccination protocols should be determined for each individual animal, giving due consideration to the seriousness of the disease, the zoonotic potential of the agent, the animal's susceptibility and exposure risk, and any legal requirements relating to vaccination. The success of mass vaccination programs depends both on the proportion of animals vaccinated and on the efficacy of the vaccine. Neither of these factors will reach 100%, so it is essential to target the vaccine effectively. It is also the case that vaccines do not confer immediate protection, so the strategy employed will depend on the rate of spread of an infection.

HERD IMMUNITY

The main purpose of vaccinating animals, especially companion animals, is to protect each individual animal. It is expected that clinical disease will be minimized. It is also expected that vaccinated animals will shed fewer pathogens. In an animal population such as a herd or flock, the benefits of vaccines result from the collective impact of the procedure on all individuals and the collective decline in pathogen shedding. This decline in shedding, together with collective immunity, contributes to herd immunity (Fig. 8.4).

When vaccines are used to control disease in a population of animals rather than in individuals, herd immunity must be considered. Herd immunity refers to the resistance of an entire group of animals to a disease as a result of the presence of many immune animals in that group. Herd immunity reduces the probability of a susceptible animal meeting an infected one so that the spread of disease is slowed or prevented. If it is acceptable to lose individual animals from disease while preventing epizootics, it may be possible to do this by vaccinating only a proportion of the population. Veterinarians should seek to ensure that as many animals as possible are vaccinated to maximize herd immunity.

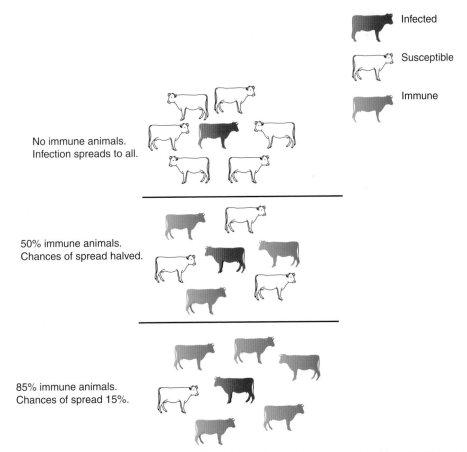

Fig. 8.4   The principle of herd immunity. This figure is based on an infectious agent that is highly efficiently transmitted. If the agent has a low R_0, herd immunity need not be 100% for its transmission to be completely blocked.

The spread of an infectious disease is, of course, dependent upon the close proximity of susceptible individuals. Solitary animals are much less likely to encounter other infected individuals. On the other hand, animals living in herds, flocks, or shelters will encounter numerous individuals. If all these other animals lack immunity, then there is nothing to prevent the spread of infection. If all these other individuals are soundly immune then the infection cannot spread. This is not, however, an all-or-nothing phenomenon. If most of the animals in the herd are immune then the chances of an infected animal encountering a susceptible one are reduced and the chances of the disease spreading is drastically reduced.

The most important factor that influences herd immunity is the basic reproductive number of the disease, termed R_0 and pronounced "R nought". R_0 is the expected number of secondary cases resulting from each primary case in a completely susceptible population. In other words, the probability of transmission of an infectious agent.

R_0 is not a constant. For example, it will vary according to population density, animal behavior, and seasonality. An R_0 of 1 indicates that each individual primary case generates one secondary case and the prevalence of the disease will remain static. An R_0 of less than 1 means that one case will on average, generate fewer secondary cases. As a result, the prevalence of disease will decline. Conversely, an R_0 greater than 1 means that each primary case will generate an increased number of secondary cases, then the numbers of such cases will increase. The higher the R_0 the more difficult it is to prevent an infectious disease. R_0 depends on the effective contact rate between individuals over time, the size of the population, and the duration of infectivity. Thus R_0 will vary as a result of stocking density, environmental effects, any biosecurity practiced, the introduction of susceptible animals, and the nature of the production system.

Vaccines, by reducing the number of susceptible animals in a population, reduce the number of contacts between infectious and susceptible animals. This reduction will be determined by the efficacy of the vaccine in reducing transmission and the amount of vaccination coverage within the population. As a result, the "effective population density" of susceptible animals is reduced and the quantity of pathogen available to infect the nonvaccinated animals decreases. Each vaccinated individual therefore contributes to herd immunity and a reduction in the effective reproductive number, R will occur. R is similar to R_0 but does not assume complete susceptibility in a population. It is not necessary for all the animals in a herd to be protected in order for R to be reduced to less than 1 and so result in disease elimination. R may be calculated by multiplying the R_0 by the proportion of susceptible animals. For example, if a vaccine protects 80% of a herd then the organism can only infect the unprotected 20% and R will drop by 80%. If there are insufficient susceptible animals in a population, R may drop to less than 1, transmission will be interrupted, and the disease will be eliminated.

The level of herd immunity needed to bring R to this level is called the "herd immunity threshold (HIT)" and is calculated by HIT $= 1 - 1/R_0$. The HIT is useful in that it provides a target for vaccination coverage. The HIT has been calculated for the major human infectious diseases. It ranges from 90% to 95% for measles and rubella, to about 85% for rubella and diphtheria, to 70% to 80% for smallpox. It has not been widely calculated for animal diseases. A figure of 70% is widely quoted for canine rabies (Box 8.1).

Although vaccination is a powerful tool for the control of infectious disease, its potential to prevent the spread of or eliminate a disease depends on selecting the correct control strategies. If an infectious disease outbreak, such as one caused by foot-and-mouth virus, is to be rapidly controlled by vaccination, it is vitally important to select the correct population to be vaccinated. The success of any mass vaccination program depends both on the proportion of animals vaccinated and on the efficacy of the vaccine. Neither of these factors will reach 100%, so it is essential to target the vaccine effectively. It is also the case that vaccines do not confer immediate protection, so the strategy employed will depend on the rate of spread of an infection. Vaccines may thus be given prophylactically, in advance of an outbreak, or reactively, in response to an existing outbreak.

BOX 8.1 ■ Herd Immunity and Rinderpest

As the great Rinderpest eradication program gathered momentum it became essential to determine what fraction of the cattle population had to be vaccinated to eliminate the disease. Mathematical modeling of infected, unvaccinated herds showed a R_0 for rinderpest ranging from 4–5 to 1.2–1.9 depending on the virus strain. This determined that the herd immunity thresholds ranged from 77% to 33%. It was also determined that the disease could only be sustained in cattle populations greater than 200,000. Great effort was therefore put into vaccinating at least 80% of the cattle in these populations. It worked and rinderpest was eradicated.

(From Mariner, J.C., McDermott, J., Heesterbeek, J.A., Catley, A., Roeder, P. (2005). A model of
   lineage 1 and lineage 2 rinderpest virus transmission in pastoral areas of East Africa. *Prev Vet Med*,
   69, 245–263.)

Both strategies have advantages and disadvantages. In general, prophylactic vaccination greatly reduces the potential for a major epidemic of a disease such as foot-and-mouth disease by reducing the size of the susceptible population. The effectiveness of this approach can be greatly enhanced by identifying high-risk individuals and ensuring that they are protected in advance of an outbreak.

It is generally not feasible to vaccinate an entire population of animals once a disease outbreak has occurred. However, two effective reactive vaccination strategies are *ring vaccination,* which seeks to contain an outbreak by establishing a barrier of immune animals around an infected area, and *predictive vaccination,* which seeks to vaccinate the animals on farms likely to contribute most to the future spread of disease. Reactive vaccination in this way can ensure that an epidemic is not unduly prolonged. A prolonged "tail" to an epidemic commonly results from the disease "jumping" to a new area. Well-considered, predictive vaccination may prevent these jumps. Thus a combination of prophylactic and reactive vaccination will likely yield the most effective results.

Safety and Efficacy

The two major factors that determine vaccine use are safety and efficacy. We must always be sure that the risks of vaccination do not exceed those associated with the chance of contracting the disease. Thus it may be inappropriate to use a vaccine against a disease that is rare, is readily treated by other means, or is of little clinical significance. Because the detection of antibodies is a common diagnostic procedure, unnecessary use of vaccines may complicate diagnosis based on serology and perhaps make eradication of a disease impossible. On the other hand, serologic tests may make it possible to determine animal susceptibility and rationalize vaccine usage. The decision to use vaccines for the control of any disease must be based not only on the degree of risk associated with the disease, but also on the availability of superior alternatives.

The second major consideration is vaccine efficacy. Vaccines may not always be effective. In some diseases, such as equine infectious anemia, Aleutian disease in mink, and African swine fever, poor or no protective immunity can be induced and vaccines are not available. In other diseases, such as foot-and-mouth disease in pigs, the immune response may be transient and relatively ineffective, and successful disease control is sometimes difficult to achieve.

As a result of these considerations, animal vaccines should be ranked based on their importance. The first category consists of core "essential" vaccines—those that are required because they protect against common, dangerous diseases and because a failure to use them would place an animal at significant risk of disease or death. In other words, a high benefit/risk ratio. Determination of which vaccines are core will vary based on local conditions and disease threats. A second category consists of optional vaccines. These are directed against diseases for which the risks associated with not vaccinating may be low. In many cases, risks from these diseases are determined by the location or lifestyle of an animal. The use of these optional vaccines should be determined by a veterinarian on the basis of exposure risk. A third category consists of vaccines that may have no application in routine vaccination but are only used under special circumstances. These are vaccines directed against diseases of little clinical significance or vaccines whose risks do not significantly outweigh their benefits. Of course, all vaccine use should be conducted on the basis of informed consent. An animal's owner should be made aware of the risks and benefits involved before seeking approval to vaccinate. This is especially important if using a vaccine in a manner different from that recommended by the manufacturer.

COMBINED AND POLYVALENT VACCINES

It is increasingly uncommon for vaccines directed against a single agent to be employed in domestic species. In practice, it is usual to employ complex mixtures of organisms within single vaccines. For example, in dogs, distemper vaccine is combined with canine adenovirus 2, canine parvovirus, canine parainfluenza, coronavirus, leptospirosis, and *Borrelia burgdorferi* vaccines. In controlling the respiratory disease complex of cattle, bovine virus diarrhea vaccines may be combined with infectious bovine rhinotracheitis, parainfluenza 3, bovine respiratory syncytial virus, leptospirosis, *Campylobacter fetus, Histophilus somni, Pasteurella multocida,* and *Mannheimia hemolytica* vaccines. These vaccine combinations protect animals against several diseases with economy of effort. However, it can also be wasteful to use vaccines against organisms that may not be causing problems. When different antigens in a mixture are inoculated simultaneously, competition occurs between antigens. Manufacturers of combined vaccines take this into account and adjust their components accordingly. Vaccines should never be mixed indiscriminately because one component may dominate the mixture or interfere with the response to the other components.

Some have questioned whether the use of complex vaccine combinations leads to less than satisfactory protection or increases the risk for adverse side effects. They are concerned that the use of 5- or 7-component vaccines in their animals will somehow overwhelm the immune system, forgetting that our animals encounter hundreds of different antigens in daily life. The suggestion that these combined vaccines can overload the immune system is unfounded, nor is there any evidence to support the contention that the risk for adverse effects increases disproportionately when more components are added to vaccines. The success of a 15-component bluetongue vaccine in sheep or a 23-component pneumococcal vaccine in acquired immunodeficiency syndrome patients, should serve as a reassurance that multiple component vaccines are not overwhelming. Certainly such vaccines should be tested to ensure that all components induce a satisfactory response. Licensed vaccines provided by a reputable manufacturer will generally provide satisfactory protection against all components.

Administration

VACCINE STORAGE AND HANDLING

Always check the package insert or the manufacturer's recommendations regarding storage. Vaccines should be stored in a refrigerator or freezer as appropriate. Refrigerated vaccines should be stored between 2°C and 8°C with a mid-range of about 5°C (40°F). Ideally check the temperature twice daily with a max/min thermometer. A signed log recording this should be maintained to ensure that this is not ignored. Make sure that vaccines do not warm or freeze inadvertently by storing them in the middle, not the front or back of the shelves. Do not store in vegetable drawers or in the door where temperature variation may be considerable. Liquid vaccines that contain an aluminum adjuvant will lose potency if frozen. Never store food in a refrigerator holding vaccines. Do not overstock a refrigerator because this may affect temperature control. A study of farm refrigerators in the United Kingdom suggests that most failed to store vaccines under the recommended conditions. Many (40%) inadvertently froze the vaccine, and 59% had a temperature that rose above 8°C at least once. This part of the cold chain is very vulnerable.

A designated person should be the vaccine coordinator, to oversee receipt of vaccines, their storage, and handling. This individual should maintain a vaccine inventory log that documents the details of each vaccine batch: name, manufacturer, lot number, expiration date, vendor, quantity, and arrival condition.

All other appropriate staff members should also receive training. A practice should have documented standard operating procedures available with respect to storage and handling posted close to the vaccine storage units and make sure that the staff knows where they are. All new employees should be trained and then refreshed annually. Make sure that staff members are instructed when recommendations are updated or when new vaccines are added.

Vaccines must be organized according to their expiration date so that the oldest products are used first. Obviously, the refrigerator should be reliable and should it fail promptly move them to a working one or to a refrigerated container. Discard vaccines that have been exposed to temperatures outside the manufacturers recommended range, whether too high or frozen. When transporting vaccines to clients make sure they are carried in a refrigerated container with a thermometer to ensure the vaccines do not warm. A cool pack may not be sufficient to maintain cold temperatures over a full day in a hot climate.

Always store vaccines in their original packages with lids closed until ready for use. Protect them from light. Store diluent with the corresponding vaccine. Clearly label where each type of vaccine and diluent are stored.

INJECTION

Most vaccines are administered by injection. Care must be taken not to injure or introduce infection into any animal. All needles used must be clean and sharp and of the appropriate size. Dirty or dull needles can cause tissue damage and infection at the injection site. The skin at the injection site must be clean and dry, although excessive alcohol swabbing should be avoided. Vaccines are provided in a standard dose, and this dose should not be divided to account for an animal's size. Vaccine doses are not yet formulated to account for body weight or age. There must be a sufficient antigen to trigger the cells of the immune system and provoke a protective immune response. This amount is not related to body size. Vaccination by subcutaneous or intramuscular injection is the simplest and most common method of administration. This approach is obviously excellent for small numbers of animals and for diseases in which systemic immunity is important.

Although this may seem obvious, it is essential that proper aseptic technique should always be followed when administering vaccines. Always follow manufacturer's instructions because these are based on the actual methods employed when the vaccine was shown to be efficacious. The site of injection should be cleaned as much as possible. Each animal should be vaccinated with a new needle and a new needle should be used for each vaccine product to ensure that they are not cross contaminated when the needle is inserted into the vaccine vial. A new needle also prevents the possible transmission of blood-borne pathogens. Vaccines must only be given by their approved route. For example, intranasal vaccines should never be injected. To facilitate treatment of any sarcomas that may arise, cats should not be vaccinated subcutaneously into the interscapular furrow in the neck (Chapter 10). Always observe the meat or milk withdrawal period of vaccines in food-producing animals. This is commonly 21 days, but sometimes it is considerably longer.

Draw up vaccines only at the time of administration because once the vaccine is inside syringes, it may be difficult to identify. Syringes are not designed for storage. Remember that once reconstituted, vaccines should be administered within 1 hour. Any reconstituted vaccines held for longer than an hour should be discarded. Do not rely on preservatives to prevent contamination of multidose vaccine containers. Never mix vaccines with other medicines and follow all manufacturer's instructions. Always dispose of used needles in a sharps box. If a vaccine is spilled, clean off the fur with alcohol swabs and disinfect any surfaces.

If an animal cannot be approached closely, it may be injected by the use of a jab stick or syringe pole. This is in effect a syringe at the end of a long (15–50 inch) rod to provide extended reach. They may simply be push rods where the syringe is pushed into the animal and the plunger continues to be pushed to inject the vaccine. Alternatively, the plunger may be pushed using a thumb-operated trigger that does not exert additional pressure on the animal. Anesthetized animals should not be vaccinated because of the risks of hypersensitivity and vomiting.

Proper documentation of vaccination is essential. Permanent medical records should include the date, the identity of the animal vaccinated, the administering veterinarian, the type and proprietary name of the vaccine(s) administered, batch number, expiry date, manufacturer, route, and the site of inoculation. Veterinarians should also offer the owner of a vaccinated animal, a vaccination certificate also containing this data. Ideally the recommended date of revaccination should also be on this certificate in addition to the details of the administering veterinarian and the practice.

Mucosal Vaccination

Most infectious agents invade the body through mucosal surfaces, especially the respiratory and digestive tracts. It makes sense therefore for vaccine antigens to be administered by the same route. Presumably, by mimicking the natural route, vaccines will trigger immune responses on these surfaces and ideally, block pathogen invasion.

When a systemic immune response is triggered by injected antigen, effector T cells in the spleen are activated. The spleen is a central lymphoid organ not associated with any body surface. As a result, splenic T cells have a "promiscuous" homing pattern and travel to many different sites including mucosal surfaces. Because most current vaccines are delivered parenterally, they rely on generating this strong systemic response. In such cases, protection of the mucosa is mediated by a migration of T cells into mucosal tissues or by antibodies entering damaged areas once the pathogen has breached the mucosal barrier. This indirect protection may work, but direct immunization of the mucosal lymphoid tissues is expected to be much more efficient. It is therefore logical to prevent such infections by administering vaccines in such a way that they either stimulate the intestinal or the nasopharyngeal lymphoid tissues.

ORAL VACCINATION

By far the greatest numbers of immune cells are associated with the gastrointestinal tract. The immune system functions on the basis that microorganisms that invade the body must be eliminated before they cause damage. Organisms that penetrate the epithelial barriers are promptly detected, attacked, and destroyed by both innate and adaptive mechanisms (Fig. 8.5). Immunoglobulin (Ig)A antibodies predominate in surface secretions. At least 80% of all plasma cells are found in the intestinal lamina propria, and together they produce more IgA than all other immunoglobulin isotypes combined. IgA is found in enormous amounts in saliva, intestinal fluid, nasal, and tracheal secretions, tears, milk, colostrum, urine, and the secretions of the urogenital tract.

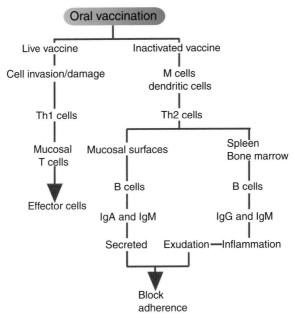

Fig. 8.5 The mechanism of action of oral vaccines. *Ig,* Immunoglobulin.

When animals are vaccinated against organisms that invade the intestinal or respiratory tracts, it makes sense to stimulate a mucosal IgA response. Because of the abundant intestinal microbiota however, intestinal IgA responses also have a high threshold, tend to lack memory, and fade rapidly. The body tightly regulates antigen import across epithelial cells. Regulatory effects on IgA production constantly adapt the IgA response to the intestinal microbiota. Once a protective IgA response has been generated, other difficulties may arise. For example, secondary immune responses are sometimes difficult to induce on surfaces, and multiple doses of vaccine may not increase the intensity or duration of the local immune response. This is not caused by any intrinsic defect but occurs because high levels of IgA can block antigen absorption and so prevent it from reaching antigen-presenting cells and memory cells.

To trigger an IgA response, the vaccine antigen can simply be ingested or inhaled. Unfortunately, such vaccines are not always effective. Inactivated antigens administered orally fail to trigger an IgA response because they are immediately washed off or simply digested when applied to mucous membranes. The only way a significant IgA response can be triggered is to use live vaccines, in which the vaccine organism can invade mucous membranes. The vaccine must persist for a sufficient time to trigger an immune response yet not cause significant damage.

The nature of the intestinal immune responses to enteroinvasive organisms depends on the sites of invasion. Enteropathogenic viruses can be divided into two broad types (type 1 and type 2) depending on their infection site in the intestine. Thus immunity to viruses that specifically attack the superficial villous enterocytes is largely mediated by specific IgA-mediated immunity in the gut lumen and within the villi. Examples of these type 1 organisms include transmissible gastroenteritis virus, porcine epidemic diarrhea virus, and rotaviruses. On the other hand, viruses that infect enterocytes deep within the crypts, designated type 2 organisms such as the parvoviruses, are controlled by both systemic and mucosal immunity. It follows therefore that type 2 organisms may be blocked by the use of parenteral vaccines whereas type 1 organisms will probably be best controlled by oral vaccines.

Systemic vaccination against surface infections may provide adequate immunity (as in human influenza and polio vaccines) because IgG may diffuse from serum to the mucosal surface. Indeed, many available vaccines simply work by stimulating high levels of IgG antibodies in blood. These are effective because once an invading organism causes tissue damage and triggers inflammation, the site of invasion is flooded by IgG. Nevertheless, this is not the most efficient way of providing immunity.

Ruminants present specific problems when considering oral vaccination. The presence and large capacity of the rumen mean that ruminal microorganisms may destroy antigens before they reach the intestine or be simply highly diluted. On the other hand, if antigen can be expressed in a fibrous plant such as alfalfa, then it will be carried to the oral cavity during rumination and thus presented to the nasopharyngeal mucosa. For example, cattle fed recombinant alfalfa hay engineered to express the leukotoxin of *Mannheimia haemolytica* increased their production of antileukotoxin IgA.

Orally delivered poxviruses, as used when vaccinating wild animals against rabies, are effectively targeted to the mouth rather than lower down the intestinal tract. The poxviruses presumably exploit small cuts and abrasions to establish lesions. Excipients that can prolong the time in the oral cavity or abrade the oral mucosa may help this process. Generally, these oral vaccines stimulate a strong humoral response.

Despite the obvious desirability of using mucosal vaccines, few effective ones have been developed. In humans there are only five: poliovirus, rotavirus, *Salmonella typhi*, *Vibrio cholera*, and the intranasal influenza vaccine. These vaccines in general do not promote long-lasting protection and all require boosting after two years.

Oral vaccines for animals may be administered in the feed or drinking water, as is done with *Lawsonia intracellularis* and *Erysipelothrix rhusiopathiae* vaccines in pigs and against Newcastle disease, infectious laryngotracheitis, and avian encephalomyelitis in poultry. Plague vaccine-coated candy has been fed to prairie dogs in the western United States and effectively prevents this disease (Fig. 20.3).

INTRANASAL VACCINATION

The intranasal route of administration has advantages over oral administration in that the vaccine is not significantly diluted by nasal fluids, and not exposed to a low pH or to digestive enzymes. It is also more appropriate to administer a vaccine at the site of the organism's potential invasion route (Fig. 8.6). Nasal associated lymphoid tissue is extensive. The collection of oronasal pharyngeal lymphoid tissue (Waldeyer's ring) includes all the tonsillar tissue, cervical lymph nodes, in addition to M cells and intraepithelial dendritic cells capturing antigen in the nasal mucosa. Intranasal vaccines are available for infectious bovine rhinotracheitis, parainfluenza 3, and respiratory syncytial virus of cattle; for *Streptococcus equi* infections in horses; for feline herpesvirus, *Bordetella bronchiseptica*, coronavirus, and calicivirus infections; and for canine parainfluenza and *Bordetella* infection. Intraocular vaccines used in poultry have a similar mechanism of action and stimulate antibody production in the harderian gland. Intranasal and intraocular administration requires that each animal be dealt with on an individual basis and may not be cost effective.

When animal numbers are large, other methods must be employed. Spray application of vaccines enables them to be inhaled by all the animals in a group. This technique is employed in vaccinating against canine distemper and mink enteritis on mink ranches and against diseases such as Newcastle disease in poultry (Chapter 19).

Novel Techniques

Although syringes and needles are simple and relatively economical, they have obvious disadvantages. Not only are they painful, but they also deposit vaccine antigens in the wrong place.

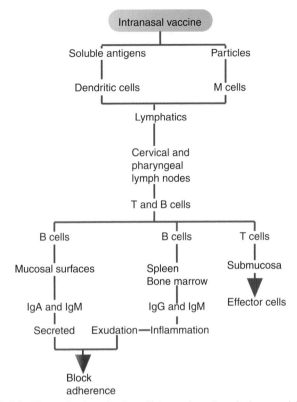

Fig. 8.6 The mechanism of action of intranasal vaccines. *Ig,* Immunoglobulin.

Antigen processing dendritic cells are relatively uncommon in the subcutis and even in skeletal muscle. The densest population of these cells is found in the dermis where there is a web of Langerhans cells and dermal dendritic cells. This means that a dose of vaccine delivered at this site will require less antigen to trigger a strong response than at other locations. Alternative methods of vaccine administration that are in development and increasingly employed in humans and animals such as pigs include intradermal vaccination using needle-free injection devices, microinjection, or topical skin application through patches or nanoparticles.

Needle-Free Injection Devices

Needle-free injection devices (transdermal jet injectors) generate a very fine stream of liquid under very high pressure. When they are held firmly against the skin the liquid stream can penetrate the epidermis. They thus deposit vaccine in the dermis and subdermis where antigen-processing dendritic cells are present in high numbers. These devices may be powered by compressed gas, batteries, or springs. Both battery and spring-powered devices are compact and relatively cheap, but exert minimal force. Gas powered units can exert much higher forces but tend to be cumbersome. They use air, nitrogen, or CO_2 cartridges attached to the injector by a tubing system. The injector is held against the skin and a stream of vaccine (with a velocity >100 meters/sec) is forced through a tiny orifice, 76 to 360 μm in diameter (about the diameter of a 36 gauge needle), and penetrates the skin in a fraction of a second (<0.3 sec). Injectors generate pressures of 130 to 1800 psi depending upon the desired depth of penetration, but higher pressures are more painful than low pressures. The fluid is delivered in three stages. An initial high-pressure stream penetrates the skin, a second delivery stage is followed by a drop-off stage as the pressure reduces. These needle-free devices are precise and very reliable. At one time these injectors were favored for mass vaccination procedures in humans because they were very efficient and fast to use. They fell out of favor because they could cause bleeding. The blood could contaminate the injector creating the possibility of disease transmission. Cases of hepatitis B transmission by jet injectors were documented. As a result, multi-use-nozzle jet injectors are no longer used in humans in the United States. They continue to be used for mass vaccination purposes in livestock, especially pigs, but many now have disposable nozzle faces that can be easily replaced as needed. Transdermal jet injectors are also employed to administer a DNA plasmid vaccine against canine oral melanoma (Oncept, Boehringer Ingelheim). These injectors are generally much less painful than needles and thus also reduce animal fear and distress. They reduce the risks of needlestick injuries, broken needles, and improper reuse. They cause less tissue damage and fewer injection site lesions because the vaccine is distributed over a wider area, and are a reliable way of delivering the correct dose. They also deliver a consistent amount of vaccine. Because these devices deliver antigen to the dendritic cell-rich environment of the dermis they generally require a smaller volume of vaccine to generate a protective immune response. The resulting immune responses are equivalent to those caused by needle injection (Chapter 18). Despite these advantages, adoption of these devices has been slow because of the cost of purchase and maintenance, required infrastructure and complexity, and also the need for training in their use.

Microneedles

Microneedle patches are adhesive patches containing an array of micron-sized needles that can be applied by pressing the patch against the skin. The patches contain a single vaccine dose. They do not require reconstitution, simplify storage, and waste disposal, and improve vaccine immunogenicity.

Microneedles are long, thin, square, or round cones tens to hundreds of micrometers in length, and about one-hundredth of the diameter of a standard hypodermic needle. They can target dendritic cells in the dermis without causing sufficient damage and producing significant pain. Four types of microneedle have been found to work well with vaccines: solid microneedles that simply make holes through which liquid vaccines can diffuse, vaccine-coated microneedles, soluble dissolving microneedles, and hollow microneedles. Dissolvable microneedles simply dissolve in tissue fluid, so releasing the vaccine within them into the dermis. Hollow implantable dissolving microneedles contain vaccine within their core. Although microneedle applications have been investigated for many virus vaccines, including rabies, most studies have focused on influenza vaccines. In general, microneedle patches stimulate greater immunogenicity, a stronger systemic response, and a better Th1 (type 1 helper cell) response, in addition to the need for much lower doses of vaccine.

Pellets

In the United States, a Moraxella vaccine for calves is available for implantation in pellet form. Two pellets are inoculated at one time under the skin. One is designed for immediate antigen release; the other pellet rehydrates slowly and releases its antigens over a two- to three-week period.

Ballistic Vaccination

It is possible to vaccinate animals from a distance using a blowpipe. The maximum effective range for blowpipe vaccination is up to 60 feet. These are especially useful in vaccinating large exotics and the animals need not be confined. Blowpipes are virtually silent and as a result do not disturb other animals in a herd unlike the ballistic vaccines that are shot from rifles (Chapter 20).

Sources of Additional Information

Albas, A., Fontolan, O.L., Pardo, P.E., et al. (2006). Interval between the first dose and booster affected antibody production in cattle vaccinated against rabies. *J Venom Anim Toxins*, 12, 476–486.

Balakrishnan, S., Rekha, V.B. (2018). Herd immunity: An epidemiological concept to eradicate infectious diseases. *J Entomol Zool Studies*, 6, 2731–2738.

Benn, C.S., Netea, M.G., Selin, L.K., Aaby, P. (2013). A small jab—a big effect: Nonspecific immunomodulation by vaccines. *Trends Immunol*, 34, 431–439.

Bernath, S., Fabian, K., Kadar, I., et al. (2004). (2004). Optimal time interval between the first vaccination and the booster of sheep for *Clostridium perfringens* Type D. *Acta Vet Brno*, 73, 473–475.

Delamater, P.L., Street, E.J., Leslie, T.F., et al. (2019). Complexity of the basic reproduction number (R_0). *Emerging Inf Dis*, 25, 1–4.

Johnson, N., Cunningham, A.F., Fooks, A.R. (2010). The immune response to rabies virus infection and vaccination. *Vaccine*, 28, 3896–3901.

Kwon, K.M., Lim, S.M., Choi, S., Kim, D.H., Jin, H.E., Jee, G., Hong, K.J., Kim, J.Y. (2017). Microneedles: Quick and easy delivery methods of vaccines. *Clin Exp Vaccine Res*, 6, 156–159.

Logomasini, M.A., Stout, R.R., Marcinkoski, R. (2013). Jet injection devices for the needle-free administration of compounds, vaccines, and other agents. *Int J Pharm Compd*, 17, 270–280.

Nalin, D.R. (2002). Evidence-based vaccinology. *Vaccine*, 20,1624–1630.

Plotkin, S.A. (2010). Correlates of protection induced by vaccination. *Clin Vaccine Immunol*, 17, 1055–1065.

Shwiff, S.A., Kirkpatrick, K.N., Sterner, R.T. (2008). Economic evaluation of an oral rabies vaccination program for control of a domestic dog-coyote rabies epizootic: 1995–2006. *J Am Vet Med Assoc* 233, 1736–1741.

Weyer, J., Rupprech,T. C.E., Nel, L.H. (2009). Poxvirus-vectored vaccines for rabies: A review. *Vaccine*, 27, 7198–7201.

Williams, P.D., Paixao, G. (2018). On-farm storage of livestock vaccines may be a risk to vaccine efficacy: A study of the performance of on-farm refrigerators to maintain the correct storage temperature. *BMC Vet Res*, 14, 136.

Failures in Vaccination

Vaccines are imperfect. They are never 100% effective. Even when administered appropriately, they will not induce immunity in every animal that receives the vaccine. This simply reflects biological variation within the vaccinated animal population. In analyzing the reasons why a vaccine may fail to protect, it is possible to attribute this to one of three different problems. One may blame the vaccine, the vaccinator, or the animal. It may be that the vaccine is to blame. For some reason it failed to work—vaccine failure. Alternatively, perhaps the vaccine was just fine, and the lack of response was the animal's fault as the animal simply failed to respond—animal failure. Or perhaps the vaccine was not administered correctly—administration failure (Fig. 9.1).

Administration Failure

At least some cases of vaccine failure result from unsatisfactory or incomplete administration of the vaccine or noncompliance with manufacturer's recommendations. For example, a live vaccine may have died as a result of poor storage, the use of antibiotics or disinfectants in conjunction with live bacterial vaccines, the use of chemicals to sterilize the syringe, or the excessive use of alcohol swabs on the skin. Sometimes animals given vaccines by unconventional routes may not be protected. When large flocks of poultry or mink are to be vaccinated, the vaccine can be administered as a spray or in drinking water. If the spray is not evenly distributed throughout a building, or if some animals do not drink, some may fail to receive sufficient vaccine. Premature vaccination of young animals before loss of maternal antibodies remains a problem. Animals that subsequently develop disease may be interpreted as cases of vaccine failure.

Even animals given an adequate dose of an effective vaccine may fail to be protected if the vaccine is given at the wrong time. Animals require several days after vaccination before immunity develops. If an animal is already incubating the infection, clinical disease may develop and this may be interpreted as either vaccine failure or attributed to the vaccine virus.

For automated procedures such as those employed in the poultry and fish industries it is essential to ensure that the automatic injectors are functioning correctly. For obese animals, injection into adipose tissue may drastically reduce vaccine efficacy. Vaccines may be administered by the wrong route, an inadequate dose may be given, or the wrong diluent may be used. Animals may receive an incomplete vaccination series and failure may be because of a lack of recommended booster doses.

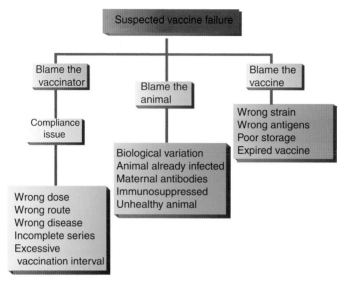

Fig. 9.1 Possible ways by which vaccination failure may occur.

INCORRECT STORAGE OR EXPIRED VACCINES

Given the wide diversity of vaccine types, and especially the different properties of inactivated and modified live vaccines, it is critical that the manufacturer's storage and handling instructions be completely followed. These may be product specific. Vaccinators must read and follow the manufacturer's recommendations for each product regarding: storage temperature, exposure to light during storage, and shaking of the product to assure uniform vaccine suspension (Chapter 8).

Many vaccines, especially modified live products, are very temperature sensitive. They may lose potency very rapidly if warmed. Thus it is essential that the cold chain be maintained all the way from the manufacturer and vendor to the veterinarian and administration to the patient. Failure to do this can result in a significant decline in vaccine efficacy, an increased rate of vaccine failures, and possibly an increased prevalence of postvaccinal adverse events.

As described in Chapter 8, it is essential that vendors, veterinarians, and ranchers carefully manage their vaccine inventory and storage to ensure that they remain effective. Should the vaccine be exposed to temperatures outside the recommended range, or if it changes color or if it is exposed to ultraviolet radiation in sunlight, consult with the manufacturer before seeking to use it.

WRONG VACCINE

The vaccine may contain the incorrect strain of organisms or the wrong (nonprotective) antigens. For many bacteria and viruses there may be many different strains, substrains, and variants that can cause disease. Immunity may, however, be strain specific. This appears to be a greater problem with killed/inactivated vaccines where nonspecific innate protective responses are less than in modified live vaccines. In vaccines directed against highly changeable viruses such as influenza, escape variants may lead to apparent vaccine failure. Examples of such strain-specific vaccines also include those directed against bovine campylobacter and porcine pleuropneumonia (Actinobacillus).

LAPSES IN VACCINATION

It is unfortunately not uncommon that a vaccination schedule is not followed, especially in the case of vaccine shortages. Lapsed vaccination should not be confused with a breakdown in vaccine effectiveness. The persistence of memory cells after antibodies have disappeared in addition to their rapid reactivation after re-exposure to antigens implies that an immunization schedule should never be started all over again. It should continue where interrupted regardless of the duration of the lapse. The consequences of vaccination lapses depend on several factors. Lapses are of greater significance during a primary course of vaccination than in older animals with a history of receiving multiple doses of vaccine. They also depend on the nature of the vaccine used. Some antibacterial vaccines give relatively short-lasting immunity even under ideal circumstances. Thus failure to boost may well result in loss of protection. In general, modified live viral vaccines give the longest immunity. If multiple vaccinated animals in a group have lapsed vaccinations, then herd immunity may drop to unsafe levels. The significance of this will depend on the risk of exposure to infected animals. In the case of a vaccine shortage, veterinarians may have to find alternative, perhaps more expensive products. Every failure in the established vaccination schedule is a matter of concern for both the individual and the herd. Regardless of how long an animal is overdue for a vaccine, administration of a single does will reactivate the immune system and regenerate protective immunity. There is no necessity to begin a vaccine series all over again.

Animal Failure

FAILURE TO RESPOND

Vaccine failures may be attributed to the animal being vaccinated. Preexisting infection is probably the most common cause of apparent vaccine failure. Alternatively, an animal may simply fail to mount an immune response. The immune response, being a biological process, never confers absolute protection and is never equal in all members of a vaccinated population. Because immunity is influenced by many genetic and environmental factors, the range of immune responses in a large random population of animals follows a normal distribution (Figs. 9.2 and 9.3). This means that most animals respond to vaccines by mounting an average immune response, whereas a few will mount an excellent response, and a few will mount a poor immune response. These

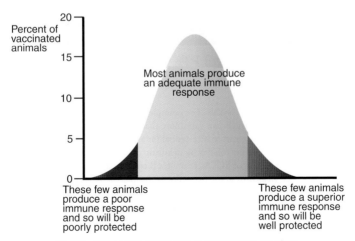

Fig. 9.2 The normal distribution of responses to vaccines.

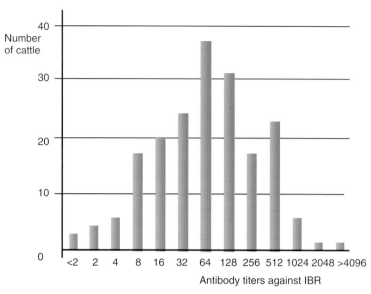

Fig. 9.3 An example of the normal distribution of antibody titers to a vaccine in a herd of cattle immunized against infectious bovine rhinotracheitis (*IBR*). (Courtesy of Dr. T. Hairgrove.)

poor responders may not be protected against infection despite having received an effective vaccine. It is impossible to protect 100% of a large outbred population of animals by vaccination. The size of this unreactive portion of the population will vary between vaccines, and its significance will depend on the nature of the disease. For highly infectious diseases against which herd immunity is poor and in which infection is rapidly and efficiently transmitted, such as foot-and-mouth disease, the presence of even a few unprotected animals can permit the spread of disease and disrupt control programs. Likewise, problems can arise if the unprotected animals are individually important, such as companion animals. In contrast, for diseases that are inefficiently spread, such as rabies in dogs, 70% protection may be sufficient to effectively block disease transmission within a population and provide significant herd immunity (Box 9.1).

BOX 9.1 ■ The Microbiota Influences the Response to Vaccines

The intestinal microbiota sends many signals to the immune system. They range from endotoxins and other microbial products to digestive products such as short-chain fatty acids (SCFAs). These signals play a key role in shaping the functions of the immune system and affect responses to both orally and parenterally administered vaccines.

The immune response is highly variable. For example, yellow fever vaccine 17D is very successful and highly effective, yet antibody levels can vary more than 100-fold between individuals. Sensing of flagellin from the gut microbiota appears to be essential for a successful influenza response. Recognition of muramyl peptide from the gut microbiota by dendritic cells is necessary for optimal responses to intranasal antigens. The production of SCFAs promotes B cell responses. Many of these positive effects are abrogated in antibiotic treated or germ-free animals. Animals heavily treated with antibiotics may have impaired vaccination responses.

(From Lynn, D.J., Pulendran, B. (2018). The potential of the microbiota to influence vaccine responses. *J Leukocyte Biol*, 103, 225–231.)

TABLE 9.1 ■ **When Not to Vaccinate**

Condition	Reason
Immunosuppression	Suffering from immunosuppressive cancers such as leukemia
	Suffering from immunosuppressive diseases such as canine distemper
	Immunosuppressed by drugs or radiation
	Receiving high dose corticosteroids
Hypersensitivity	Allergic to vaccine components
Pregnancy	Avoid certain modified live vaccines
Age	Presence of maternal antibodies
Current illness	Heavy parasite loads such as demodecosis or gastrointestinal worms
	Has a fever or other evidence of concurrent infection

Another type of vaccine failure occurs when the normal immune response is suppressed as a result of immunodeficiency. For example, heavily parasitized or malnourished animals may be immunosuppressed and should not be vaccinated (Table 9.1). Some virus infections induce profound immunosuppression. Animals with a major illness or high fever should not normally be vaccinated unless for a compelling reason. Stress may reduce a normal immune response, probably because of increased steroid production; examples of such stress include fatigue, malnutrition, and extremes of cold and heat. Most notably transportation stress is associated with the development of shipping fever and the bovine respiratory disease complex. Studies have shown that surgical neutering at or near the time of first vaccination does not impair the antibody responses of kittens. The most important cause of vaccine failure of this type is premature vaccination of the very young and resulting suppression by the presence of maternal antibodies. Very old animals may also be significantly immunosuppressed.

Analysis of an outbreak of influenza in racehorses has shown some interesting and important factors that appeared to determine vaccine effectiveness in this species. When the effect of age was analyzed, it was found that two-year-old horses were less susceptible to influenza than other animals. Further analysis suggested that this increased resistance resulted from recent vaccination of this age cohort despite horses in other age groups possessing similar antibody levels. There was evidence of gender differences in resistance (62% of females and 71% of males were infected). There was also some evidence that vaccination at less than 6 months of age in the presence of maternal antibodies to influenza had detrimental long-term effects on protection when compared with foals first vaccinated between 6 and 18 months of age.

Recent studies have also analyzed data from 10,483 dogs of all ages and breeds vaccinated against rabies to determine the factors that influence seroconversion. It was found that a strong relationship exists between a dog's size and its antibody response (Fig. 9.4). Smaller dogs produced higher antibody titers than large dogs. Vaccine effectiveness also varied among breeds. Thus significant failure rates were seen in German Shepherds and Labrador retrievers. Young animals vaccinated before one year of age produced lower antibody titers than adults. The highest antibody titers were generated in dogs aged three to four years at time of vaccination. Primary vaccination of aged animals showed lower antibody levels and increased failure rates. Gender had no effect on failure rate or titer. Failure rates varied greatly between vaccines. They ranged from 0.2% in the worst case to 0.01% in the best, and some vaccines showed significant batch-to-batch variation in efficacy. Of the variation in antibody titers observed, 19% were the result of vaccine differences, 8% were attributed to breed differences, 5% were attributed to size differences, and 3% to other differences. It is likely that similar variables influence the responses of animals to other vaccines. Perhaps vaccines should be reformulated to take these age, size, and breed differences into account.

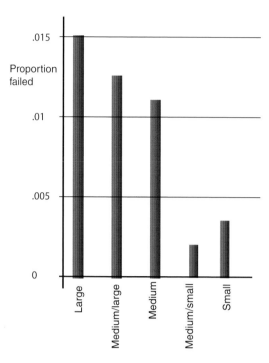

Fig. 9.4 The effect of dog size on the failure rates of rabies vaccine. This probably reflects a dose effect. Some large dogs may have received an insufficient dose of vaccine. (From Kennedy, L.J., Lunt M, Barnes A, et al. (2007). Factors influencing the antibody response of dogs vaccinated against rabies. *Vaccine*, 25, 8500–8507. With permission.)

An Australian study has investigated the causes of vaccine failure in dogs vaccinated against canine parvovirus (CPV). Investigators examined whether vaccine strain or vaccination protocol was associated with failure. Vaccine strain had no significant effect. On the other hand, there was a strong correlation of failure with the age at administration of the last vaccine dose. The older a puppy was when it received its last vaccination, the lower the risk of vaccination failure. It was concluded that a puppy should receive its last dose of vaccine when it was at least 16 weeks of age. Giving the last vaccine dose before that age predisposes to vaccine failure. Presumably, the persistence of maternal antibodies was a major contributor to CPV vaccine failure in these puppies.

Vaccine Failure

Occasionally, a vaccine may actually be ineffective although more commonly, vaccines from different manufacturers have different levels of effectiveness (Fig. 9.5). Primary failure such as a failure to seroconvert needs to be distinguished from secondary failure when immunity wanes rapidly. Some reasons for primary failure are that the method of production may have destroyed the protective epitopes, or there may simply be insufficient antigen in the vaccine. Batch variations or quality defects do occur and may cause vaccine failures. Problems of this type are uncommon and can generally be avoided by using only vaccines from reputable manufacturers (Box 9.2).

VACCINATION EFFICACY AND EFFECTIVENESS

Vaccine efficacy is measured in preclinical trials to obtain licensure. Effectiveness, in contrast, is determined by the vaccine success when used in the field.

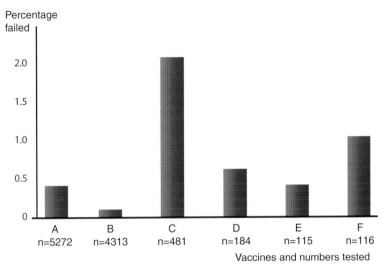

Fig. 9.5 Variations in the efficacy of different vaccines against rabies. Do not assume that all vaccines are equal. It is important to point out, however, that even the poorest vaccine protected 98% of dogs. (From Kennedy, L.J., Lunt M, Barnes A, et al. (2007). Factors influencing the antibody response of dogs vaccinated against rabies. *Vaccine,* 25, 8500–8507. With permission.)

BOX 9.2 ■ Vaccine Resistance

A highly significant issue affecting the control of infectious diseases is the development of antimicrobial resistance (AMR). The development of antibiotic and other drug resistance has resulted in a growing death toll in both humans and animals, and the problem is expected to worsen. The development of new antibiotics has slowed whereas the development of AMR is accelerating. The use of new and improved vaccines is one strategy to target AMR pathogens. Vaccination can directly reduce the incidence of diseases caused by both sensitive and resistant organisms. It can reduce the use of antimicrobials as demonstrated by the aquaculture industry. It can also preserve the microbiota from the damage caused by antibiotics. In general, the development of antibiotic resistance is inevitable and thus requires the continual production of new antibiotics. Vaccines however can largely (but not totally) prevent the evolution of resistant strains. There are several reasons for this. Most obviously, vaccines are used for disease prevention and administered when there are few if any, pathogens present in an animal, and thus are unlikely to enhance the appearance of organisms with resistant mutations. Conversely, antibiotics are used in diseased individuals where there may be very large populations of pathogens, and resistant mutations are much more likely to appear. Second, although antibiotics usually target a single metabolic pathway, vaccines generally act through multiple epitopes and induce both antibody- and T cell-mediated responses so that multiple mutations would be needed to confer resistance to a vaccine. Because animals differ in their immune responses, an organism that is vaccine resistant in one animal may be completely susceptible in another.

Although very rare, there have been instances where antivaccine resistance has been suspected and disease outbreaks have occurred in vaccinated animals. Possible examples include enteric redmouth disease caused by *Yersinia ruckeri* in farmed salmon, avian metapneumovirus infections in turkeys, and Marek's disease in chickens. It is also possible that the use of new, highly specific vaccines that contain very few antigenic components may permit the appearance of vaccine resistant strains.

(From Kennedy, D.A., Read, A.F. (2018). Why the evolution of vaccine resistance is less of a concern than the evolution of drug resistance. *Proc Natl Acad Sci USA,* 115, 12878–12886.)

When a vaccine has been developed and its efficacy experimentally determined, it is usual to first vaccinate the animals and subsequently challenge them. The percentage of vaccinated animals that survive this challenge can then be measured. It is important, however, to determine the percentage of nonvaccinated control animals that also survive the same challenge. The true efficacy of a vaccine, called the preventable fraction (PF), is calculated as follows:

$$PF = \frac{(\% \text{ of controls dying} - \% \text{ of vaccinates dying})}{\% \text{ of controls dying}}$$

For example, a challenge that kills 80% of controls and 40% of vaccinates shows that the PF of the vaccine is as follows:

$$PF = \frac{80 - 40}{80} = 50\%$$

Good, effective vaccines should have a PF of at least 80%. Obviously, less effective vaccines are acceptable if safe and if nothing better is available. In determining vaccine efficacy, however, large challenge doses may overwhelm any reasonable level of vaccine-induced immunity. It is also important to determine what degree of protection is desired. It may be much easier to prevent deaths rather than illness or infection.

After a vaccine has been licensed and experience gained with its use in the field, then its odds ratio may be determined. This is a measure of the association between vaccination and protection. It represents the odds that disease will occur in vaccinated animals compared with the outcome in nonvaccinated animals. These odds ratios can be determined by cohort studies or case-control studies. In general, an odds ratio of 1 indicates no difference between the groups. A ratio greater or less than 1 denotes a difference between the odds.

Cohort studies are prospective studies. In a cohort study, groups of vaccinated animals (cohorts) and groups of unvaccinated animals are followed prospectively for a period of time after vaccination. They are then evaluated for the outcome of vaccination, in this case, development of disease. If the vaccine is effective it would be expected that the incidence of disease would be less in the vaccinated cohort. The disadvantages of cohort studies are that the cohorts must be very carefully matched to ensure that they are separate but similar. This is not a randomized trial and it may take a significant time for the results to become apparent.

Case-control studies are retrospective studies. In a case-control study, disease occurrence in vaccinated animals is compared retrospectively with the occurrence in animals that were not vaccinated (controls). These are purely observational because no attempt is made to induce the disease. They are simply designed to estimate odds. The odds of a vaccinated animal developing disease are compared with the odds of an unvaccinated animal developing disease. If the odds of disease in the vaccinated group are significantly less than the odds of disease in the unvaccinated group then the vaccine is considered effective. This methodology is good for studying rare occurrences. It can be done rapidly because vaccination has already occurred. On the other hand, it may be difficult to find a suitable control group.

It is useful to define vaccination failures based on the probability of failures occurring. Confirmed clinical vaccine failure requires that the animal be shown to have been appropriately vaccinated, taking into account the disease incubation period and the normal delay before vaccine-induced immunity comes into play. There can be many degrees and clinical relevance of confirmed vaccine failure. Suspected clinical vaccine failure occurs when there is suspicion that the infection is not caused by the organism vaccinated against, such as influenza. Immunological vaccine failure reflects the failure of a vaccinated animal to seroconvert. This may also just be suspected.

CORRELATES OF PROTECTION

Obviously the function of vaccination is to provide protection from an infectious disease. This protection can of course be determined by challenging the animal and seeing if it is actually protected. This is quite impractical, and as a result we look for other methods of determining whether a vaccinated animal is actually protected. We look for an immune response whose presence is correlated with protection against a specific agent. This correlation may be absolute so that a test result provides assurance of protection, or, more commonly, the correlation is relative and provides at least some assurance of protection. Given the diversity of infectious agents and the immune responses mounted against them it is clear that no single test system can measure protection in all cases. Likewise, the measure of protection will depend on disease pathogenesis be it toxin or viral neutralization, bacterial killing or opsonization, macrophage activation, or T cell-mediated cytotoxicity. Measurement of correlates of protection is essential if we are to assess vaccine effectiveness and the risks associated with vaccinating or not vaccinating an animal.

For diseases caused by microbial toxins such as tetanus or botulism, neutralizing antibodies correlate well with protective immunity. For other vaccines and diseases, however, both B and T cells contribute to protection. The relative contribution of each will differ between diseases. Antibody levels are relatively easy to measure but T cell contributions are much more difficult to assess. Unlike serologic assays, T cell assays require many species-specific reagents that may not be available or are very expensive.

On the other hand, measurement of some correlate of protection will provide assurance that each new batch of vaccine is working in an anticipated and effective fashion and can be expected to protect animals when used in the field. This is also important if we are to provide effective vaccines and avoiding terminal challenge experiments in animals. It is also obvious that measurement of such correlates is critical in assessing human vaccine potency.

In practice, we rarely use T cell assays as correlates of protection. Conversely, serologic assays are widely employed and have proved useful in most cases. For example, commercial poultry breeder flocks are routinely sampled and tested for antibodies to the common poultry pathogens. This is usually done by using enzyme-linked immunosorbent assays (ELISAs) and hemagglutination tests. Should a vaccine fail then this testing will provide early warning of a problem and enable a producer to solve it before a disease outbreak occurs. As described in Chapter 13, it is increasingly common (and recommended) that pets be tested for serum antibodies against common pathogens before making revaccination decisions. It is recognized that these serologic assays do not measure T cell mediated protection, but they at least provide a surrogate of protection.

Sources of Additional Information

Heininger, U., Bachtiar, N.S., Bahri, P., Dana, A., Dodoo, A., Gidudu, J., Santos, E.M. (2012). The concept of vaccination failure. *Vaccine,* 30, 1265–1268.

Meeusen, E.N., Walker, J., Peters, A., Pastoret, P.P., Jungersen, G. (2007). Current status of veterinary vaccines. *Clin Microbiol Rev,* 20, 489–510.

Schlingmann, B., Castiglia, K.R., Stobart, C.C., Moore, M.L. (2018). Polyvalent vaccines: High-maintenance heroes. *PLoS Pathog,* 14(4). e1006904.

Teshale, E.H., Hanson, D., Flannery, B., et al. (2008). Effectiveness of 23-valent polysaccharide pneumococcal vaccine on pneumonia in HIV-infected adults in the United States, 1998–2003. *Vaccine,* 26, 5830–5834.

Adverse Consequences of Vaccination

Vaccination is the only safe, reliable, and effective way of protecting animals against the major infectious diseases. Society does not remember the devastating toll taken by infectious diseases before the development of modern vaccines. Exaggerated fear of negative side effects has discouraged owners from having their pets (and themselves) from being vaccinated. The rise of the Internet and the development of social media have enabled those who oppose vaccination to spread their opinions. Those who resist vaccination for themselves or their children are unlikely to be enthusiastic about vaccinating their pets. Much of this resistance is a result of adverse events and controversy regarding effectiveness associated with the earliest vaccines. In spite of the fact that these problems have long been solved, it takes a considerable time before confidence is restored. There is a lack of awareness of the rigorous safety tests that modern vaccines must undergo before they are marketed. Good manufacturing practices and the quality control procedures used by the biologics industry, together with rigorous regulatory controls, serve to minimize the occurrence of these events. Past issues have been corrected and vaccine safety has steadily improved. Modern vaccines are safe to use and overwhelmingly beneficial. Adverse events associated with vaccination that might compromise the health of an animal are usually rare, mild, and transient. Hypothetical, speculative, or historical adverse effects sometimes dominate perceptions. Nevertheless, it has been truly said, "The most dangerous vaccine is the one not given." In reading this chapter the reader should be aware that the events described here are rare, somewhat historical, and relatively unimportant when compared with the benefits of vaccination.

Drivers of vaccine usage differ significantly between companion animals and commercial livestock. Owners of companion animals are concerned for the health and well-being of their pets and are intolerant of any adverse events that cause discomfort, pain, or sickness. Livestock producers in contrast vaccinate to maintain livestock health, prevent disease spread, maximize economic return, and to minimize zoonotic disease risks. Vaccines that cause a drop in milk production, decreased feed conversion, increased time to market, or a decline in carcass quality may have significant economic consequences and will not be used.

ADVERSE EFFECT PRINCIPLES

In determining whether a vaccine causes an adverse effect, the following three principles should apply. First, is the effect consistent? The clinical responses should be the same if the vaccine is given to a different group of animals, by different investigators, and irrespective of the method of investigation. Second, is the effect specific? The association should be distinctive and the adverse event linked specifically to the vaccine concerned. It is important to remember that an adverse event may be caused by vaccine adjuvants and components other than the major antigens. Finally, there must be a temporal relationship. Administration of the vaccine should precede the earliest manifestations of the event or a clear exacerbation of a continuing condition.

The US Centers for Disease Control and Prevention (CDC) has classified adverse events as follows:

1. Vaccine-induced events: These are events that would not occur in the absence of vaccination and are therefore attributed to the vaccine. An example would be an allergic response to a vaccine component such as egg protein.
2. Vaccine potentiated reactions: These are events that might have occurred anyway but may have been precipitated by the vaccine. One possible example is purpura hemorrhagica in horses.
3. Programmatic error: Events that occur in response to technical errors in vaccine storage, preparation, handling, and administration.
4. Coincidental events: These are simply events that happen by chance or result from some underlying illness.

Adverse Events

The use of vaccines is not free of risk, and an owner has reason to be upset if their healthy animal is sickened by the administration of a vaccine. Residual virulence and toxicity, allergic responses, disease in immunodeficient hosts, neurological complications, and harmful effects on the fetus are potential risks associated with the use of vaccines (Table 10.1). Veterinarians should use only licensed vaccines, and the manufacturer's recommendations must be carefully followed. Before using a vaccine, the veterinarian should consider the likelihood that an adverse event will happen, and also the possible consequences or severity of this event. These factors must be weighed against the benefits to the animal. A common but mild complication requires a very different consideration than a rare, severe complication (Table 10.2).

The issue of the risk associated with vaccination remains in large part a philosophical one because the advantages of vaccination are well documented and extensive, whereas the risk for adverse effects is poorly documented, and in many cases, largely speculative. Nevertheless, established facts should be recognized, unsubstantiated allegations rebutted by sound data, and uncertainties acknowledged. For example, there is absolutely no evidence that vaccination itself leads

TABLE 10.1 ■ **The Classification of Adverse Events**

Classification	Features
Certain	Event with appropriate time course
	No other explanation
	Consistent definitive signs
Probable	Reasonable time relationship
	Unlikely to be caused by something else
Possible	No other reasonable explanation
	Reasonable time relationship
Unlikely	No reasonable time relationship
	Other plausible explanations
Unknown	Insufficient data
	Cannot be verified

TABLE 10.2 ■ Frequency of Adverse Reactions as Defined by the European Medicines Agency

	Frequency
Very common	More than 1 in 10 animals showing adverse reactions (>10%)
Common	Greater than 1 but less than 10 animals per 100 animals vaccinated (1%–10%)
Uncommon	More than 1 but less than 10 animals per 1000 animals vaccinated (0.1%–1%)
Rare	More than 1 but less than 10 animals per 10,000 animals vaccinated (0.01%–0.1%)
Very rare	Less than 1 animal in 10,000 reported (<0.01%)

BOX 10.1 ■ Canine Autism and Vaccination

Autism spectrum disorder is a chronic developmental disorder in children. Its causes are largely unknown. It usually becomes apparent in young children over one year of age at around the same time they receive their initial vaccinations. In a paper published in 1998, a physician studied 12 children with autism. He asked the parents if the children had been vaccinated, with the measles, mumps, and rubella vaccine, within the previous two weeks. Eight said yes, so the author went on to assert in his paper that this vaccine caused autism. He postulated that autism resulted from measles infection. The paper was eventually retracted and the author lost his medical license. Subsequent population-based studies have failed to demonstrate any link between vaccination and autism. Thousands of children are vaccinated every year and large amounts of data are available for analysis. All these show the same thing. There is no link between vaccination and autism risk. However, the word was out. The Internet and Twitter spread the word. Additionally, pet owners began to claim that their dog's behavior had changed after vaccination— canine autism. The British Veterinary Association felt obliged to issue a statement regarding these claims.

"There is currently no reliable scientific evidence to indicate autism in dogs or a link between vaccination and autism. Vaccinations save lives and are an important tool in keeping our pets healthy. All medicines have potential side-effects but in the case of vaccines, these are rare and the benefits of vaccination in protecting against disease far outweigh the potential for an adverse reaction."

---

to ill health. Although difficult to prove, a negative, competent statistical analysis has consistently failed to demonstrate any general adverse effect of vaccination.

Identification of an adverse event is based on the clinical judgment of the attending veterinarian and is therefore subject to bias. Standard case definitions of a vaccine-associated adverse event are not yet available. It still is often difficult to distinguish association from causality (Box 10.1).

Traditionally, adverse events resulting from vaccine administration have been reported by veterinarians to manufacturers or government agencies. The resulting numbers have been difficult to analyze satisfactorily for two major reasons. First, reporting is voluntary, so significant underreporting occurs. Adverse events are often regarded as insignificant, or it may be inconvenient to report them. Second, very little data has been available on the number of animals vaccinated. Although manufacturers know the number of doses of vaccine sold, they are unable to measure the number of animals vaccinated.

It has, however, proved possible by examining the electronic medical records of a very large small animal general practice, to determine the prevalence of vaccine-associated adverse events in over a million dogs. The use of a standardized reporting system within a very large population has permitted objective analysis of the prevalence of adverse events occurring within three days of vaccine administration. Out of 1,226,159 dogs receiving 3,439,576 vaccine doses, 4678 adverse events were recorded (38.2/10,000 dogs); 72.8% of these events occurred on the same day the vaccine was administered, 31.7% were considered to be allergic reactions, 1.7% were classified as anaphylaxis, and 65.8% were considered "vaccine reactions" and were likely caused by innate immune responses. Three dogs died. The lowest rate of such events was associated with *Bordetella* vaccination and the highest rate with Lyme disease vaccine. Additional analysis indicated that the risk of adverse events was significantly greater for small dogs than for large dogs (Fig. 10.1); for neutered than for sexually intact dogs; and for dogs that received multiple vaccines on one occasion. Each additional vaccine dose administered increased the risk of an adverse event occurring by 27% in dogs under 10 kg and by 12% in dogs heavier than 12 kg (Fig. 10.2). High-risk breeds included dachshunds, pugs, Boston terriers, miniature pinschers, and Chihuahuas.

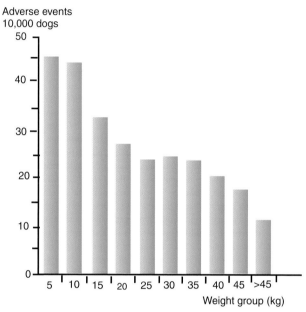

Fig. 10.1   The mean vaccine associated adverse event rates occurring within 3 days of vaccination in dogs of different weights. This survey was undertaken using data from 1,226,159 dogs at 360 veterinary hospitals in 2002 and 2003. Small dogs receiving a relatively higher vaccine dose react accordingly. (From Moore, G.E., Guptil, L.F., Ward, M.P., et al. [2005]. Adverse events diagnosed within three days of vaccine administration in dogs. *JAVMA*, 227, 1102–1108. Fig. 1. With permission.)

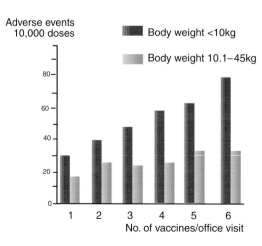

Fig. 10.2   The increase in adverse events associated with multiple vaccines given at a single office visit. This survey was undertaken using data from 1,226,159 dogs at 360 veterinary hospitals in 2002 and 2003. Presumably this reflects the additive effects of these vaccines on the innate immune response. (From Moore, G.E., Guptil, L.F., Ward, M.P., et al. [2005]. Adverse events diagnosed within three days of vaccine administration in dogs. *JAVMA*, 227, 1102–1108. Fig. 4. With permission.)

Overall, the increased prevalence of adverse events in young adult, small-breed, neutered dogs and their relationship to multiple dosing suggests that veterinarians should look carefully at the practice of giving the same vaccine dose to all dogs irrespective of their size.

In another report, from Japan 351 dogs showed an adverse event out of 57,300 vaccinated (62.7/10,000 doses). (Vaccines used included canine parvovirus, canine distemper, canine adenovirus 2, canine coronavirus, and leptospirosis.) Of these 351 dogs, 1 died, 41 had anaphylaxis, 244 developed dermatological signs, and 160 showed gastrointestinal signs. About half the anaphylaxis events occurred within 5 minutes of vaccination. Additional analysis of these anaphylaxis cases reported 87% collapse, 77% cyanosis, and both collapse and cyanosis in 71% of affected dogs. Breeds affected included miniature dachshunds (50%; these accounted for about 30% of all the anaphylaxis cases), Chihuahuas (10%), mixed breeds (5%), and toy poodles (5%). Miniature Schnauzers also appeared to be unusually prone to anaphylaxis. The highest frequency of adverse reactions occurred in dogs under 5 kg. Most adverse events were observed within 12 hours after vaccination. The adverse event rate in Japan as reported here (62.7/10,000 doses) is much higher than in the United Kingdom (0.093/10,000 doses), or in the United States (38.2/10,000 dogs).

INNATE IMMUNE REACTIONS

Vaccines may elicit mild transient injection site reactions as a result of inflammation. These inflammatory responses may manifest themselves within two to three days. As pointed out in Chapter 2, some degree of inflammation is required for the efficient induction of protection. This may cause pain or pruritus. The sting produced by some vaccines may present problems, not only to the animal being vaccinated, but also to the vaccinator, if the animal reacts violently. Lethargy, anorexia, soreness, minor behavioral changes, and tenderness at the vaccine site are normal postvaccinal responses and should resolve within 12 to 24 hours. Swellings may develop at the reaction site less commonly. These may be firm or edematous and may be warm to the touch. They appear within 24 hours and can last for about a week. Unless an injection-site abscess develops, these swellings leave little trace.

Vaccines containing killed gram-negative bacteria may be intrinsically toxic owing to the presence of pathogen-associated molecular patterns such as endotoxins, lipids, muramyl peptides, and porins that can bind to pattern recognition receptors and provoke cytokine release. In extreme cases this may lead to anorexia, and fever. Although such reactions are usually only a temporary inconvenience to male animals, they may be sufficient to provoke early embryonic deaths in pregnant females. It may be prudent to avoid vaccinating pregnant animals unless the risks of not giving the vaccine are considered to be too great. Vaccination with either immune-stimulating complex (ISCOM) vaccines or live recombinant vectored vaccines against influenza and tetanus may induce an acute-phase response in horses.

Innate immune responses may reduce an animal's growth rate and diminish its feed efficiency. This growth suppression can be mimicked by injection of interleukin (IL)-1 and tumor necrosis factor (TNF)-α. These cytokines act on the brain to reduce appetite while at the same time, causing degradation of skeletal muscle.

Intranasal vaccines such as those containing *Bordetella bronchiseptica* and some viruses may cause transient cough or sneezing. This simply reflects the mild innate response triggered as the vaccine organisms invade the upper respiratory tract.

Hypersensitivity Responses

TYPE I HYPERSENSITIVITIES

Vaccines have the potential to cause rare but serious allergic reactions (type I hypersensitivity). For example, allergic responses may occur when an animal produces immunoglobulin (Ig)E in

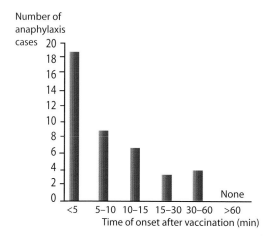

Fig. 10.3 The time of onset of vaccine-associated anaphylaxis in Japanese dogs. A total of 359 dogs showed vaccine-associated adverse events. The great majority develop within 10 minutes reflecting an immediate hypersensitivity whereas 299 occurred within 12 hours. (From Miyaji, K., et al. [2012]. Large-scale survey of adverse reactions to canine non-rabies combined vaccines in Japan. *Vet Immunol Immunopathol*, 145, 447–452. With permission)

response, not only to the immunizing antigen, but also to other components in vaccines. The most significant allergens are often vaccine excipients. For example, reactions are most likely to occur after injection of vaccines that contain trace amounts of fetal calf serum (specifically bovine serum albumin), egg proteins (ovalbumin), or gelatin. (Gelatin and serum albumin are added to vaccines as stabilizers to protect the vaccine antigens during the freeze-drying process.) Some vaccines may also contain antibiotics such as neomycin to which an animal may be sensitized. Severe allergic responses have been associated with the use of killed foot-and-mouth disease, rabies, and contagious bovine pleuropneumonia vaccines in cattle. Signs include angioedema, affecting mainly the head and ears, urticaria, pruritus, acute-onset diarrhea, vomiting, dyspnea, and collapse. All forms of hypersensitivity are more commonly associated with multiple injections of antigens and therefore tend to be associated with the use of killed vaccines.

It is important to emphasize that a type I hypersensitivity reaction is an immediate response to an antigen and occurs within a few minutes after exposure to an antigen (Fig. 10.3). It is good practice to keep an animal in the clinic for 15 to 25 minutes after vaccination to ensure that any immediate problems can be promptly recognized and treated (Box 10.2). Reactions occurring more than two or three hours after administration of a vaccine are likely not type I hypersensitivity reactions.

TYPE II HYPERSENSITIVITIES

In type II hypersensitivity reactions, antibodies directed against an animal's own cells act together with complement to cause cell lysis. These antibodies are usually induced by the presence of animal cells in the vaccine.

Hemolytic Disease of the Newborn

Natural hemolytic disease of the newborn (HDN) in calves is very rare, but it has resulted from vaccination against anaplasmosis or babesiosis. These vaccines contain pooled red cells from infected calves. In the case of *Anaplasma* vaccines, for example, the blood from infected donors is pooled, freeze-dried, and mixed with adjuvant before being administered to cattle. The vaccine against babesiosis consists of fresh, infected calf blood. Both vaccines cause infection, and consequently, the development of immunity in recipients. They also stimulate the production of antibodies against the injected red cells. If cows sensitized by these vaccines are then mated with bulls

---

BOX 10.2 ■ The Treatment of Acute Anaphylaxis

Anaphylaxis is a life-threatening medical emergency. Deterioration can occur very rapidly and time is of the essence. Initiate treatment immediately. If an animal is undergoing acute anaphylaxis take the following steps:

1. Stop administering the vaccine.
2. In the case of dogs and cats, administer epinephrine 1:1000 at 0.01 mg/kg intramuscularly. Repeat every 5–15 minutes if necessary. If very severe and shock has developed, place an intravenous catheter and administer 0.1 mg/kg of 1:10,000 epinephrine by slow intravenous infusion and monitor blood pressure and perfusion. Alternative routes of administration include intracardiac or intratracheal. Avoid subcutaneous administration because epinephrine is a potent vasoconstrictor and absorption is delayed.

   In the case of foals administer epinephrine 1:1000 at 0.01 to 0.02 mg/kg (0.5–1ml for a 50 kg foal) given slowly intravenously or intramuscularly. In adult horses administer epinephrine at 0.01 mg/kg (3–8 ml for a 450 kg horse) slowly intravenously. If the condition is mild, this dose may be administered intramuscularly. Repeat every 10–20 minutes if necessary.
3. Secure the airway, intubate if necessary, and administer oxygen to animals showing respiratory symptoms.
4. Provide isotonic shock crystalloid fluids (normal saline or lactated Ringer solution) intravenously to help restore adequate blood pressure in hypotensive animals. The volume required depends on the animal's response, but may be as high as 90ml/kg for dogs and 60ml/kg for cats.
5. Administer an H1-antihistamine such as diphenhydramine every 8–12 hours if necessary.
6. Once the animal is stabilized consider administering a fast acting glucocorticosteroid by the slow intravenous route to prevent late-phase responses.

---

carrying the same blood groups, they can transmit these antibodies to their calves through colostrum. The calves that drink this colostrum may then develop hemolytic disease. HDN in piglets had a similar pathogenesis when sows were immunized with a hog cholera vaccine containing pig blood.

Bovine Neonatal Pancytopenia

Beginning in 2007, multiple outbreaks of an unexplained hemorrhagic disease in newborn beef calves were reported from many countries in Western Europe. Affected calves showed sudden onset bleeding including nasal hemorrhage, petechiation on mucus membranes, and excessive bleeding from minor wounds such as injection, or ear-tag sites. The disease appeared 7 to 8 days after birth and affected calves could die within 48 hours. It is now called bovine neonatal pancytopenia (BNP). Investigation showed an early drop in platelets, monocytes, and neutrophils was followed by drops in erythrocyte and lymphocyte numbers. The net result was a profound pancytopenia. The bone marrow could be completely aplastic. Mortality was as high as 90% in severely affected calves, but there were also many subclinical cases.

Because this disease only occurred in suckled calves and developed within hours of first suckling, it appeared to result from the consumption of colostrum. Further investigations showed that the colostrum from these cows contained antibodies directed against the major histocompatibility complex (MHC) class I molecules expressed on neonatal leukocytes and bone marrow stem cells. Cells of the thrombocyte, lymphocyte and monocyte lineages, and precursors of neutrophil, erythrocyte, and eosinophil lineages were affected.

Further investigations showed that the disease was triggered by administration of a specific vaccine against bovine virus diarrhea (BVD). This vaccine—Pregshure—contained inactivated bovine viral diarrhea virus (BVDV) grown in bovine kidney cells. A potent, oil-in-water emulsion adjuvant containing Quil A, cholesterol, and mineral oil was then added. Immunization with this

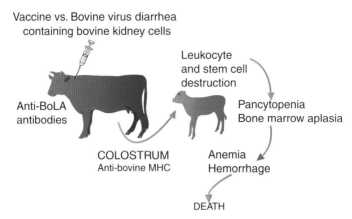

Fig. 10.4 The pathogenesis of bovine pancytopenia. Inoculation of a vaccine containing bovine kidney cells results in the production of antibodies against MHC antigens. When ingested by drinking colostrum, these antibodies destroy bone marrow stem cells in their calves. This results in a loss of all their white blood cells including platelets. *MHC,* Major histocompatibility complex.

vaccine induced antibodies against the bovine kidney cells in some cows. These antibodies, when transferred to calves via colostrum, bound to their leukocytes and bone marrow stem cells, killed them, and so induced pancytopenia (Fig. 10.4). Not all calves born from cows that received this specific vaccine developed clinical disease. The quantity and specificity of their antibody response determined the risk to their calves. Antibody levels remained high in some cows for many years and were boosted by each pregnancy. As a result, BNP cases occurred for many years after Pregshure was removed from the market in 2010.

TYPE III HYPERSENSITIVITIES

Type III hypersensitivity reactions (immune-complex-mediated) may be induced by vaccination. The deposition of immune-complexes in tissues may cause local inflammation or cause a generalized vasculitis such as purpura. Some rabies vaccines may also induce a local complement-mediated vasculitis in the skin resulting in ischemic dermatitis and local alopecia. This may occur at the injection site or at remote locations such as the ear tips, footpad, tail, or scrotum. This vasculitis is most often seen in small dogs such as dachshunds, miniature poodles, bichon frises, and terriers.

Blue Eye

In dogs infected with canine adenovirus-1 (CAV-1, infectious canine hepatitis), an immune-complex-mediated uveitis and a focal glomerulonephritis both develop. The uveitis, commonly called "blue-eye," is seen both in dogs with natural infections and in those vaccinated with live attenuated CAV-1 vaccine (Fig. 10.5). The uveitis results from the formation of virus-antibody complexes in the anterior chamber of the eye and in the cornea with complement activation and consequent neutrophil accumulation. The neutrophils release enzymes and oxidants that damage corneal epithelial cells, leading to edema and opacity. The condition resolves spontaneously in about 90% of affected dogs. Replacing CAV-1 with CAV-2 in vaccines has largely eliminated this problem.

Purpura Hemorrhagica

See Chapter 15.

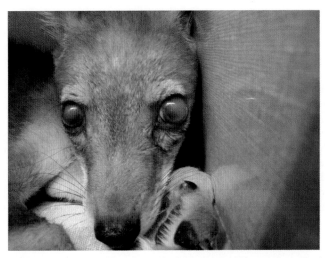

Fig. 10.5 Blue-eye in a coyote puppy. This is a form of type III hypersensitivity reaction to Canine adenovirus-1. (Courtesy of Dr. G.J. Costanzo)

TYPE IV HYPERSENSITIVITIES

Type IV hypersensitivity (delayed) reactions are T-cell-mediated inflammatory responses. They may occur at the injection site in response to vaccination, but a more common reaction is local granuloma formation. This may be in response to persistent adjuvants containing alum or oil. Vaccines containing a water-in-oil adjuvant produce larger and more persistent lesions at injection sites than vaccines containing alum or aluminum hydroxide. These lesions may develop into sterile abscesses and if the injection site is dirty, these abscesses may become infected. Injection site lesions are of major concern in the meat industries.

Residual Virulence

Modified live vaccines must be able to establish themselves transiently in a vaccinated animal yet at the same time not cause disease. They must be safe in animals and their human companions. They must be as stable as possible to enable long-term storage. They must be environmentally safe. It may be possible to achieve minimal virulence with maximal immunogenicity, but this may be unattainable in animals with any defects in their immune function. The normal distribution of immunological competence in an outbred population is such that some animals will inevitably be susceptible to an otherwise avirulent organism. This immunosuppression may result from minor stresses, but equally important some common viral infections such as canine distemper, feline pancytopenia, or feline leukemia also cause immunosuppression to a degree that an animal may become susceptible to otherwise avirulent vaccinal agents.

It is also appropriate to point out that modified live vaccines are attenuated for a specific target species for administration by a specified route. If administered to the wrong species or in the wrong way residual virulence may cause disease. Thus some modified live vaccines may retain the ability to cause disease. A good example is *Brucella abortus* strain 19. Although highly immunogenic in cattle, S19 can cause severe reactions in vaccinated cows. Swelling, fever, anorexia, depression, and a drop in milk yield have been reported. S19 can also cause abortion in pregnant cows and orchitis in bulls and humans. Safer attenuated Brucella vaccines are now available. Similar residual virulence hazards are associated with the soremouth vaccine and the sheep

Toxoplasmosis vaccine. Some modified live herpes vaccines or calicivirus vaccines given intranasally may spread to the oropharynx and result in persistent infection. In these cases, the vaccine virus may infect (and protect) other animals in contact.

Because live vaccine strains may be released into the environment, safety issues involving not only the animal but also its environment must be addressed. Are there changes in the tissue tropism of the virus? Are there changes in the carrier through the incorporation of new foreign genes? Is there reversion to virulence through the incorporation of complementation genes? Is there exchange of genetic information with other wild type or vaccine strains of the carrier? Will the carrier spread unwanted genes such as antibiotic resistance into the environment? These questions are highly relevant in the aquaculture industry where modified live vaccine viruses may escape into the aquatic environment (Chapter 21).

Postvaccinal canine distemper encephalitis is a rare complication that may develop in dogs and ferrets after administration of modified live canine distemper vaccines. Affected animals may show neurologic signs such as aggression, incoordination, and seizures, or die suddenly. The pathogenesis of this condition is unclear. It may be the result of residual virulence, increased susceptibility, or triggering of a latent paramyxovirus by the vaccine.

FETAL ABNORMALITIES

Vaccination during pregnancy carries uncertain risks, especially when live vaccines are used. The fetal immune system may not have developed sufficiently to defend itself against the vaccine strain of the virus. MLV bluetongue virus vaccine has been reported to cause malformations in the offspring of ewes vaccinated while pregnant. The severity of the lesions depends upon the stage of pregnancy at vaccination. For example, MLV bluetongue administered to ewes between 50 and 100 days of gestation has caused hydranencephaly and retinal dysplasia in lambs. Live *Erysipelothrix rhusiopathiae* vaccines have been reported to cause abortions in sows. The stress from this type of vaccination may also be sufficient to reactivate latent infections; for example, reactivation of equine herpesviruses has been triggered by vaccination against African horse sickness. A modified live virus (MLV) parvovirus vaccine administered during pregnancy has been reported to cause hydranencephaly and cerebellar hypoplasia in kittens.

IMMUNOSUPPRESSION

Many viruses promote their own survival by suppressing their host's immune system. Although immunosuppression is greatest in virulent strains, some MLVs may remain somewhat immunosuppressive. For example, some MLV canine parvovirus strains may depress T cell responses to mitogens in puppies for two to five weeks following administration, or even cause a lymphopenia. Similarly, MLV canine distemper may cause immunosuppression and thrombocytopenia. In view of this it may be best to avoid performing elective surgery on dogs for at least one week postvaccination.

MLV bovine viral diarrhea (MLV-BCD) vaccines may suppress neutrophil functions and lymphocyte blastogenesis in vaccinated calves. As a result, they may potentiate intercurrent infections. MLV-BVD may also induce mucosal disease 7 to 20 days after vaccination. Vaccination with an MLV-BHV1 vaccine has been shown to exacerbate the lesions of experimental Moraxella-induced pinkeye (Chapter 16).

Several vaccine combinations may also result in transient immunosuppression. For example, a combination of distemper and adenovirus vaccines can reduce canine lymphocyte counts and their responsiveness to mitogens, although the individual components are not detectably immunosuppressive. This T cell suppression may be accompanied by simultaneous enhancement of

B cell responses and raised immunoglobulin levels. Many of these cases of "immunosuppression" attributed to vaccines may however simply reflect alterations in the Th1/Th2 balance or transient alterations in lymphocyte recirculation patterns. They are rarely of clinical significance.

REVERSION TO VIRULENCE

As pointed out in an earlier chapter, older vaccine viruses were attenuated by prolonged passage in tissue culture or eggs. In some cases, it is possible to reverse the attenuation process by back-passage through their natural hosts. For example, attenuated distemper strains cannot grow in canine lung macrophages. Back-passage of the canine distemper virus (CDV) Rockborn strain for as few as three passages in puppies resulted in the virus regaining this ability. By four passages the virus could cause weight loss. By five passages, immunosuppression returned. The virus that had been back-passaged six to seven times had regained its virulence. The use of genetically defined, gene deleted attenuated vaccines has largely eliminated this type of problem.

OTHER ISSUES

AUTOIMMUNE DISEASE.

Louis Pasteur's first rabies vaccine contained dried rabbit brain tissue. When injected into patients it induced antibodies against myelin basic protein and an acute demyelinating encephalomyelitis developed in about 0.1% of recipients. Rabies vaccines have had an undeserved bad reputation ever since. In 2011, it was proposed that a new syndrome existed that linked diverse human autoimmune diseases with the use of adjuvanted vaccines. It was called autoimmune/autoinflammatory syndrome induced by adjuvants (ASIA). This syndrome has been investigated to determine whether it is an insignificant clinical term or whether there is an underlying mechanism that links adjuvants to autoimmunity. Aluminum-containing adjuvants were claimed to be the "cause" of ASIA. However, patients receiving allergen-specific immunotherapy receive up to 500 times more injected aluminum than regular vaccine recipients and have a lower incidence of autoimmune disease. Current data does not support the causation of ASIA by vaccine adjuvants. There is a lack of any reproducible evidence for any link between adjuvants and autoimmunity. One obvious problem with this proposed syndrome is that vaccination is so commonplace whereas autoimmunity remains uncommon. After all, huge numbers of people receive influenza vaccines annually without untoward effect.

There is a single animal study that appears to show that a link might exist between vaccination and the development of autoimmunity. A retrospective analysis of the history of dogs presenting with immune-mediated hemolytic anemia (IMHA) showed that 15 of 58 (26%) dogs with IMHA had been vaccinated within the previous month, compared with a randomly selected control group of 70 dogs in which 5% had been vaccinated. Dogs with IMHA that developed within a month of vaccination differed in some clinical features from dogs with IMHA unassociated with prior vaccination. Some studies using very large databases have tended to confirm this effect, in that they showed an approximately three-fold increase in diagnoses of autoimmune thrombocytopenia, and a two-fold increase in diagnoses of IMHA in dogs in the 30 days following vaccination, compared with other time periods. Other studies have failed to show any association between vaccination and IMHA. The overall prevalence of these diseases remains low, and they can be diagnosed at times not temporally associated with vaccination. Vaccination may therefore serve as a trigger for these diseases in some dogs—a vaccine potentiated reaction.

Contaminating thyroglobulin found in some vaccines (usually from the presence of fetal bovine serum) may lead to the production of antithyroid antibodies in vaccinated dogs. Lymphocytic thyroiditis has been found in 40% of Beagles on necropsy, but there was no association detected between vaccination and the development of this thyroiditis.

In the 1970s, a swine influenza vaccine induced Guillain-Barré syndrome (an autoimmune polyradiculoneuritis) in about 1 case per 100,000 human recipients. (Current influenza vaccines have a risk of about 1:1 million. It appears that the older influenza vaccine was unique in this respect.) Cases of this syndrome in dogs have been rarely reported. In some animals, the administration of potent, adjuvanted vaccines may stimulate the transient production of autoantibodies to connective tissue components such as fibronectin and laminin.

VACCINE-ASSOCIATED OSTEODYSTROPHY

Vaccination of some Weimaraner puppies may lead to the development of a severe hypertrophic osteodystrophy. The disease appears within 10 days of administration of MLV canine distemper vaccine. Systemic signs include anorexia, depression, fever, and gastrointestinal, nervous, and respiratory symptoms, in addition to symmetrical metaphyseal lesions with painful swollen metaphyses. Radiological examination shows radiolucent zones in the metaphyses, flared diaphyses, and formation of new periosteal bone. It is possible that the condition is triggered by the vaccine in genetically susceptible animals. These dogs may have a preexisting immune dysfunction with low concentrations of one or more immunoglobulin classes, recurrent infections, and inflammatory disease. It has been suggested that Weimaraners are especially susceptible to this condition and that they therefore receive only killed virus vaccines.

A mild transient polyarthritis has been reported in some dogs following vaccination. The dogs show a sudden onset of lameness with swollen and painful joints within two weeks of vaccination. The dogs recover within two days. No specific breed or vaccine has been associated with this problem. Vaccination against calicivirus has been associated with polyarthritis and a postvaccination limping syndrome in cats.

OVERVACCINATION

A search of web sites regarding vaccination of pets reveals that a large number express great concern regarding the practice of overvaccination. By this is meant the use of unnecessary vaccines and by implication a significant threat to the health of pets. Conversely a search of PubMed, the NCBI web site, reveals only a single scientific paper regarding this subject. The paper describes renal disease in a spaniel that received seven doses of vaccine from its owner, one vaccine per month, in the absence of any veterinary supervision. As a result, the dog developed immune-complex lesions in its kidney glomeruli. This was very likely a type III hypersensitivity nephropathy.

Clearly administration of excessive and unneeded vaccines is inappropriate. There are no health benefits and each additional dose of vaccine carries with it the chances of an untoward event. As pointed out throughout this text, the risk/benefit assessment of any vaccination procedure must be a subject for discussion between a veterinarian and the pet owner. There are many reasons why a veterinarian may suggest that it may be beneficial to vaccinate an animal and it is inappropriate to blame those vets who choose to vaccinate animals more frequently than currently recommended without a full knowledge of each specific case. This is called clinical judgment.

INJECTION SITE SARCOMAS

These are discussed in Chapter 14.

Errors in Manufacture and Administration

VACCINE CONTAMINATION

Modified live vaccines cannot contain preservatives (except antibiotics in viral vaccines). As a result, occasional cases of vaccine contamination have occurred. These have been a major issue in the past when viral identification required culturing. Modern identification techniques such as the polymerase chain reaction have made such contamination a thing of the past. There are numerous examples of such contamination. For example, Mycoplasma contamination was a feature of many live virus veterinary vaccines. The pestivirus of Border disease contaminated some soremouth and pseudorabies vaccines; bovine leukemia virus has contaminated bovine blood vaccines such as those against babesiosis and anaplasmosis. Bluetongue virus has contaminated some canine vaccines.

INJECTION SITE LESIONS

Injection site selection should include consideration of potential adverse reactions in addition to the hypersensitivity reactions described earlier. For example, injection in the gluteal muscles/hip region of cattle should be discouraged because gravitational drainage along fascial planes can occur. Should an abscess develop, considerable tissue damage may occur and result in eruptions in undesirable locations with lesions that require prolonged time to heal. They may result in unacceptable blemishes in meat destined for human consumption (Chapter 16).

Human Illness

Veterinarians and other vaccine users may be inadvertently exposed to animal vaccines as a result of unintended inoculation or spraying. Some of these vaccines may cause sickness. Veterinarians, their assistants, and other animal handlers should be especially careful when administering injectable vaccines to avoid needle-stick and eye injuries. If an individual is accidentally self-injected with a mineral oil-adjuvanted vaccine, seek immediate medical treatment regardless of the dose injected. With the notable exception of Brucellosis, these events are rarely reported. Nevertheless, accidents do occur and veterinarians should be fully aware of these risks.

Brucellosis is an existential hazard to veterinarians. The CDC has established a passive surveillance registry. In the two years 1998 to 1999, 21 individuals reported needlestick injury related exposure to the Brucella vaccine strain RB51, five were splashed in the eye, and one was splashed into an open wound. Although most received antibiotics, 19 reported clinical disease. Approximately 4 to 5 million doses of Brucella vaccines were administered annually in 1997 to 2000. It is estimated these would have resulted in at least 8000 needle-stick injuries, suggesting that exposure to RB51 is substantially under-reported.

A vaccinia recombinant rabies vaccine bait has been air-dropped across many states in the United States to vaccinate wildlife. Several instances of human exposure to these baits have been reported. (The vaccine baits have toll-free numbers printed on them.) In Ohio, there were 160 reports of bait contact and 20 of these involved contacts with the vaccine. One individual developed a severe vaccinia infection and had to be hospitalized.

Bordetella bronchiseptica causes respiratory disease in dogs and atrophic rhinitis in pigs. Infection of humans is rare but has been documented. In at least one case a young boy was inadvertently sprayed in the face with a "kennel cough vaccine." He had been holding his dog but the dog moved. He developed a pertussis-like respiratory disease that lasted several months despite antibiotic treatment. There have been reports of clients experiencing respiratory difficulty following administration of an intranasal vaccine to their dogs.

Needle-stick injuries are not uncommon and many involve vaccines. A woman was inadvertently inoculated with the Sterne anthrax vaccine while vaccinating her horse. She did not develop anthrax but did develop a local reaction within 24 hours. Serious inflammatory reactions are associated with injected *Mycobacterium paratuberculosis* vaccine. Self-injections appear to be a major issue in the aquaculture industry where workers have to work fast to vaccinate slippery fish.

Reporting

Veterinarians are encouraged to report all adverse reactions to the vaccine's manufacturer and the regulatory authorities. This provides both with the critical information that is used to evaluate and monitor vaccine safety in the field. In this way vaccine safety can be progressively improved.

Adverse reactions should be reported to the vaccine manufacturer first. After that, they should be reported to the appropriate regulatory authorities.

UNITED STATES

In the United States, adverse vaccine events should also be reported to the US Department of Agriculture APHIS Center for Veterinary Biologics at 1-800-752-6255. They have an online electronic report form. Reports can also be made by fax or mail. Vaccine lot and serial numbers should be noted in vaccination records because this will facilitate an investigation. The use of standardized reporting systems is encouraged.

Web: http://www.aphis.usda.gov/animal_health/vet_biologics/vb_adverse_event.shtml

Fax or mail: Download the PDF form at http://www.aphis.usda.gov/animal_health/vet_biologics/publications/adverseeventreportform.pdf and fax to (515) 337-6120 or mail to the Center for Veterinary Biologics (CVB), 1920 Dayton Avenue, PO Box 844, Ames, Iowa 50010, USA. Telephone: (800) 752-6255

In Canada, suspected adverse events (SAE) should be reported to the Canadian Center for Veterinary Biologics (CCVB) in Ottawa at 1-855-212-7695. As stipulated by the Health of Animals Regulations, all reports that indicate "serious expected" or "serious unexpected" adverse events related to the use of a veterinary biologic, including lack of efficacy, must be reported to CCVB within 15 days of that information becoming known to the permit or license holder. Follow-up reports, including case conclusions, must be submitted to CCVB in a timely manner. All other reports should be investigated by the license/permit holder, summarized in a summary update report, and submitted to CCVB every six months. Summary update reports should be submitted within 60 days of the end of the reporting period. SAE related to veterinary biologics are categorized as one of the following: adverse event (AE), serious AE, unexpected AE, and lack of efficacy. A causality assessment should also be assigned to each SAE. Each case should be classified as probable, possible, unlikely, or unknown.

Form CFIA/ACIA 2205, Notification of Suspected Adverse Events to Veterinary Biologics, may be found at http://inspection.gc.ca/english/for/pdf/c2205e.pdf.

UNITED KINGDOM

In the United Kingdom adverse events should be reported to the Veterinary Medicines Directorate. Forms can be obtained at their website at www.vmd.defra.gov.uk or by calling their Pharmacovigilance team at 01932 338427. The Veterinary Medicines Directorate (VMD), an agency of the Department for Environment, Food, and Rural Affairs, is responsible for the Suspected Adverse Reaction Surveillance Scheme (SARSS) for veterinary medicines. Adverse reactions in animals in the United Kingdom should be reported at http://www.vmd.defra.gov.uk/adversereactionreporting/default.aspx.

Suspected human reactions to veterinary medicines in the United Kingdom should be reported at http://www.vmd.defra.gov.uk/adversereactionreporting/default.aspx, or contact the VMD at Freepost KT4503, Woodham Lane, New Haw, Addlestone, Surrey, KT15 3BR, UK. Telephone: 01932 338427 Fax: 01932 336618

AUSTRALIA

In Australia, adverse events should be reported to the Australian Pesticides and Veterinary Medicines authority on their website at https://apvma.gov.au/node/309.

NEW ZEALAND

In New Zealand adverse event reports should be made to the Ministry for Primary Industries, PO Box 2526, Wellington, 6140, or online at ACVM-adverseevents@mpi.govt.nz.

Sources of Additional Information

Ashford, D.A., di Pietra, J., Lingappa, J., et al. (2004). Adverse events in humans associated with accidental exposure to the livestock brucellosis vaccine RB51. *Vaccine*, 22, 3435–3439.

Berkelman, R.L. (2003). Human illness associated with use of veterinary vaccines. *Clin Infect Dis*, 37, 407–414.

Broaddus, C.C., Balasuriya, U.B.R., White, J.L.R., et al. (2011). Evaluation of the safety of vaccinating mares against equine viral arteritis during mid or late gestation or during the immediate postpartum period. *J Am Vet Med Assoc*, 238, 741–750.

Davis, G., Rooney, A., Cooles, S., Evan, G.S. (2013). Pharmacovigilance: Suspected adverse events. *Vet Rec*, 173, 573–576.

Edwards, D.S., Henley, W.E., Ely, E.R., Wood, J.L.N. (2004). Vaccination and ill-health in dogs: A lack of temporal association and evidence of equivalence. *Vaccine*, 22, 3270–3273.

Fritsche, P.J., Helbling, A., Ballmer-Weber, B.K. (2010). Vaccine hypersensitivity—update and overview. *Swiss Med Wkly*, 140, 238–246.

Gershwin, L.J. (2018). Adverse reactions to vaccination: From anaphylaxis to autoimmunity. *Vet Clin North Am Small Anim Pract*, 48, 279–290.

Hawkes, D., Benhamu, J., Sidwell, T., Miles, R., Dunlop, R.A. (2015). Revisiting adverse reactions to vaccines: A critical appraisal of autoimmune syndrome induced by adjuvants (ASIA). *J Autoimmun*, 59, 77–84.

Huisman, W., Martina, B.E., Rimmelzwaan, G.F., et al. (2009). Vaccine-induced enhancement of viral infections. *Vaccine*, 27, 505–512.

Knobel, D.L., Arega, S., Reininghaus, B., Simpson, G.J.G., Gessner, B.D., et al. (2017). Rabies vaccine is associated with decreased all-cause mortality in dogs. *Vaccine*, 35, 3844–3849.

Meyer, E.K. (2001). Vaccine-associated adverse events. *Vet Clin North Am*, 31, 493–515.

Miyaji, K., Suzuki, A., Shimakura, H., Takase, Y., et al. (2012). Large-scale survey of adverse reactions to canine non-rabies combined vaccines in Japan. *Vet Immunol Immunopathol*, 145, 447–452.

Moore, G.E., DeSantis-Kerr, A.C., Guptill, L.F., et al (2007). Adverse events after vaccine administration in cats: 2,560 cases (2002–2005). *J Am Vet Med Assoc*, 231, 94–100.

Moore, G.E., Guptill, L.F., Ward, M.P., et al. (2005). Adverse events diagnosed within three days of vaccine administration in dogs. *J Am Vet Med Assoc*, 227, 1102–1108.

Moore, G.E., HogenEsch, H. (2010). Adverse vaccinal reactions in dogs and cats. *Vet Clin Small Anim*, 40, 393–407.

Moore, G.E., Ward, M.P., Kulldorff, M., Caldanaro, R., et al. (2005). A space-time cluster of adverse events associated with canine rabies vaccine. *Vaccine*, 23, 5557–5562.

Murakami, T., Inoshima, Y., Sakamoto, E., Fukushi, H., et al. (2013). AA amyloidosis in vaccinated growing chickens. *J Comp Pathol*, 149, 291–287.

Ohmori, K., Masuda, K., Maeda, S., et al. (2005). IgE reactivity to vaccine components in dogs that developed immediate-type allergic reactions after vaccination. *Vet Immunol Immunopathol*, 104, 249–256.

Ortloff, A., Moran, G., Olavarria, A., Folch, H. (2010). Membranoproliferative glomerulonephritis possibly associated with over-vaccination in a cocker spaniel. *J Small Anim Pract*, 51, 499–502.

Ramsay, J.D., Williams, C.L., Simko, E. (2005). Fatal adverse pulmonary reaction in calves after inadvertent intravenous vaccination. *Vet Pathol*, 42, 492–495.

Shmuel, D.L., Cortes, Y.. (2013). Anaphylaxis in dogs and cats. *J Vet Emerg Crit Care*, 23, 377–394.

Srivastav, A., Kass, P.H., Mcgill, L.D., Farver, T.B., Kent, M.S. (2012). Comparative vaccine-specific and other injectable-specific risks of injection-site sarcomas in cats. *J Am Vet Med Assoc*, 241, 595–602.

Strasser, A., May, B., Teltscher, A., et al. (2003). Immune modulation following immunization with polyvalent vaccines in dogs. *Vet Immunol Immunopathol*, 94, 113–121.

Production, Assessment, and Regulation of Vaccines

Given their critical importance in controlling infectious diseases, it is essential that there be a reliable, consistent supply of safe and effective vaccines available to veterinarians and animal producers. Veterinary vaccines constitute about a quarter of the global market for animal health products. Infectious diseases are highly diverse, and the significance and benefits of vaccination obviously depend on the disease. The potential economic returns on animal vaccines are generally much less than for human vaccines with lower prices and smaller markets, so there must be a lower investment in research. On the other hand, there are less stringent regulatory requirements and the cost of preclinical studies is much less. It usually takes a shorter time to take an animal vaccine to market and thus to deliver a return on investment. Additionally, veterinarians can determine the effectiveness of a vaccine in the appropriate target species rather than extrapolate from results in rodents.

Vaccine Categories

The term vaccine encompasses all products designed to induce active immunity in animals against disease. Both live and inactivated vaccines may also contain adjuvants, stabilizers, preservatives, and diluents. Products generated by recombinant DNA technology do not differ fundamentally from conventional products. The use of modern molecular and genetic techniques has generated new and improved vaccines. For administrative and regulatory purposes, these vaccines are conveniently divided into four categories.

Category I: Antigens Generated by Gene Cloning

Gene cloning can be used to produce large quantities of pure antigen in culture. In this process, DNA coding for an antigen of interest is first isolated from the pathogen. This DNA is then inserted into a plasmid and then into a bacterium or yeast in such a way that it is functional and the recombinant antigen is expressed in large amounts. Category I vaccines are not viable and present no unusual safety concerns.

Category II: Genetically Attenuated Organisms

It is possible to alter the genes of an organism so that it becomes irreversibly attenuated. These are live organisms modified by adding or deleting a gene. The added genes can encode marker antigens. The deleted genes reduce virulence. It is critical that these genetic modifications do not increase the virulence, pathogenicity, or survivability of the agent.

Category III: Live Recombinant Organisms

Genes coding for protein antigens can be cloned directly into a variety of organisms, especially DNA viruses. These live viral vectors may carry one or more foreign genes. The recombinant organism itself may then be used as a vaccine. Safety issues need to be determined for each vaccine.

Category IV: Polynucleotide Vaccines

DNA or RNA encoding protective antigens may be used as vaccines. In the case of DNA, it is inserted into a bacterial plasmid that acts as a vector. The vaccine antigen gene is placed under the control of a strong mammalian promoter sequence. When the engineered DNA-plasmid is injected intramuscularly into an animal, it is taken up by host cells. It is usual to incorporate an antibiotic resistance gene into these plasmids to serve as a marker.

Vaccine Production

Vaccine manufacturing is a challenging task. The most basic steps required to produce a safe, effective, and consistent vaccine can be difficult to execute. There is a high cost to establishing complex processes. The variability in the starting materials, the infectious agent itself, environmental conditions, the manufacturer's expertise, and also the basic production steps all add to the complexity. Many of the assays required to validate each step also have high inherent variability. Inability to manage these risks can result in vaccine failure and costly recalls.

The production of both live attenuated and inactivated vaccines requires the generation of large quantities of pathogens, both viruses and bacteria. This results in a significant time elapsing between the start of production and vaccine delivery. It requires specialized facilities that if they fail, may expose both the operators and the environment to unacceptable risks.

Regulatory authorities in the United States issue licenses for general sale and distribution of biologics manufactured domestically. Biologics manufactured outside the United States that meet all regulatory requirements are issued permits for general sale and distribution. Biologics have to meet minimum standards of potency, safety, purity, and efficacy in accordance with their label claims.

Regulatory authorities license not only the specific biological product, but also the processes by which that biologic is produced, tested, and released. Minor changes in the production process may significantly alter the final product. Clinical trials may be required to validate any new processes. These risks make vaccine manufacture more challenging than many pharmaceuticals. Additionally, as emphasized throughout this book, the commercial realities of vaccine usage, especially in the food animal industries place severe pressures on profit margins. This is one reason why the number of major animal vaccine manufacturers remains relatively small—it is not a job for amateurs.

Conditional licenses are used to meet emergency situations or other special circumstances. Products released conditionally need only a "reasonable expectation" of efficacy, but they must meet the same safety and purity standards as other vaccines. These licenses are usually issued for one or two years, but may be renewed.

KEY STEPS

The production of approved, licensed, or permitted vaccines requires strict adherence to key steps in vaccine production that can be collectively classified as quality assurance (Fig. 11.1). In

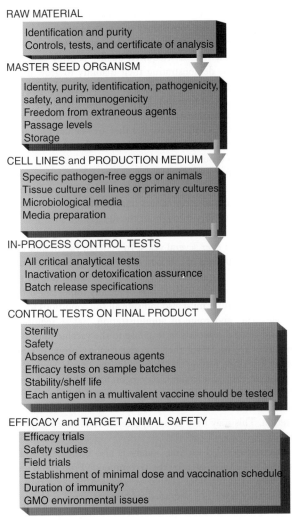

RAW MATERIAL
- Identification and purity
- Controls, tests, and certificate of analysis

MASTER SEED ORGANISM
- Identity, purity, identification, pathogenicity, safety, and immunogenicity
- Freedom from extraneous agents
- Passage levels
- Storage

CELL LINES and PRODUCTION MEDIUM
- Specific pathogen-free eggs or animals
- Tissue culture cell lines or primary cultures
- Microbiological media
- Media preparation

IN-PROCESS CONTROL TESTS
- All critical analytical tests
- Inactivation or detoxification assurance
- Batch release specifications

CONTROL TESTS ON FINAL PRODUCT
- Sterility
- Safety
- Absence of extraneous agents
- Efficacy tests on sample batches
- Stability/shelf life
- Each antigen in a multivalent vaccine should be tested

EFFICACY and TARGET ANIMAL SAFETY
- Efficacy trials
- Safety studies
- Field trials
- Establishment of minimal dose and vaccination schedule
- Duration of immunity?
- GMO environmental issues

Fig. 11.1   The key quality control steps in the vaccine manufacturing process. *GMO*, Genetically modified organism.

producing vaccines, the quality of the starting materials needs to be assured by rigorous testing. These are especially complex for antiviral vaccines. Thus a first step is characterization of the vaccine virus. A master seed virus (MSV) is prepared from a suitable strain of the virus. The identity of this virus must be confirmed, its history known, and its quality assessed by determining its purity and freedom from extraneous agents. (A major threat is the risk of transmission of spongiform encephalopathies). Not only must the master seed be tested, but also the cells in which it is grown. Known as the master cell stock (MCS), this must also be completely characterized. The cell line may also be tested for its ability to induce tumors. Thus it must be shown that both the MSV and MCS are free from mycoplasma, bacteria, fungi, cytopathic or hemadsorbing viruses, and other extraneous agents.

Only approved MSV and MCS can be used when making vaccines. In-process control tests must then be established to verify the consistency of the final product. It is usual to release the final product in batches, referred to as serials, which are then tested to confirm the reproducibility of the quality of the finished vaccine. Required quality control tests include ensuring that killed products, are nonviable by demonstrating their inability to grow in tissue culture. Safety must be tested by inoculating the reconstituted vaccine into animals. It is usual to use a greatly increased dose, usually tenfold, to confirm this. No abnormal or local reactions should occur. The potency of each batch must be demonstrated by comparing the results with previous potency tests. Efficacy must be assessed by challenge studies that are standardized for some pathogens or must be customized for other agents. Likewise, when producing live viral vaccines, the virus content should be measured and found to be within appropriate limits.

If there is no preservative in the vaccine, the manufacturer must demonstrate that it remains effective for a suitable period of time after opening the vial. If it contains preservatives, the vaccine stability and sterility in multidose containers must be demonstrated. It must also be shown that the vaccine will retain its stability throughout the designated shelf life. Many finished products require cold (4°C) or even ultra-cold (liquid nitrogen) storage to maintain stability and potency. Stability may be tested over several years. In general, vaccines in liquid and lyophilized forms are deemed to have shelf-lives of one and two years respectively. They are formulated to ensure that there will always be a minimal immunizing dose remaining by the expiration date.

All possible hazards must be indicated. This is especially important if the agent poses a risk to human health. The manufacturer must also indicate all the conditions for the correct use of the vaccine such as species, age, and route of administration. Safety requirements are absolutely critical, so any local and general reactions in response to the vaccine must be carefully examined. If the vaccine contains a live organism then the exact safety properties of the strain must be documented. These will include testing the vaccine by the recommended route in live animals known to be susceptible to natural infections. Reversion to virulence following serial passage has to be examined. Usually a minimum of four passages is required to show lack of reversion. Living vaccine strains should be tested for their ability to pass from vaccinated to naïve animals through secretions and excretion. This may have to be repeated several times to provide assurance of its inability to spread.

In the case of inactivated/killed vaccines, safety is also critical. In addition to inactivation assurance, animals need to be vaccinated by the recommended route and any local and systemic reactions assessed. These local reactions should be assessed by dissection at slaughter in food animals to ensure that they have not degraded carcass quality. Local tissue reactions help to dictate the withdrawal period before slaughter and are largely dependent on the reactivity of the adjuvant.

A vaccine must be able to do what the manufacturer claims. Efficacy and potency requirements include assessment of induced immunity. The precise nature of these assays will depend on both the animal species and the nature of the claims made for the vaccine. Any claims regarding duration of immunity must also be based on the results of challenge trials and also possible serologic assays. As discussed previously surrogates of protection have not been established for many infectious diseases.

Although it is important to test vaccines in the field before they can be licensed, it is almost impossible to assess vaccine efficacy in field trials because disease outbreaks cannot be predicted, and it is very difficult to have available unvaccinated control animals held under the same conditions. Field trials are much more useful for assessing safety under field conditions.

The release of genetically modified live organisms (categories II and III) for field-testing or distribution requires additional assurances that there will be no risk to animals, humans, or the environment. Thus before release a careful risk assessment needs to be performed. This should analyze such issues as the characteristics of the vaccine organism; human health risks; animal health risks for target and nontarget species; and environmental persistence including the possibility of increased virulence. If any environmental effect is anticipated then an environmental impact statement must be prepared.

VACCINE EXCIPIENTS

To improve the antigenicity of a vaccine it is often necessary to add adjuvants (Chapter 7). It may also be necessary to enhance the stability of the vaccine by adding excipients. These may include, binders, preservatives, buffering agents, emulsifiers, wetting agents, nonviral vectors, and transfection facilitating compounds. In general, no preservative is used in single dose vials or syringes. Preservatives are, however, required in multidose vials of vaccines. Because of perceived (but unsubstantiated) health risks the organic mercury compound thiomerosal (Merthiolate) is no longer widely used as a preservative in human vaccines, but it remains in use in some veterinary vaccines. An alternative vaccine preservative is 2-phenoxyethanol (2-PE). It is both stable and effective.

Some vaccines are unstable in aqueous solutions, especially if they cannot be held in uninterrupted cold storage. Vaccines containing live viruses are susceptible to heat inactivation, but are much more resistant when lyophilized. As a result, many vaccines are stored as a lyophilized powder. They store well but should be kept cool and away from light and should only be reconstituted with the diluent provided by the manufacturer.

However, lyophilization may also alter the product pH and solute concentration and may denature the vaccine antigens. Thus stabilizers must be added to the vaccine. These can include sugars and sugar alcohols, which encase the proteins and stabilize them. Other polymers and amino acids may also be added to improve stability. Remember, however, that intense sunlight and heat can destroy even lyophilized vaccines.

Because the living organisms or antigens found in vaccines normally die or degrade over time, it is necessary to ensure that they will be effective even after storage. Therefore it is usual to use an antigen in excess of the protective dose under laboratory conditions, and its potency is tested both before and after accelerated aging. Vaccines that contain killed organisms, although more stable than living ones, contain an excess of antigens for the same reason. Vaccines approved for licensing on the basis of challenge exposure studies must usually show evidence of protection in 80% of vaccinated animals, whereas at least 80% of the unvaccinated controls must develop evidence of disease after challenge exposure (the 80:80 efficacy guideline). The route and dose of administration indicated on the vaccine label should be scrupulously heeded because these were probably the only routes and doses tested for safety and efficacy during the licensing process. Vaccines usually have a designated shelf-life, and although properly stored vaccines may still be potent after the expiration of this shelf-life, this should never be assumed, and all expired vaccines should be discarded. Adverse reactions should always be reported to the appropriate licensing authorities in addition to the vaccine manufacturer (Chapter 10). Because modified live virus vaccines carry the risk of residual virulence and of contamination, some countries will not approve their use.

Inactivated vaccines are commonly available in liquid form and usually contain suspended or emulsified adjuvant. These should not be frozen, and they should be shaken well before use. The presence of preservatives will not control massive bacterial contamination, and multidose containers should be discarded after partial use.

COST/BENEFITS OF VACCINATION

Economics is a key consideration when deciding whether to vaccinate livestock. The agricultural sector is price sensitive so that vaccines need to be produced at low cost in large quantities. When considering vaccination costs, economic benefits must also be considered. Control of disease by vaccination will result in savings on veterinary care, reduced animal husbandry labor, improved animal health, and survival reflected in faster growth and improved feed conversion, protection of unvaccinated animals through herd immunity, and reduction in uncertainty about future outcomes. Costs will include the cost of purchasing, storing, and administering vaccines.

Vaccination against zoonotic diseases has both direct and indirect benefits. Indirect benefits include increased productive time and income, and also reduced pain and suffering. Direct benefits include the reduced costs for medical services. For example, rabies is an expensive disease. If an unvaccinated animal bites a human, costs include postexposure vaccination of the victim in addition to quarantine or euthanasia of the biting animal. The brain of the animal must be examined for the presence of the virus. These costs, of course, do not account for the stress and worry associated with this disease. In Texas, aerial vaccination by dropping vaccinia-vectored rabies vaccine enclosed in food bait has been employed to vaccinate coyotes against rabies. The costs of this were the total expenditures of the program—vaccine, food, planes, fuel, and so forth. The benefits were the savings associated with human postexposure prophylaxis, and animal rabies tests within the affected area. The calculated cost of the rabies vaccination program is about US$26 million. The benefits were estimated at between US$89 million and US$346 million. Depending on the frequency of postexposure prophylaxis and animal testing, the cost/benefit ratio therefore ranged from 3.38 to 33.13.

Many other analyses have been conducted into the benefits and costs of animal vaccines. For example, a study on vaccination against paratuberculosis in dairy cattle in North America indicated that vaccination cost US$15/cow, and the returns minus costs were US$142 per cow.

The consolidation of large livestock enterprises has resulted in fewer and bigger farms. Animal health decisions may now involve thousands of animals. The cost of an incorrect decision is so large that guessing is not an option. In general, the cost of a vaccine and its administration are relatively easy to calculate. For example, poultry vaccines sell for US$0.01 to US$0.05 per dose. Cattle vaccines cost about 20 to 30 times this, and human vaccines sell for 100 to 500 times the cost of a poultry vaccine. The benefits of vaccination are more difficult to calculate. The prime benefit expected will be improved productivity, but reduced treatment costs are also important. Measures of productivity would typically include, mortality, average daily gain and feed conversion (Feed conversion is critical, given that feed is by far the largest cost in intensive livestock systems.) Once productivity is determined this needs to be translated into revenues, costs, and profits. A benefit/cost ratio of greater than 1 indicates that the benefits exceed the costs.

COMBINED/POLYVALENT VACCINES

The development of effective combined (many different organisms) and polyvalent (many strains of the same organism) vaccines also presents manufacturing issues. Usually bulk lots of monovalent vaccines are produced and then combined into a single product. Alternatively, the individual components may be stored separately and combined just before administration. In each case both the monovalent lots and the final combined product have to undergo quality testing. Thus these vaccines require an increased investment in resources and facilities. Manufacturers must demonstrate that there are no differences in the physical, chemical, and immunological properties for the individual lots and the combined product. Likewise, vaccines that are polyvalent and combine different strains must be balanced to maximize infectivity and immunogenicity. Antigens, adjuvants, and preservatives must be compatible. For example, preservatives or buffers may alter vaccine potency.

Vaccine Presentation

VACCINE LABELS

Proper labeling will allow a lay person to be able to understand the correct need, administration, revaccination, and precautions that must be taken to use the product effectively and safely.

US Department of Agriculture (USDA)–approved label claims for veterinary vaccines are now based on the statistical significance of their efficacy data and their clinical relevance. Efficacy indication statements now simply state, "This product has been shown to be effective for the vaccination of a specific species of healthy animal of a specific age against a specific disease." This is accompanied by a standardized summary of efficacy and safety data. There is also a cautionary statement telling the public to consult a licensed veterinarian for interpretation of the data. These labels do not automatically carry a default recommendation for annual revaccination. Revaccination statements are based on available data. If this is unavailable the label will say so. There is also a required statement on labels referring the end-user to a website where basic, yet relevant, data regarding efficacy and safety is available. There is a single claim that carries the implication that if the product is licensed, it is efficacious and meets USDA requirements.

Vaccine Regulation

The production of veterinary vaccines is regulated by national agencies. The Animal and Plant Health Inspection Service (APHIS), Center for Veterinary Biologics (CVB) of the USDA in the United States; by the Canadian Centre for Veterinary Biologics of the Canadian Food Inspection Agency; and by the Veterinary Medicines Directorate in the United Kingdom; in addition to appropriate government agencies in other countries. In Europe, the European Medicines Agency grants licenses for human and animal use of GMOs, in collaboration with national authorities. In general, regulatory authorities have the right to license establishments where vaccines are produced and to inspect these premises to ensure that the facilities are appropriate and that the methods employed are satisfactory. All vaccines must be checked for purity, efficacy, safety, and potency.

APHIS has the responsibility for regulating vaccine production in the United States (Box 11.1). Vaccine licensure is managed by the CVB within this agency, located in Ames, Iowa. The CVB ensures that veterinary biologics (products used to diagnose, treat, and cure disease) are free from disease producing agents, especially foreign animal diseases. It develops the appropriate procedures and standards for products to be released, and the biologics receive either a license (domestically produced) or a permit (foreign manufacture) for general sale and distribution. It monitors and inspects both products and facilities and regulates field tests and the release of veterinary biologics. In essence the CVB ensures that vaccines sold to the public are pure, safe, potent, and effective. It also plays a role in the international harmonization of product regulations.

The CVB issues a catalogue of all currently licensed veterinary biological products including a summary of each product's safety and effectiveness. The catalog may also contain additional studies to support the product's effectiveness. Product summaries are published for vaccines, bacterins, and immunomodulators, but not for test kits, antibody products, or allergenic extracts.

Typically, the product summary will contain a summary of any efficacy studies for each microbial disease or agent against which the vaccine is claimed to be effective. Additional studies encompassing multiple routes of administration or multiple animal species may be added as well as any relevant data generated after the product has been licensed or permitted. There will be at least one field safety study and documentation of any specialized safety claims such as safety in pregnant animals.

These summaries are searchable at the APHIS Veterinary Biologics website at https://www.aphis.usda.gov/aphis/ourfocus/animalhealth/veterinary-biologics

---

BOX 11.1 ■ The Virus-Serum-Toxin Act

In the United States, the Virus-Serum-Toxin (VST) Act of 1913 (amended in 1985) was designed to protect farmers and ranchers by regulating vaccine production and assuring safety and efficacy. It originated as a result of issues with the production of anti-hog cholera serum. It made the Secretary of Agriculture responsible for licensing and regulating the manufacture, import, and export of veterinary biologicals. In practice, this is managed and enforced by the Animal and Plant Health Inspection Service. Border and import inspection is a function of the Department of Homeland Security.

The VST Act makes it unlawful to:
1. Prepare, sell, or ship any worthless, contaminated, dangerous, or harmful veterinary biological product in or from the United States.
2. Prepare, sell, or ship any veterinary biological product in or from the United States, unless it is prepared in a licensed establishment in compliance with US Department of Agriculture regulations.

The regulations designed to administer the VST act and control the preparation, sale and licenses of biologics and vaccines used in animals are published in Title 9, Code of Federal Regulations 9CFR 1996, sections 101–118. They define veterinary biological products as:

"All viruses, serums, toxins, and analogous products of natural or synthetic origin, such as diagnostics, antitoxins, vaccines, live microorganisms, killed microorganisms, and the antigenic or immunizing components of microorganisms intended for use in the diagnosis, treatment, or prevention of diseases of animals."

All biologicals must be manufactured in accordance with an approved outline of production so that they meet the requirements for purity, safety, potency, and efficacy. All labels and claims must also be approved.

Vaccines must be manufactured in a licensed Biologics Establishment that must be inspected before a license is issued. Each biological product must also have a specific product license.

GENETICALLY MODIFIED VACCINES

Regulations tend to be more stringent for genetically modified organisms (GMOs) because they are not always regarded as well characterized. Production methods are also highly variable, which makes it difficult to standardize procedures. GMOs must be investigated for safety to humans, animals, and the environment. Live vaccines require special attention. In many countries the release of GMOs into the environment is carefully regulated and environmental safety assessments may be required. This includes risks to both target and nontarget species. This is very important in fish vaccines that are released into water.

Regulatory Authorities

The World Organization for Animal Health known by its French name Office Internationale de Epizooties (OIE) has the responsibility to improve global animal health. OIE publishes standards for Veterinary Vaccines and the requirements for establishing a country's disease-free status. It also manages some animal vaccine banks (Box 11.2).

Most developed countries have their own regulatory requirements. In general, these are very similar and require proof of safety and efficacy. Manufacturing criteria are also defined, as are label claims. There are agreements in place for mutual recognition of licensure in many countries.

CANADA

The Canadian Food Inspection Agency (CFIA) is responsible for licensing veterinary biologics, including veterinary vaccines that are manufactured and/or used in Canada. The licensing program operates under the Health of Animals Act and Regulations and is administered by the Canadian Centre for Veterinary Biologics. Their web site is at https://www:inspection.gc.ca.

BOX 11.2 ■ Vaccine Banks

It is often considered necessary to stockpile vaccines in case of emergency. For example, some human vaccines, such as smallpox, are stored by governments in case of a bioterrorism attack. In 2006, the Office Internationale de Epizooties (OIE) set up the first vaccine bank to control avian influenza. This was originally reserved for African countries and over 62 million doses were distributed to six countries. Subsequently, a bank for foot-and-mouth disease vaccine has been established. It stores five core strains and six optional strains so that countries can obtain vaccines that correspond to their immediate needs. A vaccine bank to control peste des petits ruminants (PPR) has also been established. As a result, the OIE was able to provide 8 million doses to three African countries in 2014. A rabies vaccine bank to control canine rabies was also established to respond to urgent requests to contain an outbreak and delivered 3 million doses to ten Asian countries up to 2014.

In the United States, US Department of Agriculture maintains a National Veterinary Stockpile for emergency use. It includes vaccines against foot and mouth disease, hog cholera (classical swine fever), and highly pathogenic avian influenza. Critical supplies can be dispatched within 24 hours in an animal disease emergency. The web site for the stockpile is www.aphis.usda.gov/animalhealth-nvs.

EUROPE

In the European Union, licensing submissions are assessed and approved by the European Medicines Evaluation Agency. Vaccines can be registered in three ways. There is a centralized procedure where new vaccines are assessed and approved for all member states. There is a mutual recognition procedure where a single country is tasked to evaluate and approve a vaccine. Following approval, application can be made to have the product registered in other countries. There is also a decentralized procedure where the vaccine documentation is reviewed in multiple selected countries at the same time. They can be contacted at: https://www.ema.europa.eu/en/veterinary-medicines-regulatory-information. There is mutual recognition of some good manufacturing standards between the European Union, Australia, and New Zealand.

UNITED KINGDOM

The Veterinary Medicines Directorate regulates vaccine licensure in the United Kingdom. This is an agency within the Department for Environment, Food and Rural Affairs (DEFRA). It plays the key role in licensing and authorization of veterinary biologicals. Their web site is at https://www.gov.uk/government/organizations/veterinary-medicines-directorate.

A database of licensed products is available at http://www.vmd.gov.uk/ProductInformation Database/.

AUSTRALIA

The Australian Pesticides and Veterinary Medicines Authority regulate vaccine licensure. Their regulations are essentially equivalent to those in European and North American countries and they accept data generated by tests acceptable in these regions. They can be contacted at: www.daff.gov.au/. Once licensed, the use of each individual animal vaccine is regulated by state authorities.

NEW ZEALAND

The New Zealand Ministry of Primary Industries regulates vaccine marketing and standards for efficacy through the Agricultural Compounds, and Veterinary Medicines Group of the

New Zealand Food Safety Authority. The group has a web site on vaccine registration and licensure requirements at https://www.mpi.govt.nz/dmsdocument/20009/send.

THE AMERICAS

The harmonization of vaccine licensure requirements across the Americas is regulated by The Committee of the Americas for Veterinary Medicines. Its web site is at http://www.rr-americas. oie.int/proyectos/Camevet/in_acta.htm.

INTERNATIONAL

The Veterinary International Committee on Harmonization is made up of representatives of Japan, Europe, and the United States plus industry representatives. They serve to reconcile and harmonize each region's guidelines as much as possible. They can be contacted at www.vichsec.org.

Sources of Additional Information

A complete web-based database of available veterinary vaccines, vaccine candidates, and vaccine research is available at the Vaccine Investigation and Online Information Network (VIOLIN) at http://www.violinet .org/vevax/index

Gerdts, V., Mutwiri, G., Richards, J., van Drunen Little-van den Hurk, S., Porter, A.A. (2013). Carrier molecules for use in veterinary vaccines. *Vaccine,* 31, 596–602.

Josefsberg, J.O., Buckland, B. (2012). Vaccine process technology. *Biotechnol Bioeng,* 109, 1443–1460.

MacDonald, J., Doshi, K., Dussault, M., Hall, J.C., Holbrook, L., et al. (2015). Bringing plant-based veterinary vaccines to market: Managing regulatory and commercial hurdles. *Biotechnol Adv,* 33, 1572–1581.

Plotkin, S., Robinson, J.M., Cunningham, G., Iqbal, R., Larsen, S. (2017). The complexity and cost of vaccine manufacturing - An overview. *Vaccine,* 35, 4064–4071.

van Schaik, G., Kalis, C.H., Benedictus, G., Dijkhuizen, A.A., Hume, R.I.B. (1996). Cost-benefit analysis of vaccination against paratuberculosis in dairy cattle. *Vet Rec,* 139, 624–627.

Passive Immunization

As described in Chapter 1, it was not long after Louis Pasteur's initial discoveries that the sources of immune protection were found in the blood and were called antibodies. It was demonstrated that blood serum containing antibodies to bacterial toxins such as those from tetanus or diphtheria could be transferred from an immune animal to a susceptible individual and so confer protection (Fig. 12.1). Thus the recipient was "immunized" without mounting an immune response—passive immunization. Horses were the major source of these "antitoxins" because of their size and ease of management. Passive immunization was widely employed in the 1920s and 1930s against human pathogens such as *Streptococcus pneumoniae*, *Neisseria meningitides*, and *Haemophilus influenzae*, in addition to tetanus and diphtheria. With the advent of cheaper and easier to use antimicrobials and antibiotics such as penicillin and streptomycin, it fell into disuse. Passive immunization only persisted for use in toxin-mediated diseases such as tetanus and botulism, virus diseases such as rabies, and in snake envenomation (Table 12.1). It is now staging a comeback. Polyclonal antibodies generated in immunized animals and monoclonal antibodies generated in the laboratory are increasingly employed in the treatment of diverse animal and human diseases.

Immunoglobulins

The major antibody in mammalian serum is a protein called immunoglobulin (Ig)G. This is a Y-shaped protein of about 160 kDa. In passive immunization, whole or semipurified serum, or IgG obtained from an immune animal, is injected into or fed to another animal. If it is injected into an animal of the donor species then the injected antibodies will simply be removed through normal catabolic processes. If IgG is injected into an animal of a different species it will act as a foreign antigen and trigger an immune response. Such a response will result in its prompt elimination. It is therefore highly desirable to minimize the antigenicity of IgG. The simplest way of doing this is to treat the IgG with a protease such as papain or pepsin. These split the IgG molecule into two or three fragments. The first fragment to be cleaved off is the "tail of the Y" (Fig. 12.2). This fragment can be crystalized and so is called the Fc fragment. It does not contribute to toxin or virus neutralization so it can be discarded. The rest of the IgG molecule consists of the two joined arms of the Y is called Fab'2. This fragment retains the antibody activity. Further proteolytic digestion separates this into two antigen-binding fragments each called Fab. These too are functional. Elimination of the Fc region greatly reduces the antigenicity of the preparation although the smaller fragments do have a shorter half-life than intact IgG.

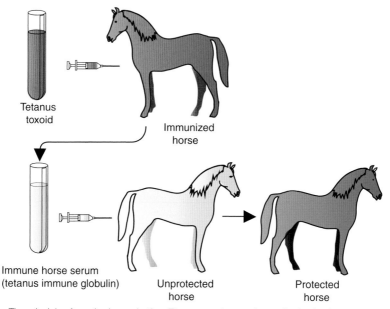

Fig. 12.1 The principle of passive immunization. Thus serum from an immunized animal contains antibodies. When injected into another animal these can confer immediate, but temporary, immunity.

TABLE 12.1 ■ Licensed Polyclonal Antibody Products for Animal Use in the United States

Function	Examples
Antibacterial	*Escherichia coli* (+K99)
	Rhodococcus equi
	Streptococcus equi
	Salmonella typhimurium
	Trueperella pyogenes
Antitoxins	*Clostridium botulinum* Type B
	Clostridium perfringens types C and D
	Clostridium tetani
	Crotalidae (rattlesnake) antivenin
Antiviral	Bovine rotavirus-coronavirus
	West Nile Virus

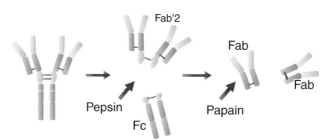

Fig. 12.2 If immunoglobulins are injected into another species they act as antigens and are removed rapidly. If fragmented by treatment with proteases and unnecessary components such as the Fc region removed, this immunogenicity is minimized.

As discussed later, modern molecular techniques also make it possible to alter the nonantigen-binding parts of immunoglobulins so that they too are identical to the recipient species and almost completely eliminating their antigenicity.

Polyclonal Antibodies

A natural immune response to a complex antigen such as a bacterium or virus activates large numbers of B cells that in turn generate a diverse mixture of antibodies, each with a different antigen-binding specificity. Most pathogens have a complex structure and present the immune system with many different epitopes. As a result, multiple B cell clones are stimulated to respond. These clones produce polyclonal antibodies. Polyclonal antibodies with their mixture of specificities can bind collectively to many different antigens. (This is in contrast to monoclonal antibodies that are derived from a single clone of B cells and bind only a single targeted epitope.)

IMMUNIZED DONOR ANIMALS

Passive immunization requires that antibodies be produced in donor animals by active immunization and that these antibodies then be given to susceptible animals to confer immediate protection. Serum containing these antibodies may be produced against a wide diversity of pathogens. For instance, they can be produced in cattle against anthrax, in dogs against distemper, or in cats against panleukopenia. They are most effective when protecting animals against toxigenic organisms such as *Clostridium tetani* or *Clostridium perfringens*, using antisera raised in horses. Antisera made in this way are called immune globulins and are commonly produced in young horses by a series of immunizing injections. The clostridial toxins are proteins that can be denatured and made nontoxic by treatment with formaldehyde. Formaldehyde-treated toxins are called toxoids. Donor horses are initially injected with toxoids, but once antibodies are produced, subsequent boosters may contain purified toxin. The responses of the horses are monitored, and once their antibody levels are sufficiently high, they are bled. Bleeding is undertaken at intervals until the antibody level drops, when the animals are again boosted with antigen. Plasma is separated from the horse blood, and the globulin fraction that contains the IgG antibodies is concentrated, titrated, and dispensed.

CHICKEN EGG YOLK

When an egg develops in the ovary of chickens, it contains a rich food source, the yolk. The yolk also contains a high concentration of chicken antibodies called IgY. IgY is the avian functional equivalent of mammalian IgG. Approximately 30% of the chicken's IgY (but only 1% of its IgM or IgA) will transfer from the plasma to the yolk. Thus a single egg yolk may contain up to 250 mg of IgY. If the hen is first vaccinated, then their eggs will contain high levels of antibodies against that antigen. If these yolk antibodies are simply fed to a mammal they will confer local immunity. Passive immunization by feeding egg yolk immunoglobulins is a relatively simple and economical method of protection against some enteric diseases. For example, chicken egg yolk antibodies can protect calves against diarrhea caused by group A rotaviruses. Seven days of IgY treatment significantly suppressed virus shedding, duration of diarrhea, and disease severity when compared with untreated calves. Similar benefits have been recorded in piglets and poultry.

Dried egg yolk powder from chickens has been administered to newborn puppies in milk replacer before closure of intestinal absorption (first eight hours after birth). Puppies supplemented in this way show significantly greater weight gain compared with controls. Weaned puppies receiving hyperimmune egg powder from chickens immunized against *Escherichia coli* and salmonella in the form of food supplementation had improved fecal quality and increased fecal

IgA. Likewise egg powder containing antibodies to canine parvovirus 2 (CPV2) protected puppies against CPV2 challenge.

BLOOD PLASMA

Spray-dried blood plasma is used as a feed additive for pigs. It contains high concentrations (20%) of immunoglobulins. It has been shown to improve weight gain and resistance to some pathogens. Thus it also protects against *E. coli* colonization. The beneficial effects appear to reside in the immunoglobulin fraction. However, it is possible that viruses such as porcine epidemic diarrhea virus may survive the spray-drying process. Pooled abattoir blood plasma is another possible source of purified IgG. Fed to piglets for seven days postweaning, it reduces the severity of postweaning diarrhea.

MILK WHEY

The major immunoglobulin in bovine milk is IgG. When casein is precipitated from milk during cheese manufacturing the liquid whey that remains contains small amounts of protein, 10% of which is IgG. However large volumes of whey are needed to obtain significant amounts of immunoglobulin for passive immunization.

Antitoxins

CLOSTRIDIUM TETANI

Antitetanus immunoglobulin (also called tetanus immune globulin or tetanus antitoxin) for veterinary use is produced in hyperimmunized healthy horses. Notwithstanding its equine origin, it can be used in cattle, sheep, pigs, dogs, and cats, as well as in horses. It is available in vials of 1500 and 15,000 units, and it contains thiomerosal and/or phenol to inhibit microbial growth. Deep, dirty wounds, especially when contaminated with soil or manure and tissues are devitalized sites where *Clostridium tetani* can grow and secrete its toxin. This toxin must be neutralized if clinical tetanus is to be avoided. Antitoxin should also be administered to nonimmune animals after castration, docking, and any surgical procedure conducted at sites where tetanus is known to be present. The half-life of equine IgG ranges from 27 to 39 days. Tetanus antitoxin given intramuscularly provides immediate immunity that lasts about 7 to 14 days in species other than horses.

To standardize the potency of different immune globulins, comparison is made to an international biological standard. In the case of tetanus immune globulin, this is done by comparing the dose necessary to protect guinea pigs against a fixed amount of tetanus toxin with the dose of the standard preparation of immune globulin required to do the same. The international standard immune globulin for tetanus toxin is a quantity held at the International Laboratory for Biological Standards in Copenhagen. An international unit (IU) of tetanus immune globulin is the specific neutralizing activity contained in 0.03384 mg of the international standard. Tetanus toxoid may also be measured in limes flocculation (Lf) units. These are determined by an in vitro flocculation test. They measure the quantity and antigenicity of a toxoid but not its potency. One Lf unit is the amount of toxoid neutralized by 1.4 IU of tetanus immune globulin.

Tetanus immune globulin is given to animals to confer immediate protection against tetanus. At least 1500 IU of immune globulin should be given subcutaneously or intramuscularly in the neck to horses and cattle; at least 500 IU to calves, sheep, goats, and swine; and at least 250 IU to dogs. The exact amount should vary with the amount of tissue damage, the degree of wound contamination, and the time elapsed since injury. Tetanus immune globulin is of little use once the toxin has bound to its target receptor and clinical disease appears. Notwithstanding this, some veterinarians seek to improve its prognosis by administering high doses of antitoxin, 10,000 to 50,000 units to horses and cattle, and 3000 to 15,000 units to goats and sheep. Animals with slow-healing puncture wounds may be given a second dose in seven days.

Although immune globulins give immediate protection, some problems are associated with their use. For instance, when horse tetanus immune globulin is given to a cow or dog, as described earlier, the horse proteins will be perceived as foreign, elicit an immune response, and be rapidly eliminated.

If repeated doses of horse immune globulin are given to an animal of another species, this may provoke IgE production and allergic reactions. Additionally, the presence of high levels of circulating horse antibodies may interfere with active immunization against the same antigen. This is a phenomenon similar to that seen in newborn animals passively protected by maternal antibodies.

Mixtures of different monoclonal antibodies directed against multiple toxin epitopes are now being tested as possible replacements for polyclonal antiserum. These are more readily standardized than polyclonal antisera.

Serum Sickness

When tetanus began to kill large numbers of soldiers during the First World War, the use of tetanus antitoxin increased dramatically. Physicians gradually increased the amount of antitoxin administered to severely wounded soldiers. However, soldiers who had received a very large dose of equine antitetanus serum developed a characteristic illness about 10 days later (Fig. 12.3). This was called serum sickness and consisted of a generalized vasculitis with erythema, edema, urticaria of the skin, neutropenia, lymph node enlargement, joint swelling, and proteinuria. The reaction was usually of short duration and subsided within a few days. A similar reaction can be produced experimentally in rabbits by administration of a large intravenous dose of antigen. The development of sickness coincides with the formation of large amounts of immune-complexes in the circulation. The experimental disease may be acute if it is caused by a single, large injection of an antigen, or chronic if caused by multiple small injections. In either case, animals develop

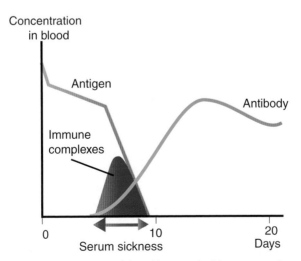

Fig. 12.3   If large amounts of foreign serum are injected into an animal, immune complexes form within a few days. These immune complexes are deposited in tissues such as the kidneys and joints to cause serum sickness.

glomerulonephritis and arteritis. For this reason, tetanus immune globulin of human origin is now preferred for the prevention of tetanus in people whenever possible.

CLOSTRIDIUM BOTULINUM

Clostridium botulinum antitoxins are commercially available. Antiserum to the type C toxin has been successfully used in ducks and mink. Type B toxin causes lethal toxicosis in foals (Chapter 15). Early administration of 30,000 IU of antitoxin intravenously has been reported to be effective in treating botulism in foals.

CLOSTRIDIUM PERFRINGENS, TYPES C AND D

This antitoxin of equine origin is given subcutaneously to prevent enterotoxemia (overeating disease) caused by *Cl. perfringens* toxinotypes C and D in calves, adult cattle, lambs, sheep, and goats, and by type C in piglets. (Type D is not known to cause disease in pigs). Protection lasts approximately 14 to 21 days. It is not standardized, and so for dosing refer to the product label. For disease treatment, the dose should be doubled.

Immune Sera

NEONATAL FOALS

Immune sera are especially useful in neonatal animals that may have failed to receive sufficient colostral antibodies. For example, commercially available horse serum, fresh frozen plasma, or horse IgG may be administered orally soon after birth or intravenously if gut closure has occurred.

Commercially available hyperimmune plasma is available to assist in the prevention of *Rhodococcus equi* pneumonia on infected farms. It should be administered as soon as possible after birth. At least 1L of licensed hyperimmune plasma should be administered to foals no older than 2 days of age. If the potential for further challenge is high, a second dose should be administered to foals between 14 and 32 days of age. This treatment reduces the severity of the disease in experimentally infected foals although it is not curative. Adult horses are susceptible to strangles caused by *S. equi* and equine antisera may be available to provide immediate protection to horses in contact. An antiserum is also available against West Nile virus.

NEONATAL CALVES

Neonatal calves that have received insufficient colostrum may be given normal bovine serum or purified IgG. They may also receive specific antisera against *E. coli, Trueperella pyogenes, Pasteurella multocida, Salmonella typhimurium,* and *Cl. perfringens* antitoxin either alone or in combination. They may also receive antibodies to bovine coronavirus and rotavirus. In general, antibodies against systemic infection are given subcutaneously, whereas antiserum against enteric disease is administered orally.

The use of commercial bovine serum is not without risks, especially if it comes from pooled random animals. Bovine virus diarrhea virus is an occasional but pervasive contaminant, whereas many other viruses may be detected by exquisitely sensitive metagenomic techniques. Ultraviolet or gamma radiation will inactivate viruses in serum, but specialized equipment is required.

NEONATAL PIGLETS

Equine antisera against *E. coli* and *Cl. perfringens* are available for use in piglets. They are given orally to treat neonatal diarrhea.

RABIES

Standard treatment of a human bitten by a rabid animal includes immediate postexposure prophylaxis. After thorough washing and flushing of the wound, local infiltration into and around the wound site or sites with rabies immune globulin (RIG) serves as a barrier to viral spread. The immune globulin will provide neutralizing antibodies at the site of exposure and prevent viral spread until the active immunization with a rabies vaccine takes effect. RIG is usually a polyvalent antiserum of human or equine origin. Human RIG is however expensive and not available in many less developed countries. Currently studies are ongoing on the use of carefully designed broad-spectrum monoclonal antibodies for this purpose.

SNAKE AND OTHER VENOMS

The primary causes of venomous snakebites in the United States are the pit vipers of the family Crotalidae—rattlesnakes, moccasins, and copperheads. Snake venom is a complex mixture and as many as 50 components contribute to its destructive properties. Collectively they cause soft tissue necrosis, vasculotoxicity, coagulopathy, cytotoxicity, and necrosis. This results in severe tissue damage, hypotension, and neurological impairment.

Administration of polyvalent crotalid antivenom is the preferred treatment for pit viper envenomation. The prompt use of this antivenom limits swelling and reverses the coagulopathy caused by the venom. Antibodies neutralize the toxin hemolysins, vasoactive, and myotoxic activities. However, these venoms contain toxins that cause immediate necrosis at the bite site so the antivenom may not prevent local tissue necrosis, especially if treatment is delayed. Early intravenous administration of the antivenom is essential when treating snake-bitten animals. Infusion should start slowly to determine if there are any immediate hypersensitivities. If all is in order then the flow rate can be increased. Ideally it should be administered within 4 hours of the bite, but it will still be beneficial if given within 24 hours. On the other hand, if the venom reaches the bloodstream, such as when an artery is pierced, then death may be inevitable despite use of antivenom.

At the present time there are two approved antivenoms available in the United States: Antivenin Crotalidae Polyvalent (ACP) (Wyeth-Ayerst) and CroFab Crotalidae Polyvalent Immune Fab (Ovine) (BTG International Inc.). ACP is minimally purified and still contains horse IgG and albumin. It is licensed for animal use. It has been used to treat humans for many years. ACP may not prevent the thrombocytopenia seen in some patients bitten by a timber rattlesnake (*Crotalus horridus*) or reverse the neurologic effects of Mojave rattlesnake (*Crotalus scutulatus*) venom. ACP generally requires the use of multiple vials depending on severity of the bite, size of the snake, and time elapsed, but cost may then be a factor. Additional doses may be given every 2 hours.

Crotalidae Polyvalent Immune Fab (Ovine) (CroFab, FabAV) is produced by immunizing sheep with 1 of 4 crotaline snake venoms: *Crotalus atrox* (Western diamondback rattlesnake), *Crotalus adamanteus* (Eastern diamond rattlesnake), *Crotalus scutulatus* (Mojave rattlesnake), and *Agkistrodon piscivorus* (Eastern cottonmouth). The IgG is then digested with papain to produce antibody fragments (Fab and Fc), and the more immunogenic Fc fragment removed. The four individual monospecific Fab preparations are then combined in equal amounts to form the final product. This product is about five times as potent as ACP. FabAV is efficacious against *Crotalus viridis* (Prairie rattlesnake), but ACP is not. As described earlier, Fab fragments are less immunogenic and less likely to induce adverse events. However, being much smaller molecules they are cleared more rapidly and thus have to be administered more frequently, perhaps as often as every six hours.

There are also two effective foreign antivenoms. One is a polyvalent product (Antivipmyn) manufactured in Mexico. The second is a polyspecific IgG product of equine origin (Polyvet-ICP) from Costa Rica. Antivipmyn, a Fab'2 antibody fragment antivenom, is cleared from the body faster than IgG but slower than the Fab fragments. One or two vials appear to be effective in the dog. Smaller dogs may require more vials. Polyvet-ICP is not specifically directed against North American pit vipers. Both anaphylaxis and serum sickness are potential complications of antivenom treatment.

HUMAN PASSIVE IMMUNIZATION

Humans have a greater diversity of passive immunization products available than animals. These include antitoxins against tetanus, botulism, diphtheria, and anthrax; immune globulins against viruses such as rabies, varicella zoster, cytomegalovirus, measles, hepatitis A and B, respiratory syncytial virus, and vaccinia; antivenoms against numerous snake species, and also black widow spiders.

Monoclonal Antibodies

Monoclonal antibodies are another potential source of passive protection for animals (Box 12.1). There are several different ways to produce them. In the original method described in 1975, they were produced from mouse plasma cell tumors—myelomas (Fig. 12.4). This was done by fusing normal plasma cells making the antibody of interest with immortal myeloma cells grown in tissue culture. The resulting mixed cell is called a hybridoma. These hybridomas divide rapidly in tissue culture. Clones that produce the desired antibody are grown in mass culture and the supernatant fluid harvested. Unfortunately these mouse antibodies are immunogenic in other species and rapidly cleared from the body.

A strategy that is used to minimize this involves the genetic manipulation of hybridomas by replacing the mouse with human or other constant regions. For example, mouse myeloma variable regions can be attached to dog constant regions to make a "caninized" monoclonal antibody for use in that species. By subsequently modifying the sequence in the V region framework regions, the monoclonal antibody may be fully caninized. A caninized monoclonal antibody, directed against interleukin-31 (Il-31) is used to prevent itch in dogs with atopic dermatitis.

Several other methods have been used to produce human monoclonal antibodies and could be readily applied to veterinary species (see Fig. 12.4). For example, phage display techniques are commonly used. In this technique, the DNA encoding variable region genes, from heavy and light chains, are prepared from blood B cells. These genes are then paired to generate Fab regions. This generates a huge library of genes that are randomly inserted into filamentous bacteriophages. The phages are then exposed to a surface covered with the target antigen. Only phages displaying antigen-binding sites of the correct specificity will bind to the target antigen. After washing to remove any unbound phages, the bound phages are eluted and amplified by infecting *E. coli*. These steps can be repeated several times, thus effectively enriching the selected phages.

BOX 12.1 ■ Nomenclature

The nomenclature of monoclonal antibodies has been approved by the World Health Organization and other national bodies. All monoclonal antibody names end with the stem *mab*, whereas polyclonal antibodies end in *pab*. The previous letter *o* identifies its species of origin as mouse, and *u* denotes human origin. The letters before that refer to the antibody's target, such as *lim* for the immune system, *ci* for the circulatory system, *ne* for the nervous system and *tum* for cancer. The stem for humanized antibodies is *zu*, and that for veterinary use is *vet*. Finally, the prefix has no special meaning, but it should contribute to an easily pronounceable name. Adalimumab is a human monoclonal antibody that acts on the immune system (specifically antiTNF).

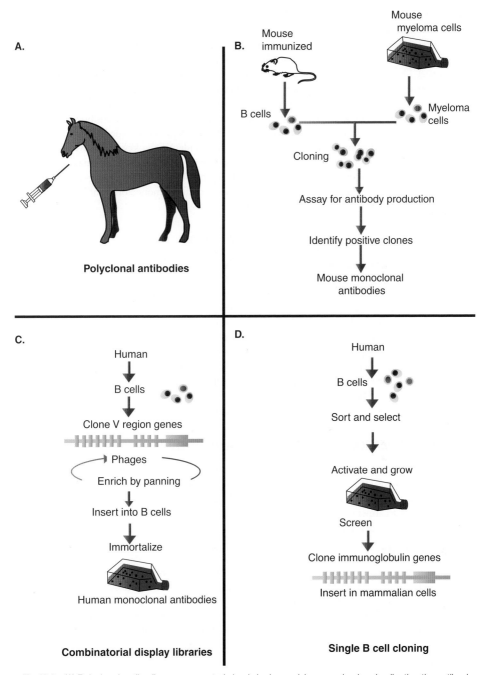

A.

Polyclonal antibodies

B.

Mouse
myeloma cells

Mouse
immunized

B cells

Myeloma
cells

Cloning

Assay for antibody production

Identify positive clones

Mouse monoclonal
antibodies

C.

Human

B cells

Clone V region genes

Phages

Enrich by panning

Insert into B cells

Immortalize

Human monoclonal antibodies

Combinatorial display libraries

D.

Human

B cells

Sort and select

Activate and grow

Screen

Clone immunoglobulin genes

Insert in mammalian cells

Single B cell cloning

Fig. 12.4 (A) Polyclonal antibodies are generated simply by immunizing an animal and collecting the antibodies produced. (B) Originally monoclonal antibodies were produced using mouse myeloma cells fused with normal plasma cells to generate hybridomas. These hybridomas produce mouse monoclonal antibodies. Recently, other methodologies have been developed that enable monoclonal antibodies to be generated in species other than mice. (C) Immunoglobulin genes are cloned into a host such as a bacteriophage, yeast, or bacterium. These are then cloned and the clones making useful antibodies are selected and enriched. (D) The B cells from an individual making polyclonal antibodies can be activated and the individual cells analyzed to determine the antibodies they are producing. Selected cells can then be cloned and immortalized.

Once isolated, the relevant gene encoding the Fab of interest can be excised, sequenced, and cloned into immortal B cells.

An alternative method is to clone antibody-encoding genes from single B cells from an immune individual. (This can be either a naturally infected and recovered individual or an immunized one.) The desired clones are identified by a single-cell polymerase chain reaction or by panning on an antigen-covered surface in a manner similar to that used for phages. It is then possible to select those cells that make the most potent antibodies, especially those that make broadly neutralizing antibodies. Memory B cells are the major source of these antibodies and they can be immortalized by infecting them with Epstein-Barr virus, an oncogenic herpesvirus. These single B cell cloning techniques have been very effective in identifying key protective antigens.

Monoclonal antibodies, because of their purity, can be used for passive immunization. Many different "humanized" monoclonal antibodies are being employed to treat cancers and suppress inflammatory and autoimmune diseases. Similar species-modified monoclonal antibodies are being increasingly employed in veterinary medicine.

ANTIMICROBIAL MONOCLONAL ANTIBODIES

Although monoclonal antibodies have not been widely employed as therapeutic agents in infectious diseases, this is an obvious future development. They would be very useful in responding rapidly to emerging viral diseases. In humans multiple monoclonal antibodies have been prepared against different strains of Ebola virus. These have great potential for the emergency treatment of infected persons. Likewise monoclonal antibodies against Zika virus might protect human fetuses from congenital Zika syndrome. Another such example would be the use of these antibodies, directed against conserved epitopes, to protect against newly emerged pandemic strains of influenza. Only one antiviral monoclonal antibody (mAb) is commercially available. It is directed against respiratory syncytial virus—palivizumab. It should be pointed out that monoclonal antibodies are very expensive to produce, (about 100 times that of a polyclonal hyperimmune globulin) and a general assumption is that they are only effective for prophylaxis, something that active vaccination may do better.

ANTIINFLAMMATORY MONOCLONAL ANTIBODIES

Among the most successful applications of monoclonal antibodies is their use to decrease unwanted inflammatory reactions. In humans these antibodies may be directed against inflammatory cytokines such as tumor necrosis factor (TNF)-α or its receptor. They have proven very effective in the treatment of diseases such as rheumatoid arthritis or systemic lupus. Many of these are now being developed for animal use.

Atopic Dermatitis

IL-31 is the major cause of the severe itching in canine atopic dermatitis. The production of IL-31 in affected skin can be neutralized by administration of a caninized monoclonal antibody—Lokivetmab (Cytopoint, Zoetis), directed specifically at canine IL-31. The antibody is injected subcutaneously. It binds to circulating IL-31 and prevents it from binding to the IL-31 receptor. In double blind, placebo-controlled trials, a single dose has provided relief from itch and a reduction in disease severity in dogs with chronic atopic dermatitis.

ANTICANCER MONOCLONAL ANTIBODIES

Monoclonal antibodies are increasingly used for the treatment of cancers. They are usually directed against specific tumor cell antigens or against immunosuppressive signaling molecules. They are discussed in Chapter 23.

Equine Serum Hepatitis

On rare occasions, horses may develop lethal, acute hepatic necrosis 30 to 70 days after receiving an immune globulin of equine origin. This is called equine serum hepatitis or Theiler's disease. Theiler noted hundreds of cases of hepatitis in horses that had received equine antiserum. It has occurred in horses that have received antiserum against tetanus, botulism, *S. equi*, anthrax, influenza, and encephalitis, and also pregnant mare serum, and equine plasma. It has also occurred after active immunization against equine encephalitis and rhinopneumonitis when the vaccines were prepared using fetal equine cells. Certain serum mixtures or just a single vaccine batch may be associated with outbreaks of the disease. Occasional cases have been described in untreated horses living with affected animals, suggesting that the disease is transmissible.

Recently four novel viruses have been identified in horses with Theiler's disease. Three are flaviviruses (nonprimate hepacivirus, Theiler disease-associated virus, and equine pegivirus) and the fourth is equine parvovirus-hepatitis (EqPV-H). Theiler's virus was identified during an outbreak of acute hepatitis in horses that had received equine botulinum antitoxin. In another example 15 out of 17 (88%) horses injected with a specific lot of immune globulin were carrying the pegivirus. The disease was severe, with 53% to 88% mortality. Clinical signs included anorexia, icterus, excessive sweating, and neurological abnormalities. Clinical chemistry confirmed severe liver damage with high liver enzyme levels, ammonia, and bilirubin. However, the pegivirus is reported to be a common infection in horses in the United States and Europe and is not hepatotropic.

In a more recent situation, a horse that died 65 days after receiving tetanus antitoxin was shown to be infected by a parvovirus. It was present in the tetanus antitoxin administered to this horse nine weeks previously. This equine parvovirus-hepatitis (EqPV-H) virus belongs to the *Copiparvovirus* genus and is related to the bovine and porcine parvoviruses. Experimental inoculation of EqPV-H into two healthy adult horses resulted in the development of acute hepatitis 80–90 days later. Subsequent studies have demonstrated that EqPV-H was present in 18 consecutive cases of Theiler's disease whereas the other viruses were not consistently present. EqPV-H appears to be endemic in some horse populations because 13% of a random sample had circulating antibodies against it. In another study 9/10 horses with Theiler's disease and 20/37 in-contact horses were positive for EqPV-H by polymerase chain reaction (PCR).

Commercial tetanus antitoxin is usually heated at 60°C for one hour, but parvoviruses are relatively heat resistant. Some antitoxins have added phenol or thiomerosal as preservatives, but these may inactivate the flaviviruses while being insufficient to inactivate EqPV-H. Producers of equine blood products must ensure that their products are free of all these viruses (Box 12.2).

BOX 12.2 ■ Bovine Antibodies

Some cattle immunoglobulin molecules are unusually large because they use a long third hypervariable polypeptide loop (CDR3), which may contain up to 69 amino acids. This length is caused by a very long germline Dh2 gene segment. As a result, these CDR3s fold into a long beta-stranded stalk supporting a disulfide-bonded "knob" domain located far from the antibody surface. The benefits of this structure to cattle are unclear.

However, cattle immunized against human immunodeficiency virus (HIV) will produce strongly neutralizing antibodies. The knob and stalk structure can block the virus CD4-binding site much more effectively than can human antibodies. These neutralizing bovine antibodies may be used prophylactically or therapeutically against HIV and other major human pathogens.

(From Sok, D., Le, K.M., Vadnais, M., Saye-Francisco, K.L., et al. [2017]. Rapid elicitation of broadly neutralizing antibodies to HIV by immunization in cows. *Nature*, 548, 108–111.)

Sources of Additional Information

Baxter, D. (2007). Active and passive immunity, vaccine types, excipients and licensing. *Occup Med (Lond)*, 57, 552–556.

Diraviyam, T., Zhao, B., Yang, Y., Schade, R., Michael, A., Zhang, X. (2014). Effect of chicken egg yolk antibodies (IgY) against diarrhea in domesticated animals: a systematic review and meta-analysis. *PLoS One*, 9, e97716.

Guglick, M.A., MacAllister, C.G., Ely, R.W., Edwards, W.C. (1995). Hepatic disease associated with administration of tetanus antitoxin in eight horses, *J Am Vet Med Assoc*, 206, 1737–1740.

Hedegaard, C.J., Heegaard, P.M. (2016). Passive immunisation, an old idea revisited: Basic principles and application to modern animal production systems. *Vet Immunol Immunopathol*, 174, 50–63.

Joao, C., Negi, V.S., Kazatchkine, M.D., Bayry, J., Kaveri, S.V. (2018). Passive serum therapy to immunomodulation by IVIG: A fascinating journey of antibodies. *J Immunol*, 200, 1957–1963.

Lukic, I., Filipovic, A., Inic-Kanada, A., Marinkovic, E., Miljovic, R., Stojanovic, M. (2018). Cooperative binding of anti-tetanus toxin monoclonal antibodies: Implications for designing an efficient biclonal preparation to prevent tetanus toxin intoxication. *Vaccine*, 36, 3764–3771.

Marston, H.D., Paules, C.I., Fauci, A.S. (2018). Monoclonal Antibodies for Emerging Infectious Diseases—Borrowing from History. *N Engl J Med*, 378, 1469–1472.

Michels, G.M., Ramsey, D.S., Walsh, K.F., et al. (2016). A blinded, randomized, placebo-controlled, dose determination trial of lokivetmab (ZTS-00103289), a caninized, anti-canine IL-31 monoclonal antibody in client owned dogs with atopic dermatitis. *Vet Dermatol*, 27, 478. e129.

Mila, H., Grellet, A., Mariani, C., Feugier, A., Guard, B., Suchodolski, J., Steiner, J., Chastant-Maillard, S. (2017). Natural and artificial hyperimmune solutions: Impact on health in puppies. *Reprod Domest Anim*, 52, 163–169.

Spaun, J., Lyng, J. (1970). Replacement of the international standard for tetanus antitoxin and the use of the standard in the flocculation test. *Bull World Health Organ*, 42, 523–534.

Tomlinson, J.E., Kapoor, A., Kumar, A., et al. (2019). Viral testing of 18 consecutive cases of equine serum hepatitis: A prospective study (2014–2018). *J vet Intern Med*, 33, 251–257.

Vega, C., Bok, M., Saif, L., Fernandez, F., Parreño, V. (2015). Egg yolk IgY antibodies: A therapeutic intervention against group A rotavirus in calves. *Res Vet Sci*, 103, 1–10.

Walker, L.M., Burton, D.R, (2018). Passive immunotherapy of viral infections: 'Super-antibodies' enter the fray. *Nat Rev Immunol*, 18, 297–308.

Witsil, A.J., Wells, R.J., Woods, C., Rao, S. (2015). 272 cases of rattlesnake envenomation in dogs: Demographics and treatment including safety of F(ab')2 antivenom use in 236 patients. *Toxicon*, 105, 19–26.

Wu, C.H.,Liu, U., Lu, R.M., Wu, H.C. (2016). Advancement and applications of peptide phage display technology in biomedical science. *J Biomed Sci*, 23, 8.

Canine Vaccines

Vaccination is widely employed to protect dogs against infectious diseases. As might be anticipated, some of these diseases are more important than others. This has led to the designations "core" and "noncore" to denote those vaccines that are essential and those that are less important. Core vaccines are those that all dogs, regardless of circumstances or location, should receive. They protect the animals from severe, life-threatening disease. The three core vaccines for dogs in North America are those against canine distemper virus (CDV), canine adenovirus 2 (CAV-2), and canine parvovirus type 2 (CPV-2). Additional vaccines may also be considered to be essential by the attending veterinarian based on their professional judgment. One obvious such example is rabies vaccine, especially in countries where rabies is endemic. Rabies vaccination is also legally required in many jurisdictions and is mandatory for international travel. Noncore vaccines are those whose use is also based upon careful risk assessment by a veterinarian in consultation with the dog owner. These risks will vary with the type of vaccine used, geographic location, local environment, degree of exposure to other dogs, and the dog's lifestyle (Box 13.1).

SPECIES CONSIDERATIONS

One unique feature of dogs is their extreme size variation. This presents problems regarding vaccine safety and efficacy. It has been conventional procedure to administer an identical dose of vaccine to all dogs irrespective of their size. Although it has long been thought that the canine immune system was somewhat indifferent to antigen dose, this is not the case. Postvaccinal antibody titers vary inversely according to a dog's body weight. For example, antibodies against CPV-2, CDV, and CAV-2 have been measured in adult dogs over a large size range, 12 months after receiving a conventional vaccine. All the dogs developed a protective level of antibodies. CPV-2 antibody titers were significantly higher in very small dogs (<5 kg) than in medium sized dogs (10–20 kg) or in large dogs (>20 kg). CDV antibody titers were significantly higher in the very light, light, and medium groups, than in the heavy group. Interestingly there were no significant differences between the size groups with respect to CAV-2 antibody titers. In another study investigating rabies vaccine failures, the proportion of dogs failing to make sufficient antibodies—their median antibody titers—decreased whereas the vaccine failure rate increased with increased dog sizes. There is also a difference in the frequency of adverse reactions to vaccination in dogs depending upon their size (Fig. 10.1). Small dogs suffer more adverse events than large dogs.

BOX 13.1 ■ Canine Vaccination Guidelines

Guidelines for Canine vaccination have been published by:

The American Animal Hospital Association (AAHA). 2017, AAHA Canine Vaccination Guidelines. Ford, R.B., Larson, L.J., Schultz, R.D., & Welborn, L.V. At: https://www.aaha.org/aaha-guidelines/vaccination-canine-configuration/vaccination-canine/

The World Small Animal Veterinary Association (WSAVA). Day, M.J., Horzinek, M.C., Schultz, R.D., & Squires, R.A. (2016). WSAVA Guidelines for the vaccination of dogs and cats. *J Small Anim Pract*, 57, 4–8. At: https://www.wsava.org/WSAVA/media/PDF_old/WSAVA-Vaccination-Guidelines-2015-Full-Version.pdf.

Other issues associated with dogs are the major differences in vaccine responses associated with different breeds. These breed differences, resulting largely from a loss of genetic variability, are reflected in differences in their responses to vaccines and also differences in their susceptibility to vaccine-induced adverse events.

Antibacterial Vaccines

BORDETELLA BRONCHISEPTICA

Bordetella bronchiseptica is a gram-negative bacterium, one of the complex mixture of agents that are associated with canine respiratory disease. Its importance was recognized in 1910 when it was wrongly believed to be the cause of canine distemper (Chapter 1). *B. bronchiseptica* is a primary pathogen because it can impair ciliary function and thus predispose to secondary opportunistic infections. It can also be a secondary invader following infection with other respiratory pathogens. Bordetella infection is associated with mild to moderate tracheobronchitis resulting in coughing, retching, sneezing, and nasal discharge. Monovalent and combined vaccines are available for administration parenterally or intranasally. Most of these are combined vaccines that contain multiple antigens against diverse respiratory pathogens.

A nonadjuvanted acellular *B. bronchiseptica* vaccine containing selected bacterial antigens may be administered by the subcutaneous route. Several different modified live intranasal *B. bronchiseptica* vaccines are also available as well as single component oral vaccines. The oral vaccines may be administered into the buccal pouch as early as 7-8 weeks of age.

Onset of immunity develops by 48 hours following oral and intranasal vaccination and the duration of immunity is 12 to 14 months so annual revaccination is recommended. These vaccines may be administered in combination with canine parainfluenza and CAV-2 vaccines. Intranasal or oral vaccines must never be delivered by parenteral injection since these live vaccines retain some virulence and may therefore cause severe adverse reactions and possibly death.

LEPTOSPIROSIS

Leptospira are aerobic gram-negative spirochetes. The taxonomy of Leptospires is complex and confusing. Three species are common animal pathogens, *Leptospira interrogans, Leptospira borgpetersenii,* and *Leptospira kirchneri*. These are each divided into multiple serogroups and serovars (Table 13.1). More than 250 serovars of Leptospira have been identified and immunity is highly serovar specific. Before the introduction of vaccination, the important serovars were considered to be canicola and icterhaemorrhagiae. Following the widespread use of vaccines against these two, the prevalence of serovars has changed. In North America, the important serovars are now considered to be Pomona, Autumnalis, Bratislava, and Grippotyphosa, whereas in Europe the important serovars are Bratislava, Grippotyphosa, and Sejroe.

TABLE 13.1 ■ A Simple Classification of the Most Common Leptospires Discussed in the Text

Species	Serogroup	Serovar
L. interrogans	Icterohemorrhagiae	Icterohemorrhagiae
		Copenhageni
	Grippotyphosa	Grippotyphosa
	Canicola	Canicola
	Australis	Australis
		Bratislava
	Pomona	Pomona
		Kennewicki
	Sejroe	Sejroe
		Hardjo
Leptospira borgpeterseni	Sejroe	Hardjo
		Hardjo-bovis
	Australis	Australis
Leptospira kirschneri	Icterohemorrhagiae	Icterhemorrhagiae
	Grippotyphosa	Grippotyphosa
	Canicola	Canicola
	Australis	Australis

Note that certain serovars such as Hardjo are found in more than one species.

Antileptospiral immunity is primarily antibody-mediated and is directed against the bacterial lipopolysaccharide (LPS). (Experimentally, polyclonal and monoclonal antibodies against this LPS can transfer immunity to susceptible animals.) However, it also appears that cell-mediated responses are required to protect against some serovars such as Hardjo in cattle. Whole, inactivated Leptospira bacterins have been used for many years but are associated with adverse reactions, in addition to serovar-specific immunity.

In the United States, dogs receive bacterins containing four serovars: Canicola, Icterhaemorrhagiae, Pomona, and Grippotyphosa. There is limited cross protection between these serovars. Some may protect against clinical disease and reduce but not prevent renal colonization and shedding. Antibodies last for about 1 year (at least 15 months in the case of Grippotyphosa). In other countries these bacterins may contain up to 8 different serovars. (Box 13.2).

BORRELIA BURGDORFERI

Borrelia burgdorferi is the cause of Lyme disease predominantly spread by the deer tick, *Ixodes scapularis*. Four different vaccines are available in North America. All induce antibodies to OspA, the antigenic outer membrane lipoprotein of the spirochete. OspA is expressed by the organisms within the tick mid-gut but is downregulated within the vertebrate host. When blood is ingested by a feeding tick, the antibodies to OspA attack the spirochetes and thus halt transmission. AntiOspA antibody titers are however not boosted by natural exposure and wane in vaccinates allowing host infection. Recently vaccines containing OspC have also been investigated. OspC is the dominant surface antigen expressed within the vertebrate host. AntiOspC antibodies and T cells induced by these vaccines may therefore eliminate organisms within the host. Available vaccines include a killed whole cell bacterin (OspA), a bacterin containing OspA and OspC, a recombinant OspA vaccine and a chimeric recombinant containing OspA plus OspC. All are administered subcutaneously. The reported efficacies of these vaccines are highly variable ranging from 50% to 100%. Vaccination of infected dogs is of no benefit so puppies should be tested to ensure that they are not infected before vaccination. Vaccination is also advisable if a dog travels from a nonendemic area to an endemic one. Vaccination must be part of a comprehensive program to reduce disease risks including adequate tick control, preferably with products that prevent tick attachment or kill ticks during early feeding.

CANINE RESPIRATORY DISEASE COMPLEX

As with other species, dogs may suffer from chronic infectious respiratory disease caused by diverse pathogens. An initial viral infection may cause tissue damage and immunosuppression leading to secondary bacterial invasion. The primary viral pathogens include canine parainfluenza, adenovirus 2, or distemper. Other viruses that may play a role include reoviruses, respiratory coronavirus, herpesvirus, influenza virus, pneumovirus, and adenovirus 1. *Bordetella bronchiseptica* may act as a primary or secondary pathogen. Other potential bacterial pathogens include Mycoplasmas, *Streptococcus equi* subspecies *zooepidemicus*, and *Chlamydophila psittaci*. Vaccines are not available against every one of these agents and the viral components are discussed in the viral section later.

Many of the available vaccines are designed to be administered intranasally. It should be pointed out that there are major differences in the nature of the immune response triggered by intranasal and injected vaccines. Thus intranasal administration with a modified live vaccine will trigger local innate responses in addition to a local immunoglobulin A (IgA) response. Parenteral immunization with an acellular vaccine will trigger a systemic immunoglobulin G (IgG) response. Both of these are protective responses. In theory, the best result may be obtained by administering the injected vaccine first and boost with the intranasal product (or vice versa). This prime boost technique has worked very well in humans vaccinated against polio. However, there is as yet, no data to support this method in dogs.

Antiviral Vaccines

CANINE DISTEMPER

Canine distemper caused by canine morbillivirus infection remains one of the most significant and lethal viral diseases of dogs. It affects the gastrointestinal and respiratory tract in addition to the nervous system.

There are currently 50 licensed distemper vaccines available in the United States; however, only one of these is directed against canine distemper virus alone. Distemper vaccine is usually combined with those against canine adenovirus 2, canine parvovirus, and canine parainfluenza. These combinations may also contain coronavirus, leptospirosis, and Borrelia vaccines. Three different types of vaccine are available to prevent canine distemper.

Inactivated CDV vaccines generally give inferior protection and are best used in susceptible wildlife species.

Modified live virus vaccines contain attenuated virus strains such as the Snyder Hill and Rockborn strains attenuated by prolonged canine cell culture, or the egg adapted Onderstepoort strain, now adapted to tissue culture. Antigenic differences between these strains are not significant and all are protective when used appropriately. Note that the modified live virus (MLV) distemper vaccines, although safe in domestic dogs, can cause disease in related wildlife such as gray foxes and the black-footed ferret. Indeed, the black-footed ferret, a highly endangered species was nearly wiped out as a result of the inappropriate use of MLV distemper vaccines (Chapter 20).

A canarypox vectored recombinant vaccine is available in some countries. The genes encoding two immunogenic CDV antigens, the hemagglutinin (HA) and fusion proteins have been inserted into an ALVAC canarypox vector (Chapter 5). This vaccine is able to overcome some maternal immunity and appears to immunize puppies about four weeks earlier than conventional MLV vaccines. The vectored vaccine has the additional advantage that it is unable to cause postvaccinal distemper encephalitis.

The recombinant and MLV vaccines perform similarly with respect to onset and duration of immunity. Measuring serum antibodies provides a reasonable assessment of protective immunity. Duration of immunity after vaccination is at least five years.

HETEROTYPIC IMMUNIZATION

Measles and canine distemper viruses are very closely related morbilliviruses; their fusion proteins are almost identical. As a result, an attenuated measles vaccine has been used for many years to provide early protection of puppies against distemper. The differences between the HA antigens of these viruses are such that maternal antibodies against distemper virus cannot completely neutralize the measles vaccine. As a result, measles vaccine may be administered somewhat earlier than distemper vaccine to effectively immunize puppies. It is given intramuscularly between 6 and 12 weeks of age. (Use the dog vaccine, not the human one. There is not enough antigen in the human one.) It is vitally important, however, that puppies also be vaccinated using a distemper vaccine at the appropriate time. Heterotypic immunity should not be relied on after 16 weeks of age.

CANINE ADENOVIRUS 2

CAV-2 is a respiratory pathogen transmitted by the oronasal route. The virus damages bronchial epithelial cells resulting in fever, cough, nasal discharge, and pharyngitis.

Inactivated CAV vaccines are usually administered in combination with CDV and CPV.

The preferred vaccines against canine adenoviruses are modified live products. These MLV also provide immunity against infectious canine hepatitis caused by CAV-1 and against tracheobronchitis caused by CAV-2. Immunity develops about five days postvaccination with the MLV. However, CAV-2 infection or vaccination will not induce the hypersensitivity reaction known as blue-eye caused by CAV-1 (Fig. 10.5). Both injectable and intranasal forms of CAV-MLV vaccines are available. Because CAV-2 is a contributor to the canine respiratory disease complex, it is commonly used in combination with other respiratory pathogen vaccines such as those against *Bordetella bronchiseptica* and canine parainfluenza virus. The duration of immunity after vaccination is at least nine years. The presence of serum antibodies indicates protection, making serology a useful guide to revaccination.

CANINE PARVOVIRUS

CPV is one of the major causes of canine acute gastroenteritis. Young puppies two to six months of age are most susceptible, but cases are increasingly recognized in adult dogs. Clinical signs include anorexia, depression, vomiting, and diarrhea that is often hemorrhagic.

The original canine parvovirus (CPV-2) first appeared in the 1970s and was likely a host variant of feline panleukopenia or a related virus. Since then new circulating variants have appeared. For example, CPV-2a and -2b appeared in the 1980s and CPV-2c in 1996. All these variants are antigenically related so that currently available MLV-CPV vaccines are believed to protect against the variants circulating in North America.

The inactivated vaccines are not as effective and are relatively slow to induce protective immunity when compared with the MLV vaccines. As a result, they are not recommended for routine use except possibly in situations such as in an immunosuppressed dog where the use of a live vaccine may be hazardous.

In the absence of maternal antibodies, MLV parvovirus vaccines may be protective within three days. This is probably because of early interferon production rather than antibodies (Fig. 4.1). These MLV vaccines can replicate in the dog intestine and thus are intermittently shed in the feces of vaccinated dogs. This shedding occurs irrespective of the presence of antibodies. MLV-CPV vaccines should not be used in wildlife as they may be insufficiently attenuated. Inactivated vaccines are safer in other species. Duration of immunity is thought to be life-long, especially following the use of MLV vaccines.

RABIES

The use of rabies vaccines in the United States is regulated by individual states or other jurisdictions. As a result, requirements may be conflicting and inconsistent. In most, but not all states, vaccination is mandatory. It is essential that practicing veterinarians are fully aware of the appropriate legislation and regulations that govern rabies vaccination.

Although modified live vaccines have been proven safe in dogs, the World Health Organization stopped recommending these vaccines in 2004. As described elsewhere (Chapter 10), self-inoculation incidents result in an unacceptable risk to humans. No modified live rabies vaccines are currently marketed in the United States.

Inactivated rabies vaccines are commonly used in mass vaccination programs where maintaining the cold chain is less critical and safety is not an issue. These viruses are generally grown to high titer in tissue culture and then inactivated with beta-propiolactone, acetylethylamine, or binary ethyleneimine (Fig. 3.2). Once inactivated, adjuvants such as aluminum hydroxide, aluminum phosphate, or saponin are added.

Vectored recombinant rabies vaccines express the highly immunogenic rabies glycoprotein G gene. Vectors used include vaccinia, canarypox, and adenoviruses. The vaccinia and adenovirus vectored vaccines may be used in North America and Europe for wildlife vaccination. It is interesting to note that injectable rabies vaccines may be of little use in less developed countries where most cases of canine-induced rabies occur. In these countries there are large numbers of stray dogs and it is not possible to catch and vaccinate them all. In such cases, encouraging results have been obtained by distributing oral recombinant vaccines similar to those used in wildlife (Chapter 20). Blister packs containing the vaccines may simply be offered to these dogs by hand, enclosed in chicken heads, meatballs or a short segment of boiled beef or pig intestine. The vaccinator can also note that the dog has punctured the vaccine blister and recover used packs. This technique is a viable strategy to supplement parenteral vaccination in otherwise unreachable dog populations.

In many jurisdictions it is a requirement that domestic dogs, cats, and ferrets are to be vaccinated. In general, they are not considered to be vaccinated until 28 days after the initial vaccine dose. The interval between doses is determined by the manufacturer and indicated on the product label, but legally they are considered unvaccinated one day after the vaccine's official duration of immunity (one year or three years). In most (but not all) states, only a licensed veterinarian is authorized to administer rabies vaccine.

The definition of exposure to rabies also varies between states. This is determined by the state Department of Health, not by the veterinarian. Most properly vaccinated dogs are immune to rabies. Should such a dog be bitten by a rabid animal, they should be quarantined for 45 days. Unvaccinated animals should be quarantined for four months. They should be vaccinated within 96 hours of exposure on entry into quarantine.

If multiple doses of vaccines are administered to small-breed dogs (<10 kg), this may increase the risk of adverse reactions. Given the importance of the size of the dog, it has been suggested that veterinarians consider delaying administration of noncore vaccines to small dogs until two to four weeks after completion of the core vaccination process.

There is currently no data available to support the practice of reducing vaccine dose or frequency of administration in small dogs. Dose reduction increases the chances that the dog will receive an insufficient dose to confer protective immunity. Likewise, there is no data to suggest that dose reduction will reduce the incidence of adverse events. After all, if the animal is already allergic to a vaccine component, even a reduced dose may trigger a reaction.

Note that vaccination of dogs against rabies has saved millions of humans from a horrible death. This is yet another triumph for the science of immunology.

CANINE PARAINFLUENZA

Canine parainfluenza (CPiV) is a Rubulavirus in the family Paramyxoviridae. It is one of the main contributors to "kennel cough." The virus causes transient mild respiratory disease and damages local defense mechanisms in the respiratory tract by destroying ciliated epithelium. As a result, secondary opportunistic infections by viruses and bacteria are common. It is usually a component of combination vaccines. The duration of immunity to this virus is unclear and it may be less than three years.

CANINE INFLUENZA

Canine influenza was first described in 2004 when it appears to have been transmitted from horses to racing greyhounds. The original outbreak began as a severe hemorrhagic pneumonia with high mortality. Viral virulence has declined since then and the canine disease is now primarily a tracheobronchitis.

An inactivated canine influenza vaccine (H3N8) may be given subcutaneously. Immunity develops approximately seven days after the second dose although vaccinated dogs may still develop mild clinical signs. This is a noncore vaccine because this strain of influenza is largely restricted to North America.

An inactivated influenza vaccine against a second influenza strain (H3N2) is also available as is a bivalent vaccine directed against both strains. This strain of influenza is also currently geographically restricted to North America. H3N2 is shed in much greater amounts than H3N8, making it that much more contagious. Ideally dogs should receive vaccines against both strains if the veterinarian perceives them to be at risk.

Influenza viruses continue to evolve rapidly. The highly pathogenic strain of influenza, H5N1, was transmitted to dogs in Central Asia after they had been exposed to infected duck carcasses. It is essential that veterinarians be aware of the inevitability of the emergence of new strains of influenza virus capable of infecting both companion animals and their owners.

COMBINATION VACCINES

Most of the vaccines used in dogs contain combinations of antigens. These are generally administered as subcutaneous modified live or recombinant canine distemper vaccine (D) plus adenovirus 2 (A), parvovirus (P), and parainfluenza (P) vaccines (DAPP). Other vaccine combinations may include leptospira.

Other Noncore Vaccines

CANINE CORONAVIRUSES

There are two groups of canine coronaviruses. Group 1 causes enteric disease. Group 2 causes a mild self-limiting respiratory disease. Although both inactivated and modified live vaccines against the group 1 virus are available, their use is not usually recommended because this virus usually only causes a mild, self-limiting or inapparent gastroenteritis with anorexia, fever, and diarrhea. It usually affects puppies younger than six weeks old and lasts for a few days. The vaccine appears to protect dogs from disease but not from infection.

CANINE HERPESVIRUS

Canid herpesvirus 1 may produce mild upper respiratory disease and inapparent infections in adult dogs. However, it causes fatal infections in newborn puppies. This susceptibility is highly age related and puppies over two weeks of age rapidly develop resistance. The clinical disease is nonspecific. Puppies vomit, show rapid shallow breathing, and die within two days. The virus may also cause abortion, stillbirth, and infertility.

Although a vaccine is not available in North America, an adjuvanted subunit vaccine is marketed in Europe (Eurican Herpes 205, Boehringer Ingelheim). It consists of purified glycoprotein subunits (especially gB glycoprotein) of the F205 strain with an oil adjuvant. It is administered subcutaneously when the female is in heat or 7 to 10 days after mating. A second dose is given one to two weeks before whelping. Revaccination during each subsequent pregnancy is recommended. As with other such vaccines its effectiveness depends upon the puppies ingesting adequate colostral antibodies.

CROTALID VACCINE

A toxoid directed against the Western Rattlesnake (*Crotalus atrox*) venom is available. It is administered to dogs that may be exposed to Western Diamondback Rattlesnakes. There is limited cross protection against other rattlesnake species. Two subcutaneous doses are given after four months of age, and annually thereafter. Although this vaccine may mitigate the severity of the venom, snake-bitten dogs must still receive immediate veterinary attention.

Vaccination and Maternal Antibodies

Current high-quality core vaccines induce high levels of antibodies in dogs. As a result, canine colostrum also contains high antibody titers. These maternal antibodies are highly effective in blocking antibody responses in young puppies (Fig. 13.1). As a result, maternal antibodies persist

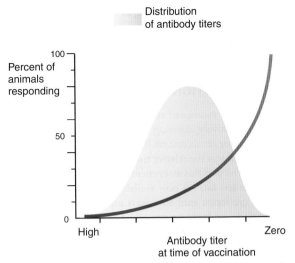

Distribution
of antibody titers

Percent of
animals
responding

100

50

0

High   Zero

Antibody titer
at time of vaccination

Fig. 13.1 The effect of maternal antibody titer on the response of newborn animals to vaccination. The presence of specific maternal antibodies profoundly suppresses the animal's immune response to a vaccine and the higher the maternal antibody titer, the greater the suppression. However, antibody titers are normally distributed so that as maternal antibody titers decline, more and more individuals will respond to the vaccine until only a few very high responders remain.

longer and many puppies cannot be primed, even by 12 weeks of age. Most puppies that have suckled successfully and received sufficient colostrum will be protected up to approximately 8 to 14 weeks of age. However, not all mothers are immune and not all puppies receive sufficient colostrum. As a result, at least three doses of the core vaccines must be administered every 3 to 4 weeks beginning between 6 and 8 weeks of age with the final dose administered on or after 16 weeks of age to ensure that a susceptibility gap does not develop between the loss of maternal immunity and vaccination. An optional fourth dose may be administered at 18 to 20 weeks of age. This is recommended if confirmed distemper or parvovirus infections have occurred in young dogs that had received the initial three-dose series.

It has been normal practice to boost puppies by vaccination at one year of age. The rationale for this is to ensure that any dog that fails to respond to the initial series of vaccines will thus be protected and the primed dogs will be boosted. It makes sense to give this vaccine at six months rather than a year. In this way the window of susceptibility of any unvaccinated dogs is reduced significantly and still providing an effective boost to their immune responses.

It is also important to point out that multiple sources of evidence support the contention that core vaccines confer a minimum duration of immunity of three years (except for one-year rabies vaccines). Vaccines are not innocuous and should consequently be given no more than necessary. Note that immunity to bacterins such as those from Bordetella, Borrelia, and Leptospira is relatively short lived, and these should be boosted annually if deemed necessary.

Management Issues

RISK FACTORS

The lifestyle of a dog should be considered when making specific vaccine recommendations. For example, how much interaction does the dog have with other dogs? Staying in a boarding kennel, attending dog shows, visits to dog parks, or living in a shelter may significantly increase a dog's risk of acquiring infections from others. Likewise, exposure to wildlife or domestic livestock and possible exposure to contaminated water sources increases risks from leptospirosis. Hunting dogs at high risk of getting bitten by ticks will be at increased risk of Lyme disease.

CORRELATES OF PROTECTION

We cannot always assume that a vaccinated animal is protected or that revaccination is necessary. We require a method of objectively assessing immunity. It is now possible to make informed decisions regarding the need for revaccination by testing animals for the presence of antibodies. A veterinarian should always assess the relative risks and benefits to an animal in determining the need for any vaccination. In the past this assessment was largely a matter of conservative tradition. Rapid, simple point-of-care test kits are now available to detect canine antibody responses. It is therefore good practice to use serum antibody assays such as rapid test ELISA kits or lateral flow assays, if available, to provide guidance on revaccination needs. Persistent antibody titers determine whether an animal requires additional protection. These tests not only identify those animals that have responded to vaccination, they can determine if an animal is a nonresponder, a problem associated with immunity to parvovirus infections. They can determine if an animal that previously suffered from an adverse event really requires revaccination. They can determine whether an animal with an undocumented vaccine history needs to be vaccinated and with which vaccines. They can determine which animals in a shelter undergoing a disease outbreak are susceptible and require vaccination. They can also determine whether revaccination is really necessary at three years. Note, however. that animals with low or undetectable serum antibody levels may still be protected as a result of persistence of memory B and T cells capable of responding rapidly to reinfection. "Blind" revaccination should be avoided if appropriate antibody assays are available. Point of care tests are usually reported as positive versus negative. In general, a negative test may indicate susceptibility. Nevertheless, false negative results do occur as a result of errors, and poor timing, and so on. Generally, however these point of care tests have been carefully standardized against gold-standard tests such as virus neutralization or hemagglutination tests.

It is known that after vaccination most dogs retain protective antibodies against CDV, CPV-2, CAV-1, and CAV-2 for many years. Thus any dog that is seronegative should be revaccinated unless contraindicated by some other problem. There is a poor correlation between antibody levels and protection after vaccination against Leptospirosis.

Studies have demonstrated that dogs receiving a modified live CDV vaccine were protected for over four years and detection of virus neutralizing antibodies implied resistance. A positive response was considered to be a two-fold increase above the assay cut-off. A negative response was considered to be an antibody titer of less than 16. However, many vaccinated dogs had a titer of less than 16 at 4 years but were still protected when challenged. In other words, a negative titer has little predictive value. Conversely all the dogs with a positive titer were also protected so its predictive value was 100% (i.e., there were no false positive results).

SHELTER-HOUSED DOGS

In general, dogs in shelters represent a random collection of dogs with no known vaccination history and a high risk of infectious diseases. The high likelihood of disease transmission demands that a comprehensive vaccination strategy be established and adhered to. All dogs entering a shelter should be vaccinated before entry with the core vaccines. It would be desirable to test dogs on admission for the presence of antiviral antibodies. In the absence of evidence of immunity or vaccination, as many dogs as possible should be vaccinated before or on admission to the

---

BOX 13.3 ■ Rabies Vaccination in Veterinary Students

A review of the rabies vaccination records of over 600 North American veterinary students has been conducted to determine the factors influencing their antibody responses. Nearly a third of the students had inadequate antibody titers two years later. These "failures" were associated with several factors such as male gender, vaccine type, a body mass index of more than 25, and an interval of more than 21 days between the first and third doses of vaccine.

(From Banga, N., Guss, P., Banga, A. [2014]. Rosenman KD. Incidence and variables associated with inadequate antibody titers after pre-exposure rabies vaccination among veterinary medical students. *Vaccine*, 32, 979–983.)

---

facility to establish herd immunity. However, remember that onset of immunity is not immediate, but intranasal vaccines may induce immunity faster than injected ones.

As elsewhere, vaccination is only one component of an infection control strategy for an animal shelter. Managers must pay attention to factors such as cleaning and disinfection protocols, personal protective equipment, segregation of susceptible animals crowding, climate management, and stressors that may influence disease resistance.

Similar considerations apply to boarding kennels (and catteries), dog or cat shows, pet day-care facilities, and any situation where these animals might gather in significant numbers.

OBESITY

It is abundantly clear from the human and mouse literature that obesity reduces the immune response to vaccination. A high body mass index in humans is associated with a reduced response to vaccines. This has been well demonstrated with respect to influenza vaccination. Obese mice mount significantly lower virus-specific antibody responses when compared with lean mice. When infected, their viral loads are much higher even after vaccination. Similar effects have been reported for hepatitis B, tetanus, and rabies vaccines. (Box 13.3) Only limited studies have been performed on obese dogs and the results did not show significant differences in responses to canine core vaccines. Nevertheless, obesity should be considered a risk factor for an inadequate vaccine response. Great care should be taken to avoid injecting antigens directly into adipose tissue.

Adverse Events

Vaccines should be administered with a minimal interval of three to four weeks between doses regardless of the vaccine or the age of the patient.

LOCAL REACTIONS

Transient injection-site reactions result from local innate immune responses. These may produce visible or palpable lumps, with pain or pruritus. Permanent hair loss as a result of ischemic vasculitis and focal skin necrosis has resulted from a vasculitis following rabies vaccination.

GENERALIZED REACTIONS

Transient nonspecific effects of the innate immune response such as lethargy, anorexia, fever, and lymphadenopathy are common in vaccinated dogs (see Fig. 13.2). They generally last for less than 24 to 48 hours.

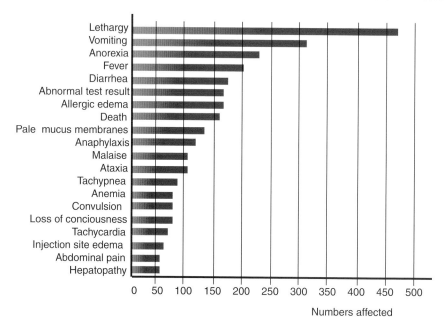

Fig. 13.2 The clinical signs of adverse events associated with administration of canine core vaccines in the UK. Note that these are the number of reports received by the Veterinary Medicines Directorate. Veterinary Pharmacovigilance in the United Kingdom, Annual Review, 2014. With permission.

Hypersensitivity reactions are the consequence of vaccination in some animals. The most important of these is a type 1 anaphylactic response. Dogs differ from the other domestic mammals in that their major shock organ is not the lung but the liver, specifically the hepatic veins. Dogs undergoing anaphylaxis show initial excitement followed by vomiting, defecation, and urination. As the reaction progresses, dogs may collapse with weakness and depressed respiration, become comatose, convulse, and die. All these signs result from occlusion of the hepatic vein because of a combination of smooth muscle contraction and hepatic swelling. This results in portal hypertension and visceral pooling, in addition to a decrease in venous return, cardiac output, and arterial pressure. This is secondary to generalized vasodilation. Identified mediators include histamine, prostaglandins, and leukotrienes. Treatment involves the prompt administration of epinephrine (Box 10.2).

TRANSIENT IMMUNOSUPPRESSION

When certain combination vaccines that contain MLV-CDV plus adenoviruses-1 or -2 are administered to puppies, there is a transient suppression of T cell responses to mitogen for several days. Some canine parvovirus-2 vaccines can cause a mild immunosuppression. This is unlikely to be clinically significant.

RESIDUAL VIRULENCE

Modified live vaccines are usually good immunogens, but their use may involve certain risks. The most important theoretical problem encountered is residual virulence. This has been a problem in the past. One serious example of this was the development of clinical rabies in some dogs and cats following administration of older strains of MLV rabies vaccine. Another example is that of the Rockborn strain of CDV that can revert to virulence in zoo and wildlife species. Postvaccinal cough or sneezing may be associated with administration of attenuated intranasal vaccines against *B. bronchiseptica* and parainfluenza. As described in Chapter 10, other adverse events associated with vaccination in dogs include postvaccinal canine distemper virus encephalitis, and vaccine-induced osteodystrophy. It should be pointed out, however, that when using modern vaccines, the risk of disease developing as a result of residual virulence is minimal.

Sources of Additional Information

Altman., K.D., Kelman, M., Ward, M.P. (2017). Are vaccine strain, type or administration protocol risk factors for canine parvovirus vaccine failure? *Vet Microbiol,* 210, 8–16.

Arent, Z.J., Andrews, S., Adamama-Moraitou, K., Gilmore, C., Pardali, D., Ellis, W.A. (2013). Emergence of novel Leptospira serovars: A need for adjusting vaccination policies for dogs? *Epidemiol Infect,* 141, 1148–1153.

Coyne, M.J., Burr, J.H.H., Yule, T.D., et al. Duration of immunity in dogs after vaccination or naturally acquired infection, *Vet Rec,* 149, 509–515.

De Cramer, K.G., Stylianides, E., & van Vuuren, M. (2011). Efficacy of vaccination at 4 and 6 weeks in the control of canine parvovirus. *Vet Microbiol,* 149, 126–132.

Ellis, J.A. (2015). How well do vaccines for *Bordetella bronchiseptica* work in dogs? A critical review of the literature. 1977–2014. *Vet J,* 204, 5–16.

Ellis, J.A., Gow, S.P., Lee, L.B., Lacoste, S., Ball, E.C. (2017). Comparative efficacy of intranasal and injectable vaccines in stimulating *Bordetella bronchiseptica*-reactive anamnestic antibody responses in household dogs. *Can Vet J,* 58, 809–815.

HogenEsch, H., Thompson, S. (2010). Effect of ageing on the immune response of dogs to vaccines. *J Comp Pathol,* 142, S74–77.

Jensen, W.A., Totten, J.S., Lappin, M.R., Schultz, R.D. (2015). Use of serologic tests to predict resistance to Canine distemper virus-induced disease in vaccinated dogs. *J Vet Diagn Invest,* 27, 576–580.

Kennedy, L.J., Lunt, M., Barnes, A., et al. (2007). Factors influencing the antibody response of dogs vaccinated against rabies. *Vaccine,* 25, 8500–8507.

Killey, R., Mynors, C., Pearce, R., Nell, A., Prentis, A., Day, M.J. (2018). Long-lived immunity to canine core vaccine antigens in UK dogs as assessed by an in-practice test kit. *J Small Anim Pract,* 59, 27–31.

Leung, T., & Davis, S.A. (2017). Rabies vaccination targets for stray dog populations. *Front Vet Sci,* 4, 52.

Pardo, M.C,. Tanner, P., Bauman, J., Silver, K., Fischer, L. (2007). Immunization of puppies in the presence of maternally derived antibodies against canine distemper virus. *J Comp Pathol,* 137, S72–75.

Pimburage, R.M.S., Gunatilake, M., Wimalaratne, O., Balasuriya, A., Perera, K.A.D.N. Sero-prevalence of virus neutralizing antibodies for rabies in different groups of dogs following vaccination. *BMC Vet Res,* 13, 133.

Schultz, R.D. (2006). Duration of immunity for canine and feline vaccines: a review. *Vet Microbiol,* 117, 75–79.

Squires, R.A. (2015). How well do vaccines against *Bordetella bronchiseptica* work in dogs? *Vet J,* 204, 237–238.

Squires, R.A. (2018). Vaccines in shelters and group settings. *Vet Clin North Am Small Anim Pract,* 48, 291–300.

Smith, T.G., Millien, M., Fracciterne, F.A., et al. (2017). Evaluation of immune responses in dogs to oral rabies vaccine under field conditions. *Vaccine.* Advance online publication. https://doi.org/10.1016/j.vaccine.2017.09.096

Twark, L., Dodds, W.J. (2000). Clinical use of serum parvovirus and distemper virus antibody titers for determining revaccination strategies in healthy dogs, *J Am Vet Med Assoc,* 217, 1021–1024.

Vogt, N.A., Sargeant, J.M., MacKinnon, M.C., Versluis, A.M. (2019). Efficacy of *Borrelia burgdorferi* vaccine in dogs in North America. *J Vet Intern Med,* 33, 23–36.

Feline Vaccines

As with other companion animal species, informed vaccination decisions for cats depend on multiple factors. In general, healthy cats should be vaccinated but mild concurrent illness may not be disqualifying. Issues such as immunosuppression by feline retroviruses, other immunodeficiencies, nutritional status, and chronic stress must be considered. The age of the cat is critical considering the persistent effects that maternal antibodies have on early vaccination, whereas old age presents other significant issues. The other key issue is, of course, lifestyle. The opportunities that a cat has to encounter other infected cats will vary greatly ranging from the housebound pet, to cats in shelters, to feral cat populations.

It is self-evident that some vaccines are of greater importance than others. The choice of a vaccine will depend not only on the factors stated earlier, but also on the prevalence and severity of a disease. Thus the core vaccines for cats in North America are considered to be those directed against feline panleukopenia caused by a parvovirus, feline rhinopneumonitis caused by feline herpesvirus-1, and feline calicivirus infection. Rabies presents a special case because its use is governed by regulation and is mandatory in certain jurisdictions. Vaccines that may be considered as noncore include those against bacterial diseases caused by *Chlamydia felis* and *Bordetella bronchiseptica*, in addition to the infections caused by feline leukemia virus (FeLV), feline immunodeficiency virus, and feline coronavirus (Box 14.1).

Antibacterial Vaccines

FELINE RESPIRATORY DISEASE

Feline respiratory disease is caused by multiple agents. The most important ones are feline herpesvirus (FHV-1), feline calicivirus (FCV), *Chlamydia felis*, and *Mycoplasma felis*, or combinations of these. As in other species it is likely that the viral infection predisposes to secondary bacterial infections such as those by *Bordetella bronchiseptica*. Licensed vaccines containing multiple antigens are most widely employed. They usually contain calicivirus, feline herpesvirus, and parvovirus. Some may also incorporate chlamydia, leukemia, or rabies vaccines.

BORDETELLA BRONCHISEPTICA

B. bronchiseptica is primarily a dog pathogen (Chapter 13), and vaccination should only be considered if there is contact between a cat and dogs with a recent or current history of respiratory disease. Routine use of this vaccine is not recommended.

> **BOX 14.1 ■ Feline Vaccination Guidelines**
>
> Guidelines for feline vaccination have been published by:
>   The American Association of Feline practitioners (AAFP) at: https://www.catvets.com/guidelines/practice-guidelines/feline-vaccination-guidelines.
>   The World Small Animal Veterinary Association (WSAVA) at: https://www.wsava.org/WSAVA/media/PDF_old/WSAVA-Vaccination-Guidelines-2015-Full-Version.pdf.
>   The Advisory Board for Cat Diseases (ABCD) at: http://www.abcdcatsvets.org/vaccines-and-vaccination-an-introduction/.

CHLAMYDIA FELIS

This pathogen is not consistently isolated from cats with respiratory disease. It should only be vaccinated against if it has been identified as a problem by a diagnostic laboratory. It is usually prevented by the use of combined vaccines containing other pathogens such as feline viral rhino-tracheitis (FVR) or feline parvovirus (FPV).

Antiviral Vaccines

FELINE HERPESVIRUS

This virus causes an upper respiratory tract infection. Symptoms include nasal discharge, rhino-sinusitis, tracheitis, conjunctivitis, keratitis, oral ulceration, fever, malaise, and loss of pregnancy. Cats of all ages are susceptible, and it is especially common in multicat households and shelters. As with other herpesviruses, infected cats become lifelong latent carriers. At times of stress, the virus may become reactivated in these latent carriers. In such cases, it may cause clinical disease or be transmitted to susceptible, in-contact animals. For example, the stress of parturition may cause queens to shed the virus.

Many inactivated adjuvanted vaccines are available against FHV, usually in combination with multiple other respiratory pathogens. These vaccines do not induce strong immunity, and as a result assessment of duration of protection is difficult.

Modified live vaccines are available for either intranasal or intraocular administration. Intranasal vaccines may be combined with a calicivirus vaccine. Owners should be warned that cats vaccinated by the intranasal route may sneeze frequently for four to seven days after vaccination. Although antibodies may be detected three years after vaccination, these antibodies do not correlate well with protection. As with all herpesviruses, cell-mediated immunity is critical. Cats at low risk may be vaccinated every three years, but cats in catteries are at high risk and may be vaccinated more frequently at the veterinarian's discretion. If a cat is to be moved to a boarding facility it should be revaccinated one to two weeks before the move, especially if its vaccines are not current.

FELINE CALICIVIRUS

Feline calicivirus is ubiquitous in cats worldwide. It causes infections that range from subclinical to oral and upper respiratory tract disease and has been considered to have high morbidity and minimal mortality. Affected cats develop oral ulcers, sneezing and a nasal discharge. Recently however, some highly virulent calicivirus biotypes have emerged. Virulent systemic feline calici-viruses strain FCV-Ari causes fever, jaundice, hemorrhage, skin necrosis, vomiting, edema, and death.

Calicivirus vaccines are usually administered in combination with vaccines against other respiratory pathogens. Multiple inactivated vaccines are available. Because of concerns regarding the antigenic diversity of calicivirus strains some manufacturers produce vaccines containing more than one strain.

Most modified live vaccines currently contain the FCV-F9 strain. Some are designed for intranasal use whereas others are injectable. Because of the genetic diversity of caliciviruses however, F9 vaccines may differ in their ability to protect against heterologous strains. Although FCV-F9 is still broadly effective against current circulating strains it may not protect well against newly emerged systemic virulent strains such as FCV-Ari. It may be necessary to add additional avirulent strains to the vaccine to maintain broad coverage. Virus neutralizing antibodies develop in about a week after vaccination and correlate well with protection. However, vaccination does not prevent infection and vaccinated cats can become persistently infected. Both cell-mediated immunity and mucosal immunoglobin (Ig)A also contribute to resistance. Duration of immunity is at least four years for inactivated products and about seven years for modified live virus (MLV) vaccines. Intranasal vaccines may induce respiratory signs such as sneezing for several days after vaccination in some individuals. This may result in shedding of the vaccine virus. However, the intranasal vaccines require only a single dose and trigger the rapid onset of immunity. They also are better able to overcome inhibition by maternal antibodies in kittens.

FELINE PARVOVIRUS

FPV causes panleukopenia. Infected cats develop a fever followed by vomiting and possibly diarrhea. They become dehydrated, followed by hypothermia, septic shock, intravascular coagulation, and death. In addition to FPV, some canine parvovirus variants (CPV-2a, -2b, and −2c) may cause disease in cats. FPV vaccines may afford some protection in these cases.

Inactivated adjuvanted FPV vaccines are invariably given with calicivirus and rhinopneumonitis vaccines. The safety of the killed FPV vaccines means that these are the preferred vaccines used in wild felids, pregnant queens, and cats immunosuppressed by retroviral infections.

Both parenteral and intranasal modified live vaccines are available in combination with the other core vaccines, FCV and FHV-1. As with other such vaccines the MLV vaccines induce protection rapidly, probably because of interferon release. They are also more effective in overcoming the blocking effect of maternal antibodies. MLV vaccines should not be administered to cats infected with the immunosuppressive retroviruses FIV and FeLV. They should not be used in pregnant queens nor should they be given to neonatal kittens (<4–6 weeks of age) to avoid possible encephalitis and cerebellar damage.

The duration of protection after natural infection is long and probably lasts at least seven years after MLV vaccination. After the preliminary series cats should be revaccinated every three years. The presence of antibodies is correlated with protection. Otherwise vaccine administration schedules are the same as for herpesvirus vaccines. (They are usually given as combination vaccines.) Feline panleukopenia virus may persist in the environment for at least a year, a fact that makes FPV vaccination absolutely essential.

RABIES

Rabies in cats is prevented by similar or identical vaccines to those used in puppies. Both inactivated and canarypox vectored recombinant vaccines are available. Because of concerns regarding the development of injection site sarcomas, many veterinarians prefer nonadjuvanted vaccines. Vaccination intervals and use may be governed by local regulations.

Other Important Vaccines

FELINE LEUKEMIA VIRUS

Before vaccinating against feline leukemia, kittens should be tested to ensure that they are not already infected. There is no benefit to vaccinating an infected cat. Although this is a noncore vaccine, it is often unknown where a young kitten may eventually be housed. It is possible that they may end-up in a high-risk environment. It is therefore recommended that kittens receive at least the initial vaccination series and their first annual booster. The protection provided by priming outweighs the risk of adverse effects. After the first year, revaccination should depend on the cat's lifestyle and risk factors. Uninfected cats in a household with infected cats should also be vaccinated. Most vaccines are directed against strain FeLV-A. There is no evidence that incorporating other strains, (FeLV-B and -C) in a vaccine provides any benefit.

A vectored vaccine is available that contains recombinant FeLV glycoprotein (gp70) plus part of the transmembrane protein expressed in an *Escherichia coli* vector. This was the first genetically engineered vaccine used in companion animals. Also available is a canarypox-vectored vaccine expressing the genes for the envelope glycoprotein, gp70, and the nucleocapsid protein, p27. Because of the great diversity in FeLV vaccines, the question of relative effectiveness is often asked. Unfortunately, few comparative studies have been performed and there have been great variations in the strains and protocols used to measure protection. Studies on available vaccines suggest that most have preventable fractions (PFs) ranging from 80% to 93%. Whole cell vaccines appear to provide the most consistent protection. Like all other vaccines, none of these are 100% protective nor do they protect against transient viremia or induce sterile immunity. However, low levels of viremia are not considered clinically important. Duration of immunity following feline leukemia vaccination appears to be about three years, therefore cats in high-risk situations should be boosted annually or every two years.

Although these are safe vaccines, with a very low prevalence (<1%) of adverse events, mainly injection site swelling or transient lethargy, FeLV vaccines are also associated with the development of injection site sarcomas.

FELINE CORONAVIRUS

Feline infectious peritonitis (FIP) is caused by feline enteric coronavirus (FCoV). FIP is a major problem in catteries but is less of an issue among pet cats. The virus causes a fatal granulomatous peritonitis of wild and domestic cats. There are two distinct genotypes of feline enteric coronavirus, avirulent and virulent. The avirulent genotype prefers to replicate within intestinal epithelial cells, whereas the virulent genotype prefers to replicate within macrophages. Macrophages also spread the virus throughout the body. FCoV tends to infect relatively young cats between six months and three years of age.

The course of the infection depends on the nature of the immune response to the virus—a phenomenon also seen in several bacterial diseases. Immunity to FCoV is entirely cell mediated, and a helper T cell 1 (Th1) response is protective. A cat that mounts a good Th1 response will become immune, regardless of the amount of antibodies it makes. Some cats, however, mount a Th2 response to the viral spike proteins. In these animals, the antibodies enhance virus uptake by macrophages. Virus-laden macrophages accumulate around the blood vessels of the omentum and serosa. Antibodies also generate immune complexes that are deposited in the serosa, causing pleuritis or peritonitis, and in glomeruli, leading to glomerulonephritis. Cats with preexisting high levels of antibodies against FCoV develop effusive FIP rapidly on challenge. Administering antiserum to FCoV before challenge may also enhance the peritonitis.

A modified live intranasal vaccine is available against FCoV (Felocell FIP, Zoetis). The vaccine contains a temperature-sensitive mutant of the FCoV strain DF2-FIPV that replicates in the upper respiratory tract and so induces a local IgA response in the mucosa. Ideally this acts in the oropharynx at the site where FCoV enters the body. This local mucosal response should prevent FCoV invasion without inducing high levels of serum antibodies. This vaccine, however, will only be effective if administered before coronavirus exposure. In highly endemic situations where kittens are infected at a young age, vaccination at 16 weeks of age may be too late to prevent infection. The American Association of Feline Practitioners does not recommend this vaccine.

FELINE IMMUNODEFICIENCY VIRUS

A vaccine containing an inactivated FIV-infected-cell associated virus containing subtypes A and D has been marketed in the United States. It gave 100% protection against FIV subtype A. However, this protection did not correlate well with antiviral antibody titers and was not effective against other FIV subtypes.

DERMATOPHYTOSIS

Superficial fungal infections—ringworm, caused by fungi belonging to the genera *Trichophyton* and *Microsporum*—occur in both companion and food animals. Under some situations these may be controlled by vaccination.

Fungi have a cellulose cell wall that is difficult for the body's immune defenses to attack or penetrate. Antibodies are ineffective against these organisms, but cell-mediated responses may be effective. Protection often correlates with a positive delayed hypersensitivity skin test. Once established, this immunity may be long lasting. Inactivated fungal vaccines are available in some countries but it is difficult to assess their efficacy. In Norway, Russia, Sweden, and other countries a systematic campaign against bovine ringworm that includes vaccination has been very successful. There are four commercially available vaccines against bovine ringworm in Europe. Three are monovalent attenuated live vaccines and one is an inactivated 3-way vaccine. The live vaccines appear to be more efficacious than the dead one. Two doses are given 10 to 14 days apart and revaccination may not be necessary. These vaccines may be used prophylactically or therapeutically. Dermatophytosis is of major concern in the fox, chinchilla, and rabbit fur industries because it drastically reduces the quality of their pelts. A modified live vaccine is available in Eastern Europe and Russia for use in these species. It is of interest to note that ringworm downgrades the quality of cattle hides as well, and ringworm scars may also reduce their price.

Both attenuated live and inactivated vaccines against ringworm in cats and dogs are available in some European countries. Unfortunately, is difficult to make an informed opinion as to their efficacy. Published articles on vaccination against both canine and feline dermatophytosis have shown mixed results. Three studies reported protection in dogs and foxes against *Microsporum canis*. A killed *M. canis*–cell wall vaccine induced both humoral and cell-mediated immunity in experimental cats, but did not protect cats against challenge. A vaccine containing killed *M. canis* fractions in adjuvant was licensed in the United States for the treatment of cats rather than prevention. However, it did not prevent the establishment of a challenge infection and did not shorten the duration of disease in vaccinated cats compared with unvaccinated controls. The product is no longer available in the United States.

Maternal Antibodies

Most feline infectious diseases are of greatest significance in kittens younger than six months of age. Therefore these are the primary targets of vaccination. Unfortunately, maternal antibodies interfere with early vaccination by neutralizing the injected antigen and inhibiting antibody synthesis in small kittens. As noted above, current high-quality core vaccines induce high levels of maternal antibodies. As a result, maternal antibodies persist for longer and many kittens will not be primed, even by 12 weeks of age. Kittens should receive at least three doses of the core vaccines between 6 and 8 weeks and 16 and 20 weeks of age. This should successfully bridge the period until maternal antibody titers decline to nonblocking levels. One of the most significant causes of apparent vaccine failure in cats is interference by these antibodies with vaccine responses, especially if the initial vaccination series is terminated prematurely.

OTHER TIMING ISSUES

It is uncommon for vaccines to be tested in pregnant queens. In the absence of such data, a decision to vaccinate a pregnant queen must be based on a risk assessment. The risks of abortion or birth defects must be weighed against the risk of death of the mother and kittens. Additionally, vaccination of pregnant queens will generate colostral antibodies. Modified live FPV vaccines should not be given to pregnant queens because this has been associated with the development of cerebellar hypoplasia in their kittens. Inactivated vaccines are much less risky.

Special Management Issues

CAT HOUSING

The risks of acquiring infection are primarily governed by population density and the degree to which a cat encounters other cats. As a result, cats living in a multiple-cat household, in boarding facilities, breeding facilities, and in animal shelters are at substantially higher risk than housebound single cats. Likewise, the introduction of a new cat into a household increases the risk of disease introduction. Stress induced by changed social structures may result in feline herpesvirus recrudescing and causing clinical disease. Conversely, single housebound cats are no longer exposed to other infections, and as a result will not be boosted by natural exposure. Periodic housing of pets at boarding facilities while owners are away also places such cats at increased risk.

In general, cats in shelters, or boarding catteries represent a random collection of cats with no known vaccination history and a high risk of infectious diseases. The most important diseases in these situations are FPV and the upper respiratory tract infections. It is essential to provide immunity rapidly and ideally cats should be vaccinated ahead of intake. The high likelihood of disease transmission demands that a comprehensive strategy be established and adhered to. All cats entering a shelter should be vaccinated with the core vaccines before entry. It would be desirable to test cats on admission for the presence of antiviral antibodies. In the absence of evidence of immunity or vaccination, as many cats as possible should be vaccinated before or on admission to the facility to establish herd immunity. Unfortunately, because of animal turnover and the constant admission of susceptible cats, herd immunity may be inefficient and unreliable. Remember too that onset of immunity is not immediate. Vaccination is only one component of an infection control strategy for an animal shelter. Managers must pay attention to many other factors such as cleaning and disinfection protocols, personal protective equipment, segregation of susceptible animals, crowding, climate management, and stressors that may influence disease resistance and viral recrudesce.

FERAL CATS

Most free-roaming feral cats lack protective antibodies against FPV, FHV-1, and rabies. If they are vaccinated when trapped to be spayed or neutered, then those antibodies should remain elevated for several months. A single rabies dose will probably protect them for several years even although the regulatory agencies only recognize protection for one year.

GERIATRIC PATIENTS

Immunosenescence is known to suppress the immune response of old animals. However, if cats have received appropriate vaccines throughout their lives, then they will most likely be immune. It is probably most appropriate to continue with vaccination in a routine fashion. Old cats have high FHV antibody levels in comparison to young animals, suggesting that revaccination at shorter intervals is not always necessary.

ASSESSMENT OF VACCINATION NEEDS

Cats are affected by two immunosuppressive retroviruses, most notably FeLV, and FIV. Data is lacking on whether cats infected with these viruses can be successfully immunized or on how this can be accomplished. Inactivated vaccines are safer in such animals than modified live virus vaccines. Vaccination against these retroviruses is of no benefit if they are already infected.

Adverse Events

Allergic reactions are always a possibility and the most extreme form is anaphylaxis. It occurs in 1 to 10 cases for every 10,000 doses of vaccine administered. In cats, the major shock organs are the lungs. Cats undergoing anaphylaxis show vigorous scratching around the face and head as histamine is released into the skin. This is followed by dyspnea, salivation, vomiting, incoordination, collapse, and death. Epinephrine is the specific antidote (Box 10.2).

The prevalence of vaccine-associated adverse events has been followed after the administration of 1,258,712 doses of vaccine to 496,189 cats. There were 2560 adverse events reported (51.6/10,000 cats vaccinated). The risk was greatest for cats one year old. For unknown reasons, this risk was greater in neutered than in sexually intact cats. Lethargy was the most commonly reported event followed by pain or swelling at the injection site, vomiting, facial edema, and pruritus (Fig. 14.1). The number of adverse events increased significantly when multiple vaccines were given during a single visit. Revaccination should be avoided in cats that have a history of vaccine-triggered anaphylaxis. (If vaccination is considered essential then cats may be premedicated with antihistamines and corticosteroids, given a different formulation vaccine, and monitored very closely for several hours.)

INJECTION-SITE SARCOMAS

When cats are vaccinated, any inflammation at the injection site usually resolves rapidly and completely. In some cats however, tumors develop at the injection sites usually between three months and three years after vaccination. These tumors are mainly fibrosarcomas, malignant histiocytomas, and osteosarcomas. Less common forms include rhabdomyosarcomas, hemangiosarcomas, chondrosarcomas, liposarcomas, and lymphosarcomas. These tumors are highly invasive and may metastasize. Successful treatment requires a combination of radical surgical excision and adjunct therapy, including radiation, immunotherapy (such as interleukin [IL]-2 treatment), and chemotherapy, but recurrence is common.

These sarcomas were first noticed following the introduction of potent, inactivated, adjuvanted vaccines such as those directed against rabies and feline leukemia. Cats with sarcomas occurring at sites where vaccines are currently administered were compared with cats that developed sarcomas at nonvaccine-injection sites. Cats receiving an inactivated FeLV vaccine were 5.5 times more likely to develop a sarcoma at the injection site than cats that had not received a vaccine. There was a twofold increase in risk with rabies vaccination. However, the risk was not enormously high. It has been calculated that 1 to 3.6 sarcomas develop per 10,000 vaccinated cats

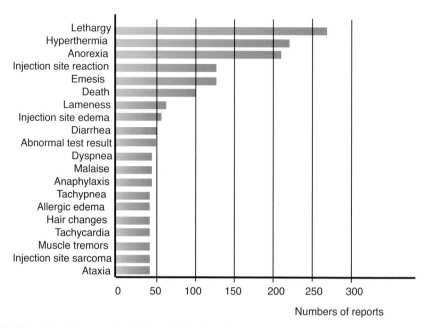

Fig. 14.1 The clinical signs associated with administration of one or more core vaccines to cats in the United Kingdom. Note that these are the number of adverse event reports received by the Veterinary Medicines Directorate. Veterinary Pharmacovigilance in the United Kingdom, Annual Review, 2014. With permission.

in the United States. (The prevalence of sarcomas in the United Kingdom is somewhat lower at 0.021 per 10,000 vaccinated cats.) The risk increased with the number of doses of vaccine administered; a 50% increase following one dose, a 127% increase following two doses, and a 175% increase following three or four vaccines given simultaneously. Vaccine-associated sarcomas tend to occur in younger animals and are larger and more aggressive than sarcomas arising at other sites. They metastasize in 25% to 70% of cases. In one study, injection site sarcomas developed on average 26 months after rabies vaccination and 11 months after FeLV vaccination. Global, web-based surveys suggest a somewhat lower prevalence of sarcomas (0.63 sarcomas/10,000 cats or 0.32 sarcomas/10,000 doses of all vaccines, or one sarcoma from 31,000 doses administered). It must be pointed out therefore that the chances of developing a sarcoma are considerably smaller than the disease risks incurred by unvaccinated cats. In addition to rabies and FeLV vaccines, injection site sarcomas have also been associated with administration of inactivated vaccines against feline panleukopenia, feline herpesvirus, and feline calicivirus. Similar vaccination-related injection site sarcomas have been reported in ferrets, dogs, and a horse. Data from the UK's pharmacovigilance reports suggest that the prevalence of these sarcomas has been dropping progressively (Fig. 14.2).

The pathogenesis of these sarcomas is unclear, but it has long been known that carcinogenesis and prolonged inflammation are linked. Indeed, it has been estimated that 15% to 20% of cancer deaths worldwide are associated with persistent infections and chronic inflammation. When first reported it was assumed that tumor development resulted from the presence of potent adjuvants in vaccines. Tumor development has however also been associated with the use of nonadjuvanted vaccines and even with injection of substances other than vaccines, including penicillin, glucocorticoids, lufenuron, cisplatin, and meloxicam, in addition to the presence of persistent suture material, a retained surgical swab, or implanted microchips. There is no evidence that feline sarcoma virus, feline immunodeficiency virus, or feline leukemia viruses cause these tumors.

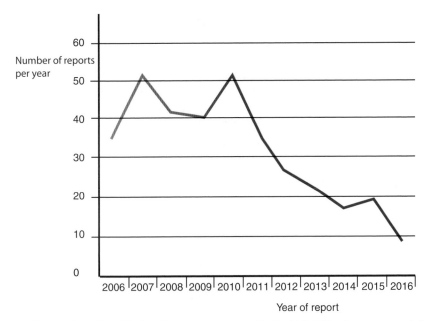

Fig. 14.2 The number of cat injection-site sarcomas reported to the United Kingdom pharmacovigilance authorities between 2006 and 2015. Veterinary Pharmacovigilance in the United Kingdom, Annual Review, 2015. With permission. (Courtesy of the Veterinary Medicines Directorate.)

Prolonged irritation will increase the activation state of the cells involved in inflammation and tissue repair. The repair process activates stem cells that can differentiate to replace damaged tissues. These stem cells are long lived and so have plenty of opportunities to accumulate mutations. Chronic, prolonged irritation leads to an increase in stem cells and the possibility that some of these may mutate (Fig. 14.3). During chronic inflammation, macrophages secrete growth factors that enhance cell growth. Oxidants released from activated macrophages may act as mutagens, especially in rapidly dividing cells. Fibroblasts proliferate at sites of chronic inflammation and wound healing. In some of these fibroblasts, the *sis* oncogene may be activated. The *sis* oncogene codes for the platelet-derived growth factor (PDGF) receptor, and vaccine-associated sarcomas have been shown to express both PDGF and its receptor. In contrast, nonvaccine-associated tumors and normal cat lymphocytes are PDGF negative. Therefore it has been suggested that lymphocytes within the vaccine-associated sarcomas secrete PDGF, which then serves as a growth factor for the fibroblasts. This combination of abnormalities could result in the loss of growth control in the fibroblasts engaged in the chronic inflammatory process.

The tumor suppressor gene *p53* encodes a protein that regulates the cell cycle. This p53 protein increases in response to cell damage. This in turn, delays cell division and allows DNA repair before the cell divides. If the cell is severely damaged, the p53 protein triggers apoptosis and so prevents DNA damage being transmitted to the next generation. Cells in which *p53* has mutated can, however, continue to divide, giving rise to abnormal and possibly malignant cells. As many as 60% of injection site sarcomas express mutated *p53*.

The key transcription factor for the innate immune system, NF-κB plays a critical role in several cancers. Activation of NF-κB is rapidly induced by viral and bacterial infections, necrotic cell products, DNA damage, oxidative stress, and pro-inflammatory cytokines. NF-κB is activated when its specific inhibitors are destroyed by enzymes in the IKK complex. Most of the

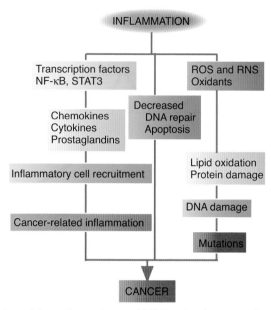

Fig. 14.3 The links between inflammation and cancer. *RNS,* Reactive nitrogen species; *ROS,* reactive oxygen species.

increased NF-κB activity that occurs in tumors is caused by the production of IKK-activating cytokines such as IL-1 and tumor necrosis factor. The loss of functional p53 also triggers NF-κB activation. This NF-κB plays key roles in the progressive steps of tumorigenesis. It is needed for the generation of reactive oxygen species that cause DNA damage and oncogenic mutations. It enhances tumor cell proliferation and survival. By chronically stimulating cancer cell proliferation, inhibiting cell death, and promoting mutagenesis, NF-κB drives malignant progression.

There is no evidence to prove that injection of less irritating vaccines can reduce the incidence of sarcomas. No specific brands of vaccine, no specific manufacturers, and no other vaccination-associated factors have been associated with an increased prevalence of sarcomas.

Feline injection site sarcomas have a poor prognosis. Most cats die as a result of local recurrence or metastases. They must be treated by radical resection, but this is often difficult, requires a long recovery period, and may cause significant disfigurement (Figs. 14.4 and 14.5). This is especially true of cats vaccinated subcutaneously in the interscapular region. The American Association of Feline Practitioners recommends that the three core vaccines against feline panleukopenia (FPV), feline herpesvirus-1, and feline calicivirus be injected subcutaneously below the elbow on the right forelimb and vaccines against feline leukemia, FIV, and rabies virus be injected below the stifle joint on the left and right hind leg respectively. Another possible injection site is in the distal tail. There are no significant differences in the cat's immune response. Both routes elicit similar antibody responses to FPV and to rabies antigens. Vaccines should be administered as distally as possible to permit amputation if required. The site of vaccine administration and the product used should be recorded for each vaccine to help in assessing risk factors. Clients should be instructed to monitor injection sites for swellings or lumps so that any developing tumors are detected and excised as early as possible.

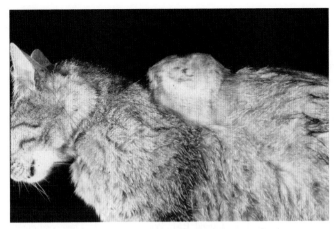

Fig. 14.4 A postvaccinal sarcoma in a cat. Note its position over the scapular groove, a convenient site for subcutaneous vaccination in cats. (Courtesy of Dr. MJ Hendrick.)

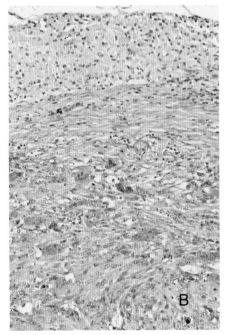

Fig. 14.5 A histological section of a postvaccinal sarcoma. This is a fibrosarcoma with the characteristic interwoven bundles of spindle cells. (Courtesy of Dr. MJ Hendrick.)

Sources of Additional Information

Afonso, M.M., Pinchbeck, G.L., Smith, S.L., et al. (2017). A multi-national European cross-sectional study of feline calicivirus epidemiology, diversity and vaccine cross-reactivity. *Vaccine*, 35, 2753–2760.

Almeras, T., Schreiber, P., Fournel, S., et al. (2017). Comparative efficacy of the Leucofeligen FeLV/RCP and Purevax RCP FeLV vaccines against infection with circulating feline calicivirus. *BMC Vet Res*, 13, 300.

Bradley, A., Kinyon, J., Frana, T., Bolte, D., et al. (2012). Efficacy of intranasal administration of a modified live feline herpesvirus 1 and feline calicivirus vaccine against disease caused by *Bordetella bronchiseptica* after experimental challenge. *J Vet Intern Med,* 26, 1121–1125.

Coyne, M.J., Burr, J.H.H., Yule, T.D., et al. (2001). Duration of immunity in cats after vaccination or naturally acquired infection. *Vet Rec,* 149, 545–548.

Day, M.J., Horzinek, M.C., Schultz, R.D. (2010). WSAVA guidelines for the vaccination of dogs and cats. *J Small Anim Pract,* 51, 338–356.

Hosie, M.J., Addie, D.D., Boucraut-Baralon, C., et al. (2015). Matrix vaccination guidelines: 2015 ABCD recommendations for indoor/outdoor cats, rescue shelter cats and breeding catteries. *J Feline Med Surg,* 17, 583–587.

Huang, C., Hess, J., Gill, M., Hustead, D. (2010). A dual-strain feline calicivirus vaccine stimulates broader cross-neutralization antibodies than a single-strain vaccine and lessens clinical signs in vaccinated cats when challenged with a homologous feline calicivirus strain associated with virulent systemic disease. *J Feline Med Surg,* 12, 129–137.

Jas, D., Aeberle, C., Lacombe, V., et al. (2009). Onset of immunity in kittens after vaccination with a non-adjuvanted vaccine against feline panleukopenia, feline calicivirus and feline herpesvirus, *Vet J,* 182, 86–93.

Jas, D., Coupier, C., Toulemonde, C.E., Guigal, P.M., Poulet, H. (2012). Three-year duration of immunity in cats vaccinated with a canarypox-vectored recombinant rabies virus vaccine. *Vaccine,* 30, 6991–6996.

Kass, P.H. (2018). Prevention of feline injection-site sarcomas: Is there a scientific foundation for vaccine recommendations at this time? *Vet Clin North Am Small Anim Pract,* 48, 301–306.

Lund, A., Deboer, D.J., (2008). Immunoprophylaxis of dermatophytosis in animals. *Mycopathologia,* 166, 407–424.

Munks, M.W., Montoya, A.M., Pywell, C.M., et al. (2017). The domestic cat antibody response to feline herpesvirus-1 increases with age. *Vet Immunol Immunopathol,* 188, 65–70.

Patel, M., Carritt, K., Lane, J., Jayappa, H., Stahl, M., Bourgeois, M. (2015). Comparative efficacy of feline leukemia virus (FeLV) inactivated whole-virus vaccine and canarypox virus-vectored vaccine during virulent FeLV challenge and immunosuppression. *Clin Vaccine Immunol,* 22, 798–805.

Reese, M.J., Patterson, E.V., Tucker, S.J., et al. (2008). Effects of anesthesia and surgery on serologic responses to vaccination in kittens. *Am J Vet Med Assoc,* 233, 116–121.

Scherk, M.A., Ford, R.B., Gaskell, R.M., et al. (2013). 2013 AAFP Feline Vaccination Advisory Panel Report. *J Feline Med Surg,* 15, 785–808.

Schultz, R.D., Thiel, B., Mukhtar, E., et al. (2010). Age and long-term protective immunity in dogs and cats. *J Comp Pathol,* 142, S102–S108.

Sparkes, A.H. (1997). Feline leukaemia virus: a review of immunity and vaccination. *J Small Anim Pract,* 38, 187–194.

Srivastav, A., Kass, P.H., McGill, L.D., Farver, T.B., Kent, M.S. (2012). Comparative vaccine-specific and other injectable-specific risks of injection-site sarcomas in cats. *J Am Vet Med Assoc,* 241, 595–602.

Equine Vaccines

There are more than 3.6 million horses in the United States, 2.5 million in Argentina, and up to 1.2 million in the United Kingdom, Germany, and France. Infectious diseases are of significant concern in all these animals, although the specific threats they face differ according to their use and location. As with other species, travel and intermingling of animals from multiple sources greatly increases infectious disease risk. Unlike other species, horses travel internationally on many occasions, especially in the racing industry. Well-considered vaccination is the most efficient method of preventing disease spread (Box 15.1). Owners should be reminded that vaccination is cheap compared with the value of a horse. In the United States, the five core equine vaccines include: tetanus, rabies, Eastern and Western encephalitis, and West Nile encephalitis.

Antibacterial Vaccines

TETANUS

Clostridium tetani is found in the intestinal tract of horses and is abundant in the soil on many horse farms. Its spores may persist in the environment for many years. *Cl. tetani* grows in the anaerobic environment of deep puncture wounds, surgical incisions, umbilical wounds in foals, and in the uterus associated with retained placenta or other trauma. It should be noted that the size or severity of the wound is not always predictive of tetanus development. As the organism grows it secretes a potent neurotoxin called tetanospasmin that is responsible for the disease.

Tetanus vaccines consist of purified, formalin-inactivated toxoids. Tetanus toxoid is a good antigen, especially when adjuvanted and it stimulates a strong, protective antibody response. Circulating antibodies alone can neutralize tetanus toxin. All horses are at risk of tetanus, and tetanus toxoid is a core vaccine for all horses. The duration of immunity is at least one year, so annual revaccination is required. It takes about two weeks for immunity to develop after vaccination. It is also essential to vaccinate pregnant mares four to eight weeks before foaling. This not only protects their foals through colostral antibodies, but also protects them against foaling related tetanus. Tetanus immune globulin should also be administered to any unvaccinated horse that requires immediate immunity as a result of a wound (Chapter 12).

BOTULISM

Botulism results from exposure to the neurotoxins of *Clostridium botulinum*. These toxins cause a flaccid paralysis by inhibiting the release of acetylcholine from motor neurons. *Cl. botulinum* can

BOX 15.1 ■ Equine Vaccination Guidelines

The guidelines for vaccinating horses in North America have been produced by the American Association of Equine Practitioners (AAEP). They are available at http://www.aaep.org/info/vaccination-guidelines-265.

produce seven different neurotoxins. Types A, B, and C are associated with botulism outbreaks in horses, but type B accounts for more than 85% of equine botulism cases in the United States. This organism is found in soil so it can contaminate wounds. *Cl. botulinum* can also cause a rapidly fatal shaker foal syndrome (toxicoinfectious botulism) as a result of ingestion of spores on vegetation. Likewise forage poisoning occurs when preformed toxin is ingested with improperly baled hay or contaminated feed.

A formalin-inactivated toxoid against botulinum toxin type B is licensed for use in horses in the United States. There are no toxoids available for types A or C. Vaccination is warranted for all horses because they may move into recognized endemic areas. It is especially recommended for horses that reside in the endemic areas in Kentucky and the Mid-Atlantic states. The horses at greatest risk are those fed baled hay, haylage, and silage in addition to foals born to unvaccinated mares. Shaker foal syndrome is a significant problem in endemic areas in foals two weeks to eight months of age.

STRANGLES

Streptococcus equi subspecies *equi* causes strangles in horses, donkeys, and mules. Clinical disease includes abrupt pyrexia, pharyngitis, and dysphagia, so that horses have difficulty swallowing and develop anorexia. Lymphadenopathy then develops, leading to abscess formation in the submandibular and retropharyngeal lymph nodes. When these abscesses burst, their contents contribute to a copious purulent and highly infectious nasal discharge. Metastatic strangles is characterized by abscesses in other lymph nodes, especially in the abdomen and thorax. Although most severe in weanlings and yearlings, horses of any age can develop the disease. As of 2017, strangles is a reportable disease in the United States. Recovery from clinical disease results in prolonged immunity that lasts for at least five years. This immunity is associated with the production of antibodies against *S. equi* M protein. Strains of *S. equi* show little genomic diversity and strangles vaccines should offer cross protection against all circulating strains of the bacteria. Vaccination is recommended where strangles is a persistent endemic problem or for horses at a high risk of exposure. Several cell-free vaccines are available in some countries. These inactivated injectable *S. equi* bacterins are associated with a relatively high prevalence of injection site reactions (soreness or abscesses at the injection site and occasional cases of purpura hemorrhagica). In addition, any protection conferred by these vaccines is short-lasting. A purified Streptococcal M-protein (Strepvax II, Boehringer Ingelheim) vaccine given intramuscularly is available in the United States. This vaccine will not prevent the disease. It will, however, reduce the severity of clinical disease and reduce disease prevalence by about 50%.

Strangvac 4 (Intervacc) is a subunit vaccine, currently under development, that contains a mixture of eight soluble recombinant streptococcal fusion proteins. The proteins were identified by analysis of the bacterial genome and studies in mice. They consist of a combination of surface and secreted proteins. The cloned proteins are generated in *Escherichia coli*, purified, and then combined. A saponin based adjuvant, Matrix C is subsequently added. This vaccine is administered intramuscularly. Strangvac 4 has DIVA (differentiate infected from vaccinated animals) capability, because none of the antigens included in diagnostic ELISA (enzyme linked immunosorbent assay) tests are present in the vaccine.

Several attenuated live vaccines are available globally. For example, a live intranasal vaccine containing a nonencapsulated strain of *S. equi* (Pinnacle, Zoetis Animal Health) is available in the United States and New Zealand. After administration, attenuated bacteria should ideally reach the lingual and pharyngeal tonsils where they stimulate local immunity. They can be isolated from vaccinated horses up to 46 days after vaccination. In some cases, the attenuated bacteria may cause the slow development of mandibular or retropharyngeal abscesses, a nasal discharge, and occasional cases of purpura hemorrhagica. These may be severe in young foals. Because this attenuated organism retains the ability to infect wounds, no other vaccines should be delivered concurrently and no invasive procedures performed at the same visit. This vaccine was generated by treating a wild-type isolate with a mutagen. It differs from the original strain by about 68 mutations, but it is not known which of these are responsible for its attenuation. Its activity depends on the production of nasopharyngeal mucosal immunoglobulins (IgG and IgA) directed against the M protein.

A second modified live vaccine (MLV), Equilis StrepE (MSD Animal Health), is available in Europe. This contains a live attenuated *aroA* deletion mutant (Strain TW928) that lacks 932 base pairs of the *aroA* gene. This vaccine is administered by submucosal injection into the inside of the upper lip, but painful reactions at the injection sites may occur. Immunity to experimental challenge persists for about three months. This vaccine is not DIVA-compatible. Because of the risk of purpura, horses known to have had strangles within the previous year and horses with high antibody levels (Titers>1:3,200) should not be vaccinated.

ANTHRAX

Anthrax is a fatal septicemia caused by *Bacillus anthracis*. The infection can be acquired by ingestion, inhalation, or wound contamination. It is restricted to certain areas in North America associated with alkaline soils. Vaccination is not required outside these endemic areas. The anthrax vaccine, the Sterne strain, is an attenuated nonencapsulated spore vaccine. It may cause injection site swelling in young foals and should not be used in pregnant mares. Anthrax is a zoonosis, therefore a physician should be consulted if the vaccine is accidentally injected or gets into human skin wounds or eyes. Because this is a live bacterial vaccine it is important to ensure that antibiotics are not given to the horse at the same time.

LEPTOSPIROSIS

Leptospirosis is a sporadic disease of horses. The leptospires cause equine recurrent uveitis, abortions, and renal disease. The bacteria are spread via the body fluids of infected horses, especially their urine. The most common serovars in horses in the United States are *Leptospira interrogans,* serovar Pomona type kennewicki, and *Leptospira kirchneri* serovar Grippotyphosa. A killed whole cell monovalent bacterin against serovar Pomona is approved for use in horses.

POTOMAC HORSE FEVER

Equine neorickettsiosis, (Potomac Horse Fever), is caused by an obligate intracellular bacterium, *Neorickettsia risticii*. It is transmitted by the accidental ingestion of insects harboring the metacercaria of an infected trematode. The infection results in abortion in mares in addition to depression, fever, leukopenia, enterocolitis with profuse diarrhea, and laminitis. A killed adjuvanted whole cell vaccine is available. It may be beneficial in endemic areas but *N. risticii* is genetically very heterogeneous, and as a result, the vaccine does not protect against all strains. Vaccination should be timed for the spring in advance of the trematode/snail season in summer and fall.

Antiviral Vaccines

EASTERN AND WESTERN EQUINE ENCEPHALITIS

Both Eastern equine encephalitis (EEE) and Western equine encephalitis (WEE) are caused by alphaviruses in the family Togaviridae. These viruses are maintained in the environment by circulating through birds and mosquitos. They are not common diseases but do occur sporadically in mid-summer and fall across the United States. Outbreaks may be especially common in very wet years when pools of stagnant water form and mosquitos thrive. Clinical EEE cases are primarily restricted to the Eastern coastal plains and the Gulf coast. Conversely WEE primarily occurs in Western and Midwestern states and the southeast. A variant of EEE (Madariaga virus) occurs in South America. Thus these diseases can be considered endemic across both North and South America. Both diseases present with fever, anorexia, and depression. Severe cases can result in blindness, ataxia, behavioral changes, convulsions, and death within two to three days. EEE is nearly always fatal in horses (75%–80% mortality) whereas WEE causes about 30% to 40% mortality. Recovered horses likely have lifelong immunity. Combined vaccines against EEE and WEE are core vaccines that should be boosted annually. In areas with a prolonged mosquito season it may be appropriate to give two doses annually, one in the spring and one in the fall. Likewise, horses that were not vaccinated in the previous year should receive two doses three to six weeks apart.

All currently available EEE/WEE vaccines are formalin-inactivated whole viral products. It has not yet been possible to produce effective modified live vaccines. These vaccines may be combined with vaccines containing antigens from tetanus, influenza, and West Nile Virus.

VENEZUELAN EQUINE ENCEPHALITIS

Venezuelan equine encephalitis (VEE), as its name implies, is endemic in tropical wet forest areas of South and Central America. It is caused by an Alphavirus, maintained in a rodent reservoir, and transmitted by mosquitos. It can cause debilitating and potentially lethal encephalitis in horses and humans. VEE has not been diagnosed in the United States since 1971. It is therefore a reportable foreign animal disease. Should VEE recur, an inactivated vaccine may be given to horses in a two dose primary series, three to four weeks apart with annual revaccination. However, there have been outbreaks of disease associated with incomplete inactivation of formalin-treated vaccines. Vaccination against EEE and WEE will induce antibodies that cross-react with VEE and may provide partial protection.

A modified live vaccine strain of VEE, C-84, is also used in horses. The vaccine must be kept cold and given as a single dose to horses over three months of age. Once reconstituted it must be used immediately. Horses should be revaccinated annually. This vaccine has been conditionally approved in the United States. Obviously, it cannot be used in the United States at the present time but would be released should a VEE outbreak occur.

WEST NILE VIRUS

West Nile virus (WNV) is the most significant insect borne encephalitis virus in North America. It is classified as a Flavivirus. WNV is now found across the entire United States and most of Canada and Mexico. WNV affects birds, humans, and horses, but horses are by far the most susceptible species, representing over 95% of clinically affected mammals. Affected horses develop ataxia and motor deficits ranging from mild symptoms to an inability to walk. Fever is not a consistent feature. About 30% of infected horses die and the survivors may show residual effects including altered gait and abnormal behavior. Because of its distribution and significance, WNV vaccination is considered essential (core). At the present time in the United States there are two licensed inactivated tissue culture adjuvanted whole virion vaccines, a canarypox recombinant vectored vaccine, an inactivated yellow fever chimera vaccine, and a DNA-plasmid vaccine.

Inactivated vaccines may not prevent infection, but they do reduce disease severity and prevent the development of a viremia.

A recombinant canarypox vectored WNV vaccine is available that will not replicate in vaccinated horses but persists for a sufficient period to stimulate a protective response. It is administered with a carbopol-based adjuvant (Chapter 7).

A chimeric vaccine, (EquiNile, Merck Animal Health) also incorporates a carbopol-based emulsion adjuvant. This vaccine consists of a vaccine strain of yellow fever (17D) with inserted West Nile premembrane (prM) and envelope (E) proteins to generate a chimeric virus-like particle. The remaining nucleocapsid proteins in addition to the nonstructural proteins and untranslated gene termini are those of yellow fever 17D virus.

A DNA-plasmid vaccine (West Nile-Innovator DNA, Fort Dodge Animal Health) has also been developed. The vaccine consists of a plasmid vector engineered to express high levels of the virus premembrane (prM) and envelope (E) proteins. In addition, the plasmid contains gene promoters and marker genes (see Fig. 6.2). Upon injection, together with a biodegradable oil adjuvant, this plasmid enters cells and causes them to express the WNV proteins.

Antibodies to WNV are detectable by 21 days postvaccination and reach maximal titers by about 4 weeks. WNV antibody titers may be somewhat lower in response to combined vaccines when compared with single antigen vaccines. Recovered horses probably develop life-long immunity.

EQUINE RHINOPNEUMONITIS

Equid herpesvirus type 1 (EHV-1) and type 4 (EHV-4) cause respiratory and neurologic disease, and abortion. They are endemic in horse populations worldwide. Many foals become infected in the first weeks or months of life, but infections also occur in when horses from different sources are mingled. Both viruses cause upper respiratory tract disease with fever, lethargy, anorexia, nasal discharge, cough, and mandibular lymphadenopathy. Both EHV-1 and EHV-4 can cause abortion in naïve mares, weak nonviable foals, or a relatively infrequent paralytic neurologic disease (equine herpesvirus myeloencephalopathy, EHM). EHV-4 causes especially severe abortion outbreaks.

Like other herpesviruses, these viruses establish latent infection in horses, which then become asymptomatic carriers. Most horses are therefore re-infected multiple times during their lifetime, usually subclinically. Viral reactivation occurs when horses are stressed, resulting in a viremia and short-term viral shedding. If this reactivation occurs in pregnant mares, they may abort.

Vaccination is required for the prevention of abortion and to reduce the severity of rhinopneumonitis in young or other at-risk horses. Although horses develop antibodies after infection, these antibodies are not correlated with protection. There is no evidence that vaccines prevent the development of EHM.

Many different inactivated vaccines are available for the control of EHV-1 and -4. These include some licensed for protection against respiratory disease alone, and two that are used for protection against both rhinopneumonitis and abortion. One inactivated vaccine is given intramuscularly for two doses, but the third dose may be given intranasally. Not all these vaccines are equally protective and immunity is generally short lasting.

A modified live EHV-1 vaccine is also available (Rhinomune, Boehringer Ingelheim). It is used for protection against rhinopneumonitis. Like other live herpesvirus vaccines, it causes rapid onset of protection as a result of interferon production. Because immunity is relatively short lasting, multiple doses may be administered annually. Even infected, recovered horses probably only remain immune for up to six months. Horses younger than five years of age, horses in contact with pregnant mares, horses that come into extensive contact with frequently moved horses, and show horses in high-risk environments should receive EHV-1 vaccines. Equestrian organizations may require such vaccination. (See section "International Vaccine Requirements".)

RABIES

Although not a common disease in horses, equine rabies is invariably lethal and is of public health significance. Rabies vaccine should therefore be considered a core requirement in horses. There are five licensed rabies vaccines currently approved for use in horses in the United States. All are inactivated and tissue-culture derived. They are given intramuscularly and are highly effective.

Some veterinarians prefer that mares be vaccinated before breeding. Given the potency of these rabies vaccines, the mare's antibody levels will remain high throughout the pregnancy and still provide sufficient colostral antibodies.

If confronted with foals from mares with an unknown vaccination history one may assume that they have been vaccinated and boost accordingly. An alternative approach is to test their serum for antibodies against rabies about 24 hours after birth at a time when it would be expected that they have received colostral antibodies. If negative, they should be treated as if the mares were unvaccinated, whereas if positive, one must assume that the mare had been vaccinated.

If a vaccinated horse has been exposed to a rabid animal then it should immediately be revaccinated by a veterinarian and then placed under observation for 45 days as directed by the regulatory authorities. If an unvaccinated horse is exposed to a rabid animal it may be euthanized immediately. If this is an unacceptable procedure, then the horse should be monitored for six months under veterinary supervision and with the approval of the appropriate authorities. This may also include isolation and immediate vaccination.

EQUINE VIRAL ARTERITIS

Equine viral arteritis is caused by equine arteritis virus (EAV), an RNA virus in the genus Arterivirus. It occurs in horses worldwide. EAV can cause abortion in pregnant mares and establish a long-term carrier state in breeding stallions. Foals infected during the first few months of life may develop edema, conjunctivitis, urticaria, and rarely, a severe pneumonia, enteritis, or pneumoenteritis. The majority of primary EAV infections are however subclinical or asymptomatic. Persistent carrier stallions are the natural reservoir of EAV. All horses should be serologically tested and a negative antibody titer should be documented by a US Department of Agriculture laboratory before vaccinating. An inactivated adjuvanted vaccine is licensed for use in certain European countries. It is prepared from virus grown in equine cell culture. This vaccine is used in breeding and nonbreeding horses. Its safety in pregnant mares has not been investigated. Interestingly, another inactivated vaccine has been developed in Japan. It is stored in case an outbreak of EVA should occur in Japan. It is not commercially available.

A modified live EAV vaccine is licensed for use in the United States and Canada. It contains a virus attenuated by multiple serial passages in primary equine and rabbit kidney cells and in equine dermal cells. It is safe and effective in stallions and nonpregnant mares. It should not be given to pregnant mares. Mild febrile reactions and transient lymphopenia do occur. However, in first-time vaccinates, the frequency, duration, and amount of vaccine virus that is shed via the respiratory tract is less than that observed with natural infection. Vaccination in the face of an EVA outbreak has been successful in controlling disease spread. When vaccinating against EVA, it is important to consult with state and/or federal animal health officials to ensure that the program is in compliance with any official control program.

Breeding stallions should receive annual revaccination against EVA no later than four weeks before each breeding season. Before initial vaccination, all stallions must undergo serologic testing and be confirmed negative for antibodies to EAV. All first-time vaccinated stallions should then be isolated for three weeks after vaccination before being used for breeding. Some countries bar entry of any horse that is serologically positive for antibodies to EAV, regardless of vaccination history. Countries that do accept EVA vaccinated horses typically require stallions or colts to have a certified vaccination history and confirmation of prevaccination negative serological status.

EQUINE INFLUENZA

Equine influenza virus (EIV) causes an acute respiratory disease in horses, donkeys, and mules worldwide. This disease, caused by the orthomyxovirus, equine influenza A type 2 (A/equine 2), is one of the most common and important infectious diseases of horses. It is highly contagious and spreads rapidly between horses as a result of coughing. It is endemic in many countries and causes major outbreaks when sufficient antigenic drift occurs and the horse population is no longer immune. It causes high morbidity with significant economic consequences. Mortality is uncommon, but the virus may kill donkeys and colostrum-deprived foals.

EIV, like other influenza viruses, undergoes continuous antigenic change (drift) as a result of mutations in its RNA genome, which result in amino acid substitutions in its hemagglutinin and consequent alterations in its structure and antigenicity. Continuous virus surveillance and characterization are essential for its control. Influenza vaccines only work when they match the circulating strains and they must be updated periodically if failures are to be avoided. This update is based on a formal review of circulating strains by an expert committee of the OIE (The World Organization of Animal Health).

Influenza viruses have two major surface proteins, the hemagglutinin (HA) and the neuraminidase (NA). The HA is the major target of neutralizing antibodies and an essential antigen in influenza vaccines. Equine influenza viruses are classified by their subtype, and also the location and year they were first isolated. For example, H7N7 was first isolated in Prague in 1956, whereas H3N8 was first isolated in Miami, Florida in 1963. H7N7 strains have not been detected since the late 1970s.

The original H3N8 equine influenza virus strain changed very little between 1963 and 1988. In 1989, however it diverged into two antigenically and genetically distinct lineages, one European and one American. The European lineage has not been isolated for many years and is believed extinct. The American lineage subsequently evolved into Kentucky, South America, and Florida lineages. The Kentucky and South American lineages have not been isolated recently. Sometime after 2000, the Florida lineage in turn diverged into two sublineages, clades 1 and 2. These are the dominant EIV lineages currently circulating internationally. Florida clade 2 viruses have predominated in Europe and Asia whereas clade 1 viruses predominate in North America. Florida clade 1 includes A/eq/Ohio/03, A/eq/Wisconsin/03, and A/eq/South Africa/03 viruses. Florida clade 2 includes A/eq/Italy /99, A/eq/Newmarket/03, and A/Richmond/07 viruses. Viruses from these two sublineages are sufficiently different antigenically as to require the presence of both in vaccines. Vaccination against one clade may not fully protect against disease caused by the other. Currently, OIE recommends that horses travelling internationally should receive vaccines containing both Florida clade 1 and clade 2 viruses. Antigenic drift continues to occur, however. and recent isolates are diverging from both clades. Newly emerged strains of clade 2 may be responsible for recent outbreaks of influenza in vaccinated horses in the United Kingdom and France.

It is clear that influenza outbreaks generally follow introduction of an infected horse into a stable where it spreads rapidly through susceptible animals. Thus quarantine of newly arriving horses and timely vaccination are required for disease control. All horses should be vaccinated regularly against influenza with the currently recommended strains. Vaccination reduces both clinical signs and viral shedding, although vaccinated infected horses may still shed some virus. Equine influenza does not infect humans, but the virus has spread to dogs (Chapter 13).

Should an outbreak of influenza occur, it may be necessary to establish a buffer zone surrounding that area. In the 2007–2008 Australian outbreak caused by the Florida clade 1 strain A/eq/Sydney/07, the disease was compartmentalized by ring vaccination that blocked viral spread.

In some countries, vaccination is mandatory for horses participating in equestrian activities under the rules of International Equestrian Organizations. Some of these organizations require biannual rather than annual revaccination because antibody levels appear to drop after four to six months. It is absolutely critical that equine influenza vaccines contain epidemiologically relevant strains because there is minimal cross-strain protection.

There are four types of EIV vaccine currently available: whole inactivated and subunit vaccines, an intranasal modified-live cold adapted vaccine, and a recombinant canarypox vectored vaccine.

The earliest flu vaccine developed consisted of whole, inactivated, products. Inactivated influenza vaccines may contain many different antigens from multiple strains of influenza A clade 2. They contain whole viruses combined with adjuvants such as carbomer, aluminum hydroxide, or ISCOM-matrix. The viruses are first grown in embryonated chicken eggs or in tissue culture and concentrated and purified before they are inactivated with formaldehyde or beta-propiolactone. They induce antibodies against the viral hemagglutinin, neuraminidase, and other conserved viral antigens. However, immunity is often short-lived. Thus most of these vaccines require two injections for priming, although three are better. They are most suitable for vaccination of pregnant mares to boost colostral antibodies.

A subunit influenza vaccine is also available (Equilis Prequenza, MSD Animal Health). It contains the purified HA and NA subunits of the European and Florida clade 1 virus, but not clade 2 virus. It is adjuvanted with ISCOM/ISCOM-matrix. It is not currently available in the United States.

A modified-live cold adapted intranasal vaccine against H3N8 is also available (Flu Avert, Merck Animal Health). A/Equine 2, Kentucky/91 was attenuated by cold adaptation in embryonated eggs. As a temperature-sensitive agent it can replicate in the upper respiratory tract, but not deeper within the body. It is approved for vaccination of nonpregnant horses over 11 months of age, followed by revaccination every 6 months. As with other live intranasal vaccines horses shed the vaccine virus. However, shedding lasts for less than a week. Onset of immunity occurs by seven days postvaccination. It is best not to use this vaccine in pregnant mares. In addition to safety concerns, this vaccine does not elicit high serum antibody levels so colostral antibodies may not be elevated. This is not entirely surprising because the intranasal immune response is primarily restricted to the mucosa. This vaccine is only available in the United States.

A canarypox-vectored vaccine encoding the hemagglutinin genes from A/eq/Ohio/03 and A/eq/Richmond/1/07 is marketed under the name Recombitek (Boehringer Ingelheim/Merial) in North America and as ProteqFlu in Europe. It contains a carbopol adjuvant and is administered intramuscularly. During the 2007 Australian outbreak it was shown to significantly reduce the severity and duration of disease and viral shedding. An accelerated vaccination schedule with only 14 days between vaccination and boosting was applied in emergency situations. Ideally it should be administered at least 4 weeks before an event. This vaccine induces high antihemagglutinin levels, so it should induce colostral antibodies in pregnant mares. The advantage of this vaccine is that it has DIVA capability. Vaccinated horses only have antibodies against the hemagglutinin whereas infected horses develop antibodies against multiple other viral antigens such as the neuraminidase.

In general, horses receive two priming doses of vaccine four to six weeks apart, followed by revaccination five to six months later. Foals should be vaccinated at six to seven months, and annually or biannually thereafter. If necessary, vaccination of foals at three months may be effective. Antibody levels appear to wane rapidly between the second and third vaccination and if the interval between these boosters is too long there may be an "immunity gap" to EIV lasting several weeks. Horses infected during this time may develop subclinical infection and shed significant amounts of live infectious virus, posing a risk to naïve contacts. Interestingly, there also appears to be a negative correlation between the number of doses of vaccine received by a horse and its antibody titers. The reasons for this are unclear, but it has been suggested that newly formed plasma cells displace older memory plasma cells resulting in a loss of preexisting antibodies. Perhaps there is an overvaccination problem. Mares have significantly higher antibody levels than stallions for reasons unknown.

Strategic vaccination may be appropriate such as timing revaccination to correspond to periods of exposure to other horses. Vaccination in the face of an outbreak may be effective if the outbreak is detected sufficiently early. In unvaccinated horses, the rapid onset of immunity that occurs after the use of the intranasal product suggests that this would be the logical vaccine to use.

ROTAVIRUSES

Rotaviruses, nonenveloped RNA viruses, are a major cause of foal diarrhea. Morbidity is often high whereas mortality is low. Rotavirus vaccination of pregnant mares results in a decrease in the prevalence and severity of foal diarrhea on infected farms probably as a result of rotavirus antibodies in mares' colostrum. An inactivated vaccine that contains rotavirus Group A is specifically licensed for use in pregnant mares to induce colostral antibodies.

Other Equine Vaccines
AFRICAN HORSE SICKNESS

African Horse Sickness is an insect-borne disease affecting all Equidae caused by an unenveloped double-stranded RNA Orbivirus related to bluetongue virus. It is transmitted by *Culicoides* midges and is confined to sub-Saharan Africa. Nine antigenically distinct viral serotypes have been identified. Both monovalent and polyvalent modified live vaccines are commercially available. These contain virus attenuated by growth in Vero cells and most provide good protection, although they have the potential to revert to virulence, undergo reassortment, and possibly be transmitted by their vectors. Some are more reactive than others and protection may be incomplete. Additionally, the currently available vaccines may cause fetal abnormalities when given to pregnant mares. Annual revaccination is required.

HENDRA VIRUS

Hendra virus is a Henipavirus in the subfamily Paramyxovirinae. It occurs in horses in Australia where it causes a high fever and severe respiratory disease with pulmonary edema. It results in a 58% death rate in humans and a 75% death rate in horses. A vaccine containing the viral G protein (required for cell attachment) is available for use by licensed veterinarians in Australia (Equivac HeV, Zoetis). It should be given to foals over four months with two boosters at three-week intervals followed by annual revaccination.

CROTALID SNAKE BITE

The risk of rattlesnake bites with envenomation may justify the use of a *Crotalus atrox* (Western diamondback rattlesnake) toxoid vaccine in horses. It may provide protection against other species of Crotalid and copperheads, but it does not protect against venom from Mojave rattlesnakes, water moccasins, or coral snakes. Three doses should be administered at one month intervals to horses over six months, and horses should be revaccinated every six months.

GONADOTROPIN RELEASING HORMONE

Gonadotropin releasing hormone (GnRH) controls the pituitary release of follicle-stimulating hormone and luteinizing hormone. These in turn regulate male and female sexual activity. Blocking of GnRH production can be accomplished by vaccination. Antibodies bind to GnRH in the hypothalamic-pituitary portal vessels and prevent the GnRH from binding to its receptor. Thus vaccination can be used to control inappropriate sexual behavior in both stallions and mares. In mares, the reduction in GnRH leads to a decline in estrogen levels so that behavioral estrus ceases. The adjuvanted GnRH conjugated to a foreign protein such as ovalbumin is given as a two dose intramuscular series four weeks apart to suppress ovarian activity and associated estrus behavior in fillies and mares that are not being bred. Antibodies peak about two weeks after the second vaccine dose. Cyclical estrus behavior will start to decline within two weeks after the second dose as the ovaries shrink. This suppression is expected to last for three to six months.

If given to young stallions the presence of antiGnRH antibodies results in decreases in testosterone, libido, sperm production, and sperm quality. Recovery from vaccination is usually complete, should a decision be made to breed with a vaccinated animal. There is however much individual variation in responses. GonaCon is a GnRH vaccine used by the Environmental Protection Agency as a contraceptive and inhibitor of sexual behavior in wild horses and burros (Chapter 20).

PRESCOTTELLA (RHODOCOCCUS) EQUI

Prescottella equi is a facultative intracellular bacterium that causes lethal bronchopneumonia and pyogranulomatous lung lesions in foals three weeks to six months in age. The organism elicits both antibody and cell-mediated immune responses in foals. (Protection is attributed to a type 1 response mediated by IgG1 antibodies.) Traditional live, killed, and attenuated vaccines have proved to be ineffective. Subunit and DNA vaccines may be somewhat better but they are not yet available. Encouraging results have been obtained when pregnant mares are vaccinated against poly-N-acetyl glucosamine, a highly conserved capsular polysaccharide. It is assumed that this immunity results from transfer of maternal antibodies in colostrum. Passive immunization with hyperimmune serum against whole bacteria or against poly-N-acetyl glucosamine may also be of significant benefit when treating infected foals (Chapter 12).

Adverse Events

Allergic reactions, although uncommon, may occur in horses in response to vaccine antigens. In severe anaphylaxis, the major shock organs of horses are the lungs and the intestine. Bronchial and bronchiolar constriction leads to coughing, dyspnea, and eventually apnea. The major mediators of anaphylaxis in horses are probably histamine and serotonin. Anaphylaxis requires prompt epinephrine treatment administered intramuscularly or intravenously (Box 10.2).

Local injection site reactions may occur, especially in response to strangles vaccines and some polyvalent vaccines. Although usually transient, they may be treated with nonsteroidal antiinflammatory drugs and also the use of warm compresses (Fig. 15.1).

The first MLV equine herpesviruses consisted of a virulent hamster adapted strain that retained significant virulence. Vaccines gradually improved and safety increased, although some strains retained the ability to cause abortion in pregnant mares. One such vaccine was associated with the development of posterior paralysis in many horses 8 to 11 days after vaccination.

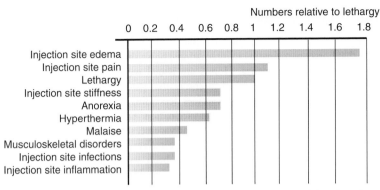

Fig. 15.1 The most common clinical signs observed in horses following the administration of one or more vaccines. (Form Veterinary Pharmacovigilance in the United Kingdom, Annual Review, 2014. With permission.)

PURPURA HEMORRHAGICA

Following exposure to *Streptococcus equi* antigens, some horses may develop purpura hemorrhagica, an acute, immune-complex-mediated vasculitis. Other triggers of purpura hemorrhagica include infections with *Corynebacterium pseudotuberculosis*, *P. equi*, equine influenza virus, and equine herpesvirus type 1. In some cases, it develops in the absence of any obvious prior infection. Clinical signs develop within 2 to 4 weeks following natural or vaccinal exposure to streptococcal antigens. There are great variations in disease severity and clinical course ranging from a mild transient reaction to fatal disease. Clinical signs include severe subcutaneous edema in all limbs and hemorrhages on the visible mucous membranes. Other signs may include depression and reluctance to move, fever, anorexia, tachycardia and tachypnoea, colic, epistaxis, and weight loss. The edema may result in skin exudation, ulceration, crusting, and sloughing. Severe edema of the head may compromise breathing and eating. Other abnormalities include anemia, and neutrophilia, hyperglobulinemia, elevated muscle enzymes (resulting from rhabdomyositis), and hyperproteinemia. The vasculitis may also affect the gastrointestinal tract, lungs and muscle. Small-intestinal intussusception may complicate the disease as does muscle infarction.

Skin biopsy shows a leukocytoclastic vasculitis. Immediate medical attention should be sought for affected horses. This usually involves the use of corticosteroids (dexamethasone and/or prednisolone). Horses may also receive nonsteroidal antiinflammatory drugs (phenylbutazone or flunixin meglumine), and antibiotics to limit secondary infections. Preexisting high serum antibody levels to *S. equi* may predispose horses to this condition. Immune-complexes are found in the serum of these horses and consist of streptococcal M or R protein complexed with IgM or IgA. These immune-complexes also trigger a glomerulonephritis leading to proteinuria and azoturia. Deposition of these complexes in blood vessel walls results in the vasculitis, vessel leakage, and hemorrhage.

Adverse reactions are inherent risks of vaccination and unpredictable. Some horses may develop transient systemic signs of innate immunity including fever, anorexia, colic, diarrhea, and tachycardia. Therefore it is recommended that horses not be vaccinated in the two weeks before shows, performance events, sales, or domestic shipment. Some veterinarians may elect not to vaccinate horses within three weeks of international shipment.

International Vaccine Requirements

The International Federation for Equestrian Sports (FEI) has a mandatory biosecurity policy that requires that horses participating in international horse show events must be vaccinated every six months against equine influenza. Horses are issued with a "passport" that records every vaccination. These passports are checked to ensure that participating horses have indeed been vaccinated. Horses may also require other vaccines depending on their environment, for example, equine herpesvirus, West Nile virus, or GnRH vaccination. These vaccines must also be recorded in the horse's passport. These include details of the vaccine, serial/batch number, date, and route of administration. All entries must be signed by the veterinarian and stamped with the veterinarian's clinic stamp. Competing horses must have been vaccinated against influenza within 6 months and 21 days of the previous booster vaccination. However, they cannot compete if they have been vaccinated within seven days of arrival. In the United States, the United States Equestrian Federation (USEF) issues the passports for FEI competition. The passport must be renewed every four years and updated when ownership changes.

Related Species

DONKEYS

There is remarkably little information available on the immune system of donkeys. In general, donkeys should receive the same core vaccines as horses, but revaccination will depend on the specific circumstances and geographic location of the animals in addition to a careful risk assessment. These vaccines may include rabies, tetanus, Eastern and Western equine encephalomyelitis, and West Nile virus. The use of other risk-based vaccines will in part depend upon their degree of contact with other equids. There is no evidence to support the use of lower doses of horse vaccines in donkeys. After all, miniature horses and foals still get the same dose.

Sources of Additional Information

Ault, A., Zajac, A.M., Kong, W.P., et al. (2012). Immunogenicity and clinical protection against equine influenza by DNA vaccination of ponies. *Vaccine*, 30, 3965–3974.

Barquero, N., Daly, J.M., Newton, J.R. (2007). Risk factors for influenza infection in vaccinated racehorses: Lessons from an outbreak in Newmarket, UK in 2003. *Vaccine*, 25, 7520–7529.

Bannai, H., Nemoto, M., Tsujimura, K., et al. (2018). Comparison of protective efficacies between intranasal and intramuscular vaccination of horses with a modified live equine herpesvirus type-1 vaccine. *Vet Microbiol*, 222, 18–24.

Boyle, A.G., Timoney, J.F., Newton, J.R., Hines, M.T., Waller, A.S., Buchanan, B.R. (2018). *Streptococcus equi* infections in horses: Guidelines for treatment, control, and prevention of strangles-revised consensus statement. *J Vet Intern Med*, 32, 633–647.

Correia, L., Martins, G., Lilenbaum, W. (2017). Detection of anti-Leptospira inhibitory antibodies in horses after vaccination. *Microb Pathog*, 110, 494–496.

Cursons, R., Patty, O., Steward, K.F., Waller, A.S. (2015). Strangles in horses can be caused by vaccination with Pinnacle I. N. *Vaccine*, 33, 3440–3443.

Cywes-Bentley, C., Rocha, J.N., Bordin, A.I., et al. (2018). Antibody against poly-N-acetyl glucosamine provides protection against intracellular pathogens: Mechanism of action and validadion in horse foals challenged with *Rhodococcus equi*. *Plos Pathog*, 14. Retrieved from e1007160,https://doi.org/10.1371/1/journal.ppat.1007160.

Giles, C., Vanniasinkam, T., Ndi, S., Barton, M.D. (2015). *Rhodococcus equi* (*Prescottella equi*) vaccines; the future of vaccine development. *Equine Vet J*, 47, 510–518.

Heldens, J.G., Pouwels, H.G., van Loon, A.A. (2004). Efficacy and duration of immunity of a combined equine influenza and equine herpesvirus vaccine against challenge with an American-like equine influenza virus (A/equi-2/Kentucky/95). *Vet J*, 167, 150–157.

Horohov, D.W., Dunham, J., Liu, C., et al. (2015). Characterization of the in situ immunological responses to vaccine adjuvants. *Vet Immunol Immunopathol,* 164, 24–29.

Horspoo,l L.J., King A. (2013). Equine influenza vaccines in Europe: a view from the animal health industry. *Equine Vet J,* 45, 774–775.

Janett, F., Stump, R., Burger, D., Thun, R. (2009). Suppression of testicular function and sexual behavior by vaccination against GnRH (Equity) in the adult stallion. *Anim Reprod Sci,* 115, 88–102.

Paillot, R., Marcillaud Pitel, C., D'Ablon, X., Pronost, S. (2017). Equine vaccines: How, when and why? Report of the vaccinology session, French Equine Veterinarians Association, 2016, Reims. *Vaccines (Basel),* 5.

Paillot, R. (2014). A systematic review of recent advances in equine influenza vaccination. *Vaccines,* 2, 797–831.

Paillot, R., El-Hage, C.M. (2016). The use of a recombinant canarypox-based equine influenza vaccine during the 2007 Australian outbreak: A systematic review and summary. *Pathogens,* 5.

Paillot, R., Prowse, L. (2012). ISCOM-matrix-based equine influenza (EIV) vaccine stimulates cell-mediated immunity in the horse. *Vet Immunol Immunopathol,* 145, 516–521.

Pouwels, H.G., Van de Zande S.M., Horspool, L.J., Hoeijmakers, M.J. (2014). Efficacy of a non-updated, Matrix-C-based equine influenza subunit-tetanus vaccine following Florida sublineage clade 2 challenge. *Vet Rec,* 174, 633.

Robinson, C., Frykberg, L., Flock, M., Guss, B., Waller, A.S., Flock. J.I., (2018). Strangvac: A recombinant fusion protein vaccine that protects against strangles, caused by *Streptococcus equi. Vaccine,* 36, 1484–1490.

Robinson, C., Heather, Z., Slater, J., et al. (2015). Vaccination with a live multi-gene deletion strain protects horses against virulent challenge with *Streptococcus equi. Vaccine,* 33, 1160–1167.

Ryan, M., Gildea, S., Walsh, C., Cullinane, A. (2015). The impact of different equine influenza vaccine products and other factors on equine influenza antibody levels in Thoroughbred racehorses. *Equine Vet J,* 47, 662–666.

Stout,T.A. (2004). Colenbrander B. Suppressing reproductive activity in horses using GnRH vaccines, antagonists or agonists. *Anim Reprod Sci,* 82, 633–643.

Bovine Vaccines

Proper vaccination is critically important for the control of infectious diseases in both beef and dairy cattle. With the growing increase in antibiotic resistance, improved vaccines are essential if bacterial diseases are to be effectively controlled. Disease prevention is of special importance in intensive feedlot and dairy operations, in addition to cow-calf operations with their high stocking density and low profit margins. Although carefully considered vaccination is important, other management issues such as nutrition, parasite control, and sanitation are also essential in controlling infectious diseases. Vaccines administered to breeding animals are designed to prevent reproductive losses, including infertility, embryonic death, abortion, and stillbirths. Vaccination of breeding cows is also critical in increasing the level of colostral antibodies and so ensuring that calves are protected. Calf vaccination is primarily designed to prevent deaths by respiratory and diarrheal diseases. As in other species, it is usual to use combined vaccines with multiple antigenic components, especially for the control of bovine respiratory disease. Core vaccine recommendations may be modified in relation to the nature of the cattle operation in addition to the degree of exposure to other cattle from multiple sources and any stresses that the animals might be under such as transportation, castration, and weaning. It should also be emphasized that not all vaccines are cost-effective. There is no point in vaccinating animals against diseases that do not occur in the herd, region, or state (Tables 16.1, 16.2, and 16.3).

Vaccine Administration

Beef quality assurance guidelines are concerned with physical damage to meat sold to the consumer. Injection site lesions such as bruising, abscesses, or broken needles, causing carcass blemishes or worse, are of major concern. Although not all such lesions are caused by vaccination, they must be minimized. Clostridial vaccines are known to be especially irritating. Intramuscular vaccination presents the greatest risk. Needle damage, deposition of foreign material, local inflammation, and scarring are all possible results. Scars may persist for up to 300 days following injection. Abscess formation with fluid or pus-filled cavities is the most obvious of these problems (Fig. 16.1). A second common form of damage is a dry, sterile, scarred woody-looking pale area in the muscle. Although mild, these lesions still require trimming at processing. They are especially important if they are located in the rump where the meat is not usually ground but used as whole meat products. In some cases, these lesions may not be detected until the consumer has cut into it. Otherwise the meat has to be trimmed to remove these lesions. Muscles from the hind legs of carcasses have been examined for the frequency of injection site lesions. These range from 60% to 35% in dairy cattle and from 31% to 20% in beef cattle. The difference is probably because

TABLE 16.1 ■ Vaccination of Calves Under 1 Year

Vaccine/Disease	Vaccine Timing	Comments
Bacterial Diseases		
Mannheimia haemolytica	Calves vaccinated under 6 months should be revaccinated after 6 months or at weaning. Ideally these vaccines should be boosted at least 2–3 weeks before weaning, shipping, or other stresses. Revaccinate on arrival.	Usually combined with the other respiratory pathogens, BVD IBR, BRSV, and PI3, and also clostridial vaccines. Withdrawal time 21 days.
Histophilus somni	Given at the same time as the *M. hemolytica* bacterin. *Vaccinate calves* 3–6 months of age. Revaccinate in 3 weeks. Calves vaccinated under 6 months should be revaccinated after 6 months or at weaning.	Usually combined with the other respiratory pathogens, BVD IBR, BRSV, and PI3. Revaccination is need based. Withdrawal time 21 days.
Leptospirosis	Vaccinate at 12 weeks. Revaccinate 4–6 weeks later and at 3–6 months of age.	Semiannual revaccination may be required. Withdrawal time 21 days.
Clostridial mixed bacterins and bacterin-toxoids.	Two doses are required 3–6 weeks apart. Vaccinate calves at marking and revaccinate at weaning (60–90 days).	Withdrawal time 21–60 days.
Brucella abortus	Vaccinate healthy heifers with RB51 vaccine between 4–12 months.	Must be given by an accredited veterinarian. Withdrawal time 21 days.
Salmonella	Vaccinate calves over 2 weeks of age. Revaccinate 2 weeks later.	Injections on opposite sides of the neck. Withdrawal time 21–60 days.
Fusobacterium necrophorum	To prevent footrot, vaccinate calves older than 6 months. Revaccinate 21 days later. For the prevention of liver abscesses vaccinate on arrival at the feedlot and revaccinate 60 days later.	Meat withdrawal time 21 days.
Infectious bovine keratitis Pinkeye: *M. bovis* and *M. bovoculi*	Vaccinate calves over 2 months of age, ideally 3–6 weeks before the fly season.	Withdrawal time 21–60 days.
Johne's Disease *Mycobacterium avium paratuberculosis*	Vaccinate calves over 35 days.	Given in the brisket/dewlap area. Only with state approval. Hazardous to humans. Meat withdrawal time 60 days.

Viral Diseases

Disease		
Infectious bovine rhinotracheitis	Vaccinate in combination with BVD and PI3 2–4 weeks before weaning at 3–6 months. Revaccinate 1 month after weaning. Calves vaccinated before 6 months should be revaccinated after 6 months.	Vaccinated on entering a feedlot or the dairy. Withdrawal time 21 days.
Bovine virus diarrhea	Vaccinate 2–4 weeks before weaning.	Withdrawal time 21–60 days.
Parainfluenza 3	Vaccinate 2–4 weeks before weaning.	Withdrawal time 21–60 days.
Bovine respiratory syncytial virus	Vaccinate 2–4 weeks before weaning.	Withdrawal time 21–60 days.
Rota and coronavirus	Vaccinate neonatal calves 30 minutes before allowing the calf to suckle because the colostral antibodies will inactivate it.	Some veterinarians prefer to vaccinate the pregnant cow and rely on colostral immunity. Withdrawal time 21–60 days.
Rabies	Vaccinate cattle between 12 weeks and 3 months.	Annual revaccination. Withdrawal time 21 days.

These tables are examples of consensus vaccination programs. Individual programs may vary greatly and reflect animal health, local environmental and housing conditions, severity of challenge and disease prevalence in addition to professional judgment. Be sure to follow the manufacturer's recommendations on the label.
All withdrawal times are for meat unless otherwise stated.

TABLE 16.2 ■ Vaccination of Adult Cattle

Vaccine/Disease	Vaccine Timing	Comments
Bacterial Diseases		
Mannheimia haemolytica	Annual revaccination if necessary.	Withdrawal time 21 days.
Histophilus somni	Annual revaccination if necessary.	Withdrawal time 21 days.
Leptospirosis	Vaccinate 30–60 days before breeding. Revaccinate at 3–4 weeks and 5 and 2 weeks before breeding. The herd should be vaccinated 60 and 30 days before the breeding season and again when pregnancy is assessed. Revaccinate in the fall with a booster 4–6 weeks later. Replacement heifers require 2 doses of Leptospirosis and Campylobacter bacterins.	Annual revaccination, but more often in endemic situations. Also use on animals entering the herd. Withdrawal time 21 days.
Clostridia	7–8-way combination. Vaccinate cattle over 6 months. Calves vaccinated under 3 months of age should be revaccinated at 6 months. Also vaccinate heifers prebreeding and precalving.	Annual revaccination. Withdrawal time 21 days.
Campylobacter (Vibriosis)	Vaccinate heifers 30 to 60 days before breeding. Revaccinate in 3–4 weeks and on entering the herd. Vaccinate bulls prebreeding.	Annual revaccination. Withdrawal time 21–60 days depending on the vaccine.
Salmonella	Vaccinate with two doses at 14–21 day intervals.	Withdrawal time 21–60 days.
Footrot and liver abscesses (Fusobacterium)	Vaccinate cattle over 6 months. Revaccinate in 3–6 weeks.	Revaccinate annually if risk persists. Withdrawal time 21 days.
Anthrax	Vaccinate using two doses in known enzootic areas 2–3 weeks apart.	Annual revaccination before the time the disease is expected. Withdrawal time 42 days.
Infectious bovine keratitis (Pinkeye)	Vaccinate cattle over 2 months of age. Revaccinate in 3–4 weeks or at weaning, ideally 3–6 weeks before the fly season.	Annual revaccination if needed. Withdrawal time 21–60 days.
Johne's Disease	Vaccinate only replacement heifers, and bull calves between 1 and 35 days of age.	Only with state approval. Withdrawal time 60 days.

Viral Diseases

Infectious bovine rhinotracheitis	Vaccinate 1 month before breeding heifers. Vaccinate replacement heifers 30–60 days before breeding. Vaccinate bulls before breeding.	Annual revaccination. Withdrawal time 21–60 days.
Bovine virus diarrhea	Vaccinate 1 month before breeding. Vaccinate replacement heifers 30–60 days before breeding. Vaccinate bulls before breeding.	Annual revaccination. Withdrawal time 21–60 days.
Parainfluenza 3	Vaccinate 1 month before breeding. Vaccinate replacement heifers 30–60 days before breeding. Vaccinate bulls before breeding.	Annual revaccination. Withdrawal time 21–60 days.
Respiratory syncytial virus	Vaccinate 1 month before breeding. Vaccinate replacement heifers 30–60 days before breeding. Vaccinate bulls before breeding.	Annual revaccination. Withdrawal time 21–60 days.

Protozoan diseases

Trichomoniasis	Vaccinate with two doses 2–4 weeks apart. Complete by 4 weeks ahead of the breeding season.	Annual revaccination. Withdrawal time 60 days.

These tables are examples of consensus vaccination programs. Individual programs may vary greatly and reflect animal health, local environmental and housing conditions, severity of challenge, and disease prevalence, in addition to professional judgment. Be sure to follow the manufacturer's recommendations on the label.
All withdrawal times are for meat unless otherwise stated.

TABLE 16.3 ■ **Vaccination of Pregnant Cows**

Vaccine/Disease	Vaccine Timing	Comments
Bacterial Diseases		
Clostridia	Vaccinate 2–3 weeks precalving.	Withdrawal time 21 days.
Campylobacter	Vaccinate breeding animals twice before the breeding season. Vaccinate bulls twice annually, 3 weeks apart, with the last dose 2 weeks before the breeding season. Cows should be revaccinated about half-way through the breeding season.	Withdrawal time 21–60 days.
Salmonella	Vaccinate cows 4–6 weeks before calving.	Withdrawal time 21–60 days.
Colibacillosis	Vaccinate cows twice with the final dose 4–3 weeks before calving.	Withdrawal time 21–60 days.
Viral Diseases		
IBR, BVD, PI3, and BRSV	To prevent IBR-induced abortion and BVD-persistently infected calves ensure that cows have been completely vaccinated before breeding. Use modified live vaccines in these immune cows only if they are approved for this purpose. Inactivated vaccines may be used without prior protection.	Withdrawal time 21–60 days.
Rota and coronavirus	Vaccinate healthy pregnant cows 3 months before calving. Revaccinate in 3–6 weeks. These may be combined with other vaccines such as *Escherichia coli* or *Clostridium perfringens*.	These may also be given to neonatal calves. Revaccination in subsequent pregnancies should be based on the presence of the infection. Withdrawal time 21 days.

These tables are examples of consensus vaccination programs. Individual programs may vary greatly and reflect animal health, local environmental and housing conditions, severity of challenge and disease prevalence in addition to professional judgment. Be sure to follow the manufacturer's recommendations on the label. All withdrawal times are for meat unless otherwise stated.

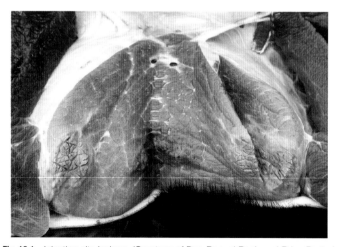

Fig. 16.1   Injection site lesions. (Courtesy of Drs. Raquel Rech and Brian Porter.)

of the fact that more dairy cattle than beef cattle are given vaccines. These lesions are estimated to cost the beef industry over US$4 million annually.

Injection site lesions are most likely to occur when cattle are injected from behind while their heads are restrained. The preferred sites for bovine vaccination are in the neck muscle in front of and behind the shoulder. Veterinarians should avoid intramuscular injections if other inoculation routes are available. Subcutaneous products should be inoculated into pinched "tented" skin. Intramuscular injections should be injected straight and deep into the muscle. Good sanitation is absolutely essential. When using killed vaccines, alcohol sponges may be used to clean needles between injections. This is not appropriate if using modified live vaccines.

Antibacterial Vaccines

BOVINE RESPIRATORY DISEASE COMPLEX

Bovine respiratory diseases (BRD) and undifferentiated fevers are estimated to cost the North American cattle industry up to US$1 billion each year. From 2011 to 2015, BRD in preweaned calves cost the US cow-calf industry about US$165 million annually. It is equally significant in other cattle-producing countries. BRD has a complex etiology and its occurrence depends upon age, weight, origins (ranch or sales barn), genetics, environmental problems, and stresses such as transportation, weaning, and overcrowding in addition to exposure to potential pathogens. In general, stress causes immunosuppression that permits viral infection that is followed by secondary bacterial invasion of the respiratory tract. The common viruses involved in BRD include bovine herpesvirus 1 (BHV-1), parainfluenza 3 (PI3), bovine respiratory syncytial virus (BRSV), and bovine virus diarrhea virus (BVDV). Other viruses that may be involved include bovine coronavirus, enteroviruses, and reoviruses. Bacterial pathogens may include *Mannheimia haemolytica*, *Pasteurella multocida*, *Mycoplasma bovis*, and *Histophilus somni*. Because of the complex pathogenesis of BRD, combined vaccines containing multiple antigens are usually used to control these pathogens. Combination vaccines may contain antigens against the five major respiratory viruses: BVD types 1 and 2, BRSV, BHV-1, and PI3. Mannheimia, Pasteurella, Histophilus, Campylobacter, and Leptospirosis antigens may also be added to these vaccine mixtures.

When calves arrive at a feedlot, the initial processing usually includes vaccination for the common bacterial and viral organisms associated with shipping fever. However, pneumonia often develops within two weeks after arrival before these vaccines have had sufficient time to confer immunity. Ideally these vaccines should be given at least two to three weeks before shipping to the feedlot. They can then be boosted on arrival.

MANNHEIMIA HAEMOLYTICA

M. haemolytica is the predominant bacterium found in bovine pneumonic lesions. This is commonly *M. haemolytica* serotype 1, but there are at least 12 other bacterial serotypes based on their capsular antigen structure. Protective immunity to *M. haemolytica* requires the development of neutralizing antibodies against its leukotoxin and its outer membrane proteins. Most *M. haemolytica* vaccines are therefore of the bacterin-toxoid type. These vaccines are also effective against the related respiratory pathogen *Bibersteinia trehalosi*.

PASTEURELLA MULTOCIDA

P. multocida subgroup A is a gram-negative bacterium commonly found in the bovine upper respiratory tract where it can act as a commensal or as a pathogen. When BRD develops as a result of environmental changes and stresses such as transportation or overcrowding, *P. multocida* is commonly isolated from the lesions. Immunity is presumed to be antibody-mediated. The bacterial leukotoxin is a major protective antigen. Available vaccines include bacterin-toxoids and a live streptomycin-dependent attenuated strain. These are usually administered as combined vaccines that also contain *M. haemolytica* and other BRD-associated pathogens.

HISTOPHILUS SOMNI

H. somni is commonly isolated from BRD cases. In addition to respiratory disease it causes septicemia with vasculitis, thrombotic meningoencephalitis, myocarditis, arthritis, and it localizes in the uterus to cause abortion. It acts synergistically with bovine respiratory syncytial virus. *H. somni* also undergoes some antigenic variation that probably explains its persistence in infections. It is an extracellular organism that can be controlled by antibodies against the bacterial outer membrane proteins. An alum adjuvanted bacterin is available against *H. somni*. This may be administered as a combined bacterin with Clostridia and diverse other respiratory pathogens (see Table 16.1). The efficacy of these bacterins is unclear because it is difficult to reproduce pure *H. somni*-mediated disease experimentally. As pointed out, calves should be vaccinated before entering the feedlot because vaccination on entry may be too late.

LEPTOSPIROSIS

This disease is caused by multiple Leptospira serovars and spreads through a herd via animal contact and contaminated water. The most important of these serovars are *Leptospira borgpetersenii* serovar, Hardjo-bovis, and *Leptospira interrogans* serovars, Hardjo and Pomona. The acute disease causes agalactia, icterus, and hemoglobinuria. The chronic disease results in abortions, stillbirths, and weak calves.

Multivalent killed adjuvanted Leptospira bacterins are available. Of the 55 licensed Leptospira combination vaccines currently available in the United States, all contain Pomona, 36 contain Hardjo, and 23 contain Hardjo-bovis. These provide immunity against disease caused by most serovars with the possible exception of serovar Hardjo. However, as with all Leptospira bacterins, the immune response is directed against the bacterial lipopolysaccharide. As a result, immunity is strain-specific and is not long lasting. Even under the best of conditions these do not provide protection for much longer than six months. Other serovars occasionally implicated in cattle include Grippotyphosa, Bratislava, and Icterohaemorrhagiae.

CLOSTRIDIAL VACCINES.

A wide diversity of clostridial vaccines are available for use in cattle (see Table 16.2). They may be administered singly or in many combinations. They may contain toxoids or bacterin-toxoids. Commercial vaccines may contain multivalent 2-, 4-, 7-, 8-way or even 9-way combinations of bacterins and toxoids. In general, these combinations contain a mixture of clostridia, especially *Clostridium tetani*, *Clostridium chauvoei* (blackleg), *Clostridium septicum* (malignant edema), *Clostridium haemolyticum* (bacillary hemoglobinuria), *Clostridium novyi* type B (black disease), *Clostridium sordellii*, and *Clostridium perfringens* types C and D (enterotoxemia). Interestingly, it is conventional to consider that these 8 organisms constitute a "9-way" vaccine, because the combination of *Cl. perfringens* types C and D also protects against *Cl. perfringens* type B toxin.

Tetanus vaccination is essential, especially when castrating older calves and using bands. It too may be administered in combination products to cattle, sheep, and goats. A common vaccine combines *Cl. tetani* with *Cl. perfringens* types C and D. Feedlot cattle may receive a 4-way vaccine combining *Cl. chauvoei*, *Cl. novyi*, *Cl. septicum,* and *Cl. sordellii* for the prevention of blackleg and malignant edema. Addition of *Cl. perfringens* will also protect against enterotoxemia and addition of *Cl. haemolyticum* will protect against necrotic hepatitis. These vaccines may cause significant local reactions so it is important to administer them subcutaneously in the neck. Pregnant cows may also be vaccinated to maximize maternal antibody levels in colostrum (see Table 16.3). These antibodies may block effective anticlostridial responses in calves until they are at least two to three months of age.

BRUCELLOSIS

Brucella abortus causes abortions, reduced milk yield, and infertility. It has been controlled in North America and Europe by a vaccination, test, and slaughter program. Brucellae are facultative intracellular bacteria and as a result they cannot be effectively controlled by antibodies alone. Antibodies may influence the initial phase of infection, but once the organisms enter cells, they can only be controlled by T cell-mediated macrophage activation. Cell-mediated immune responses are therefore essential and this means that only live organisms can serve as effective vaccines. Unfortunately, none of these live vaccines are entirely satisfactory.

Brucella Abortus Strain 19 Vaccine

Strain 19 is a very widely used modified live vaccine and the standard by which all others are judged. It is usually given to 4- to 12-month-old heifers in a single subcutaneous injection containing 7 to 10×10^9 viable bacteria; vaccination of bull calves is not recommended. A reduced dose of 3×10^8 to 5×10^9 bacteria may be given to adult cows, but they may abort and secrete the organism in their milk. The vaccine may also be given to cattle by the conjunctival route. S19 produces good immunity against moderate challenge by *B. abortus* and *Brucella melitensis*. However, it must be administered by an accredited veterinarian and vaccinated animals must be identified by an ear tag and a tattoo. The main disadvantage of S19 is that it has a smooth phenotype, and as a result induces antilipopolysaccharide antibodies. These are detected by conventional agglutination tests, and as a result it is difficult to distinguish vaccinated from infected animals.

Brucella Abortus Strain RB51

RB51 is the brucellosis vaccine strain currently licensed for the protection of cattle against Brucellosis in the United States. It is a stable spontaneous rifampin-resistant rough mutant that lacks the O-polysaccharide side chain because of a mutation in its *wboA* glycosyl transferase gene. As a result, RB51 does not induce the antibodies against the smooth polysaccharide that cause false-positive agglutination tests. It is as effective as S19 but less likely to cause abortions. Immunosuppression will not cause its recrudescence. Unfortunately, full doses of RB51 may still invade the placenta, and fetus and so cause abortions. The organism also invades the mammary gland and may be excreted in the milk. Even with a reduced dose RB51 may still be shed by a few vaccinated animals. Like S19, it must be administered by an accredited veterinarian. Vaccination of high-risk animals over 12 months of age requires special authorization from state or federal animal health officials. Vaccinated animals must be identified by an ear tag and a tattoo. Although still infectious for humans, RB51 is less virulent than S19.

CAMPYLOBACTERIOSIS

This is a sexually transmitted ascending infection caused by *Campylobacter fetus* subspecies *venerealis*. It is spread by infected bulls. *C. fetus* causes infertility, embryonic death, and abortion. The infection is usually self-limiting, but animals may remain infected for many months. Some infected cows may have a normal calf but still remain persistently infected. As a result, they may continue to infect bulls and so allow the infection to persist from year to year. Infections with *C. fetus* subspecies *fetus* also cause abortions but tend to be more sporadic.

A formalin-killed, oil-adjuvanted bacterin is available against *C. fetus*. It provokes an antibody response in the serum, uterus, and vagina. This vaccine should be given at weaning, when cows are palpated, and then revaccinated annually. Breeding bulls must also be vaccinated eight and four weeks before the breeding season and annually thereafter.

SALMONELLOSIS

Bovine salmonellosis is a matter of public health concern and also an economically important infection. Although it may affect cattle of all ages, it is of greatest significance in calves under 10 weeks of age. The most common serotypes are Typhimurium and Dublin. They are responsible for acute diarrhea in calves and multisystemic illness in adult cattle in addition to invasive septicemia. Even when not clinically apparent, Salmonellae may be carried by healthy cattle and transmitted to humans through meat or milk products. It is important therefore to control Salmonella-mediated disease in addition to the carriage and shedding of these organisms. Killed bacterins and modified live vaccines have both been employed. As expected, the live vaccines usually give better protection than the killed ones. A rough mutant of serotype Dublin (Enter-Vene-d, Boehringer Ingelheim) is the most widely employed live vaccine. An SRP vaccine using siderophore receptor and porin proteins is also available. It reduces the shedding of serotype Newport in dairy cattle.

COLIBACILLOSIS

Enteric colibacillosis caused by enteropathogenic *Escherichia coli* in neonatal calves is a significant disease and a major cause of economic loss. It commonly occurs in calves 2 to 10 days after birth but may begin as early as 12 hours. In addition to hygiene, good nutrition, and stress issues, its occurrence is linked to insufficient colostrum intake. Because of its very early onset it must be largely controlled by vaccination of pregnant cows and the induction of colostral antibodies. Available bacterins contain enterotoxic *E. coli* possibly supplemented by the addition of F5 (K99) adherence pili. These are usually administered to pregnant cows in two doses three to four weeks before calving. Revaccination is recommended at each subsequent pregnancy. A polyclonal equine anti F5 serum is available for the oral treatment of neonatal calves. Note that vaccination is only one part of a comprehensive management strategy to control calf scours.

A vaccine against *E. coli* O157 is also available for use in cattle. Its function is to reduce the carriage rate of this significant human pathogen. It is administered to cattle over five months of age. Given the importance of cattle in the transmission of this organism, the vaccine, if used, is likely to cause a significant drop in the prevalence of this infection.

ANAPLASMOSIS

Caused by *Anaplasma marginale*, a member of the order Rickettsiales, this infection results in anemia, jaundice, and sudden death. An experimental killed vaccine has been approved by US Department of Agriculture (USDA) and is used in several US states. It contains purified Anaplasma cell bodies with adjuvant and is administered subcutaneously. Because it does not contain red cell proteins it does not induce neonatal isoerythrolysis (Chapter 10).

Attenuated live vaccines are available is some countries and were marketed in the United States until 1999. These consisted of chilled or frozen infected bovine blood. They were expensive, required annual boosters, and their use raised significant safety issues, because other infections in the donor animals could be disseminated through many recipients. Because the organisms in the vaccine were live, they induced clinical reactions that had to be treated with tetracycline or imidocarb. A live frozen vaccine is currently available in California. It is given to cattle under 11 months of age.

In some countries, a related avirulent species, *Anaplasma centrale,* is used as a vaccine against *Anaplasma marginale.* In these cases, a susceptible splenectomized calf is infected and when the bacteremia is high, it is bled and its blood used as a vaccine. Because it contains bovine red cells, this vaccine has the potential to cause hemolytic disease of the newborn in calves from vaccinated cows (yellow calf disease) (Chapter 10).

FOOTROT

Bovine footrot is a bacterial infection of the hoof and interdigital skin caused by a complex of anaerobic gram-negative bacteria, including *Fusobacterium necrophorum, Porphyromonas levii,* and *Prevotella intermedia. F. necrophorum* also causes liver abscesses in cattle. A bacterin is available in North America against *F. necrophorum.* (Fusoguard, Elanco). It is used for the prevention of both footrot and liver abscesses. (See Chapter 17.) Footwarts (papillomatous interdigital dermatitis) can be a serious problem in dairy cattle. The cause is believed to be spirochetes of the genus *Serpens.* An adjuvanted bacterin is available against these organisms. It should be used in association with appropriate management procedures.

INFECTIOUS BOVINE KERATOCONJUNCTIVITIS (PINKEYE)

Pinkeye is a severe conjunctivitis caused by the bacteria *Moraxella bovis, Moraxella bovoculi,* and *Moraxella ovis.* It is not uncommon to find other bacteria in eye lesions as well. These organisms attach to the cornea through their pili and trigger severe inflammation, resulting in corneal edema, ulceration, and partial or total blindness. Consequently, there is a drop in feed intake, body condition, and milk yield. The initial attachment of *M. bovis* to corneal cells is mediated through the Q pilus, but persistent attachment is caused by the bacterial I pilus. Thus bacterins should contain both pilus antigens. An effective bacterin is available against *M. bovis* and there is a multivalent bacterin available against *M. bovoculi* as well. They may be combined with clostridial vaccines.

In the United States, a Moraxella vaccine is also available for implantation in pellet form. Two pellets are inoculated at one time under the skin at the base of the ear or in the neck. One pellet is designed for immediate antigen release to promote rapid protection. It rehydrates rapidly and begins antigen release at once. The other pellet rehydrates slowly and releases Moraxella antigens over a two to three week period. It is thus designed for prolonged antigen release, effective boosting, and longer-term immunity. Because of the diversity of bacterial strains involved, autogenous vaccines are often used for this disease.

MYCOBACTERIUM AVIUM, SUBSPECIES *PARATUBERCULOSIS*

Mycobacterium avium, subspecies *paratuberculosis* (MAP) is the cause of Johne's disease, a chronic enteritis that results in a drop in milk yield, significant weight loss, and decrease in body condition. In the United States, MAP-positive herds lose almost US$100/cow and production losses may reach US$200 to US$250 million. Many vaccines have been developed in different countries for this disease. These included heat-killed bacterins, live attenuated vaccines incorporated with oil and pumice powder, and lyophilized live attenuated vaccines combined with oil adjuvants.

A single paratuberculosis vaccine (MAP strain 18) is available in the United States (Mycopar, Boehringer Ingelheim). Interestingly the organism in this vaccine is not a MAP but *Mycobacterium avium* serovar 2. It is a whole cell bacterin suspended in oil and it is injected into the dewlap. The withdrawal time for this product is 60 days.

The use of MAP vaccines carries several risks. The oil adjuvant can induce a granulomatous reaction at the injection site—most are small and painless. Similar vaccines in other countries may be more reactogenic. Granulomas may become abscessed and leak. Accidental self-inoculation of humans may also cause severe acute reactions with tissue sloughing and chronic synovitis. If this occurs, the victim should seek immediate medical attention and the oil removed by suction or excision.

MAP vaccine may only be administered by a veterinarian who has been approved by state health officials. The herd owner and the veterinarian must enter an agreement with the state veterinarian regarding its use. Three conditions must be met before this can be done. First, it must be confirmed that the premises are actually infected with MAP either by isolating the organism or detecting it by polymerase chain reaction (PCR). Second, all the animals in the herd must have a negative tuberculin test and replacement stock must also be tuberculosis free. Third, the owner and the state animal health authorities must sign an agreement regarding its use.

Only replacement heifers and bull calves between 1 and 35 days of age may be vaccinated. Vaccinated calves must have external identification and a tattoo indicating that they have been vaccinated against Johne's disease.

Vaccinated cattle develop a delayed hypersensitivity that may result in a false positive caudal fold skin test for tuberculosis. In such cases confirmatory comparative cervical tests must be performed, using bovine and avian tuberculin. The *M. avium* response should be much greater than the response to *M. bovis*. In a large herd the cost of this can be significant and the herd must be quarantined until its true TB status is clarified. As a result, many states do not permit MAP vaccination.

Although this vaccine may not prevent new infections, much depends on the age of the cattle, the level of mycobacterial contamination, and herd management standards. It generally reduces clinical disease, fecal shedding, and MAP burden. These factors, plus an increase in herd immunity, should reduce herd transmission.

In countries such as Australia, ovine Johne's disease is a significant problem, and there is widespread use of a heat killed, mineral oil adjuvanted MAP vaccine (MAP strain F316, Gudair, Zoetis). It appears to be very effective in sheep and goats. A similar vaccine (Silirum Zoetis), is used in young farmed deer in New Zealand.

Bacille Calmette-Guerin (BCG) vaccine, an attenuated strain of *Mycobacterium bovis,* is of limited effectiveness in protecting humans against tuberculosis, but can protect cattle against *M. bovis* with 55% to 86% efficacy. Its developers, Calmette and Guerin demonstrated this in 1911. Low dose BCG (3×10^5 organisms) has been used successfully to control tuberculosis in free-ranging cattle in New Zealand. Unfortunately, the conventional dose of BCG (10^8–10^{10} organisms) sensitizes cattle resulting in positive tuberculin skin tests and cannot therefore be used routinely.

Antiviral Vaccines

INFECTIOUS BOVINE RHINOTRACHEITIS

Bovine herpesvirus 1 (BHV-1), a member of the genus Varicellovirus, subfamily *Alphaherpesvirinae,* causes reproductive, respiratory, enteric, and neurologic disease in cattle. The infection is characterized by upper respiratory tract disease with a purulent nasal discharge, hyperemia of the muzzle and conjunctivitis. Systemic disease causes abortions in nonimmune pregnant cows and may result in a loss of up to 60% of fetuses. The virus can also invade the genital tract to cause pustular vulvovaginitis. BHV-1 plays a significant role in the bovine respiratory disease complex.

Inactivated and modified live BHV-1 vaccines are available. As with all herpesvirus vaccines they can reduce clinical signs and reduce viral shedding but cannot completely prevent infection. Viral DNA persists in the sensory ganglia of its hosts for life.

Inactivated vaccines contain virus or purified viral glycoproteins and are adjuvanted. They are given subcutaneously or intramuscularly. Although inactivated vaccines do not induce a long-lasting response and vaccinated animals are slow to develop immunity, they can be given safely to pregnant cows. BHV-1 glycoprotein E or -D-deleted attenuated mutants are available and can be used as components in a DIVA strategy.

A temperature sensitive (ts), cold-adapted strain of BHV-1 is also available to be administered intranasally. This vaccine induces a rapid protective response, within 24–48 hours of administration. However, it may also induce mild respiratory disease and a drop in milk production.

An attenuated BHV-1 field strain passaged in tissue culture has generated small plaque variants. These variants proved to have lost the genes for gE and US9. These are the basis of current DIVA vaccines. A thymidine kinase deleted (TK⁻) BHV-1 vaccine has also been developed. It appears to be very safe but, like other herpesvirus vaccines, is unable to prevent latent infections.

BOVINE VIRUS DIARRHEA

Bovine virus diarrhea viruses (BVDVs) are Pestiviruses in the family *Flaviviridae*. This genus contains four important livestock pathogens: BVDV1, BVDV2, classical swine fever, and border disease virus. A new species called "HoBi-like" or BVDV3 has been identified in South America and Asia. The two BVD viruses have multiple subgenotypes (15 in BVDV1 and 2 in BVDV2). They induce enteric, respiratory, and reproductive diseases in cattle. BVDV includes two distinct biotypes: cytopathic (cp) and noncytopathic (ncp). (The name describes their behavior in cell culture, not their pathogenicity in animals.) Ncp strains suppress type I interferon (IFN) production but permit type III (IFN-λ) production by dendritic cells. The type III interferon suppresses some T cell subsets and enables the virus to cause persistent infections. Cp strains, in contrast, induce type I IFN production and do not cause persistent infections. Ncp BVD infections occurring in pregnant cows between 50 and 120 days postconception, before the fetus develops immune competence, result in asymptomatic persistent infection (PI) because the fetal calves develop tolerance to the virus. Once born, these PI calves remain viremic, yet because of their tolerance they do not make antibodies or T cells against BVDV. Some of these calves may show minor neurologic problems and failure to thrive, some die suddenly, but many are clinically normal. These persistently infected calves grow slowly and often die of opportunistic infections such as pneumonia before reaching adulthood (BVDV has a tropism for T cells and is therefore immunosuppressive). Because they are tolerant to BVDV, persistently infected calves can shed large quantities of the virus in their secretions and excretions.

The cp strains, however, can cause mucosal disease (MD), a severe enteritis resulting in profuse diarrhea, dehydration, and death. Mucosal disease results from a mutation in the gene that controls the BVDV biotype while the animal fails to produce neutralizing antibodies or T cells. The cp strain can spread between tolerant animals and lead to mucosal disease outbreaks.

Recombination may occur between persistent wild-type ncp strains and vaccine cp strains and this may also cause MD. Some of the lesions in MD are attributable to the direct pathogenic effects of BVDV, but glomerulonephritis and other immune-complex–mediated lesions also develop. Because persistently infected calves can reach adulthood and breed, it is possible for BVDV to persist indefinitely within carrier animals and their calves.

Preventing disease and limiting viral spread motivate vaccination of young cattle. Vaccination of reproductive age cattle is intended to prevent viremia and the birth of persistently infected calves. Currently almost all inactivated BVDV vaccines contain both BVDV1a, and BVDV2a. Most contain cp strains for safety reasons (they will not cause persistent infection), whereas some may also contain an ncp strain. Although very safe, these vaccines are relatively ineffective and require multiple boosters to induce protection. Inactivated vaccines usually generate antibodies by three to four weeks after a single dose and antibody levels peak by about six weeks.

Onset of immunity may be delayed in some animals for four to six weeks, resulting in a period of susceptibility. There appears to be significant variation in effectiveness of different commercially available vaccines.

Modified live vaccines (MLVs) stimulate much higher levels of antibodies than do inactivated ones, and also stimulate cell-mediated immunity. Protection may develop as soon as three to five days following vaccination with MLVs. They reduce viremia and nasal shedding in addition to preventing disease and mortality. There is little field evidence to suggest that MLV cp strains can cause mucosal disease, but a recent report described MD in cattle after vaccination with BVDV1a and -2a and the gene sequence of the isolated virus resembled the vaccine strain. At least one BVD-MLV vaccine has been shown to induce a leukopenia and suppress the lymphocyte response to mitogens as a result of a drop in T cell numbers,

Cows and replacement heifers should be vaccinated before the breeding season whereas calves should be vaccinated at weaning. Maternal antibodies to BVDV persist for 5 to 6 months or longer in dairy calves (see Fig. 8.2). (Evidence suggests that while maternal antibodies block antibody responses, calves may develop BVDV-specific memory in the presence of these antibodies.) MLV ncp vaccines should not be given to pregnant cows although some cp vaccines now carry label approval for such vaccination under certain conditions. Vaccination cannot overcome the problems caused by the presence of persistently infected animals in a herd. Thus these must be detected and removed and all introduced animals must be screened before admission.

PARAINFLUENZA 3

Parainfluenza 3 (PI3) is a ubiquitous myxovirus that causes mild or subclinical respiratory disease in mature cattle. Its main significance lies in the fact that it predisposes cattle to infectious bovine rhinotracheitis and other respiratory diseases. Thus it is considered a part of the bovine respiratory disease complex. In practice, vaccination against PI3 is usually combined with those against other respiratory pathogens such as BHV-1, BVD, and BSRV (see Table 16.1). Inactivated vaccines are available in a great variety of combinations with other antigens. Modified live vaccines are also available as are strains attenuated for intranasal use.

BOVINE RESPIRATORY SYNCYTIAL VIRUS

Bovine respiratory syncytial virus (BRSV), a pneumovirus, is the major cause of pneumonia in calves and an occasional cause of respiratory disease in nonimmune adult cows. Affected calves develop increased breathing difficulty caused by fluid accumulation in the lungs. BRSV is very common and endemic in many herds so that outbreaks typically recur every year. The disease develops around one to three months of age at a time when calves still possess maternal antibodies, and this suggests that these antibodies may not be protective. Nevertheless, pregnant cows should be vaccinated to provide some maternal immunity. Alternatively, very young animals should be vaccinated in an effort to stimulate protection by cell-mediated immune mechanisms, because helper T cell 1 responses appear to be important in conferring protection. Evidence suggests that administering an inactivated BRSV vaccine to calves in the presence of maternal antibodies may prime their T cell system and so induce partial protection. Inactivated parenteral vaccines have been difficult to assess because clinical trials have yielded equivocal results in demonstrating efficacy, and there is some evidence that they worsen the disease. Both intranasal and intramuscular modified live vaccines are also available. The intramuscular products stimulate the production of protective antibodies but may cause abortion in pregnant cows. The intranasal product can be used in pregnant animals. It can prime animals for protective immunity but the duration of this immunity is short. These vaccines are usually administered in combination with vaccines against the other major bovine respiratory pathogens.

Other Important Vaccines

BOVINE CORONAVIRUS AND ROTAVIRUSES

These viruses cause diarrhea in very young calves. As a result, they are usually controlled by a single combined vaccine that is either given to neonatal calves or to pregnant cows several weeks before calving. Two live vaccines are available for the vaccination of newborn calves. One MLV vaccine can be given orally immediately after birth. Another MLV vaccine can be administered intranasally to calves at three days. The rapid onset of immunity in calves receiving the oral or intranasal live vaccines is probably due to the production of interferon. Inactivated vaccines are also available for use in pregnant cows.

FOOT-AND-MOUTH DISEASE

Foot-and-mouth disease (FMD) is one of the most contagious of the diseases affecting cloven-hoofed animals, and the most important disease limiting the global trade in animals and animal products. Its cause is a virus of the genus Aphthovirus of the family *Picornaviridae*. Infected cattle and pigs develop vesicles on their feet, nose, mouth, tongue, and mammary glands. The mouth and nose vesicles rupture and result in excessive salivation and nasal discharge. The foot lesions located around the coronary band cause lameness. In adult sheep and goats the disease may be mild or subclinical, but in juvenile lambs and kids, mortality may reach 50%. Infected animals shed large amounts of virus, and because the infectious dose is low, the virus can spread very rapidly among susceptible animals.

FMD has the potential to cause great economic losses as a result of reduced weight gain, growth failure, reductions in milk production, and loss of traction potential. About half the infected animals remain persistently infected virus carriers. There are seven known serotypes of FMDV: A, O, C, SAT1, SAT2, SAT3, and Asia-1. In addition, there are more than 60 subtypes of FMDV, and there is no universal vaccine against all of these. Infection or vaccination with one serotype does not confer protection against the other serotypes.

The United States has been free of this disease since 1929. It is also absent from Canada, New Zealand, Australia, and most of Europe. Most disease-free countries have never vaccinated their livestock. They rely on surveillance, movement controls, and controls on the importation of animal products. Sporadic outbreaks in FMDV-free countries have been controlled by the prompt slaughter and destruction of infected animals and potential contacts. In recent outbreaks, the death of very large numbers of mostly uninfected animals has led to a public outcry and questions regarding the decision to implement depopulation policies. The disease is endemic in much of the rest of the world.

All currently available FMDV vaccines are inactivated. The first vaccines originally contained formaldehyde-inactivated virus obtained from tongue lesions. Subsequently it became possible to grow the virus in cultured tongue epithelium. It is now grown in large-scale suspension cultures using baby hamster kidney (BHK21) cells. Unwanted components and tissue culture residues are removed by ultrafiltration and chromatography. When the virus reaches its maximum yield, the culture is clarified by centrifugation and/or filtration. It is then inactivated with binary ethyleneimine and concentrated by ultrafiltration. These vaccines are then adjuvanted with a mineral oil emulsion or an aqueous adjuvant such as aluminum hydroxide or saponin. Pigs respond poorly to these vaccines, and double adjuvants, such as water in oil in water, are required to generate significant immunity in this species. FMDV vaccines must undergo efficacy testing in addition to the usual identity, sterility, safety, and freedom from contamination. In endemic countries, calves should be vaccinated every six months until two years of age and then annually thereafter.

Problems with currently available FMDV vaccines include serotype dependency, limited antigenic matching between vaccine and outbreak strains, slow development of immunity, a short duration of immunity (four to six months), vaccine instability, and the high costs incurred as a result of the need for very high-containment facilities. Although the vaccines may protect against clinical disease, they cannot prevent viral persistence in the mucosa of the nasopharynx, and as a result, vaccinated animals may become asymptomatic carriers. Local injection site reactions are not uncommon with the oil adjuvanted products. Other reactions can include fever, pain, and lethargy, and also urticarial, exudative, and necrotic dermatitis. They may also induce a temporary but significant drop in milk yield.

FMD vaccines may be classified as "standard" or "higher potency" vaccines. Standard potency vaccines contain about three PD_{50} (protective dose 50) whereas "higher potency" vaccines contain more than 6 PD_{50}. The latter are used to protect naïve animals in the presence of an outbreak. In countries where vaccination is practiced, vaccines are given twice a year because it is essential to maintain a high level of herd immunity. Immunity develops within seven to eight days. Because of the lack of cross-protection between serotypes and subtypes of FMDV the appropriate vaccine strain must be carefully selected if vaccination is to be effective.

Modified live vaccines against FMDV are not currently used owing to concerns about their stability and reversion to virulence. However, genetically modified live vaccines with massive gene deletions may be effective. One such example is the development of a leaderless vaccine (Chapter 4). The leader protein in this virus is nonstructural but determines virulence. Once this gene is eliminated the virus is attenuated and not transmissible, but it is both immunogenic and protective.

The antigenic determinants that induce protective immunity against FMDV are located on the virus capsid. This capsid is formed by 4 structural proteins, VP1 through VP4. VP1 is the most antigenic component of the virus. Several replication-defective adenovirus-5 vectors engineered to express FMD VP1 have been successfully tested in multiple species including swine. Such a vaccine could serve to differentiate vaccinated from naturally infected individuals. These AdV-5 vectors can only grow in cells that express the missing AdV-5 gene so they are very safe. Many other studies are underway seeking to improve on current vaccines including the use of virus-like particles, vectored recombinant, chimeric, and DNA-plasmid vaccines

The control of FMD is a national responsibility and vaccines may be used only with the permission of the appropriate national authority. FMD vaccine production facilities must operate under stringent containment and biosecurity procedures. There is obviously no need to use a vaccine in a country where the disease is not present. Nevertheless, countries must be prepared for a disease outbreak. Disease free countries have established strategic reserves of inactivated vaccines so that vaccines may be available in an emergency. For example, vaccines directed against serotypes O, A, and Asia are stockpiled in many Asian countries. The North American foot-and-mouth vaccine bank is located at the USDA Foreign Animal Disease Laboratory at Plum Island, New York. The bank stores many different serotypes of concentrated FMDV antigens in liquid nitrogen. There is no way of knowing ahead of time which serotype to vaccinate against. Once the causal serotype is identified, a process that takes about four days, these antigens can be rapidly formulated into vaccines. This would probably only occur should a FMD outbreak occur and should eradication fail to eliminate the outbreak. Because of the major economic consequences of this disease, rapid eradication remains the preferred method of control.

Emergency vaccination could play an important supporting role should a FMD outbreak occur in the United States. Currently two strategies are employed to block disease spread. Both employ vaccination of animals located in the area surrounding the disease outbreak. Once the disease is eliminated then the vaccinated animals may then be killed. This is called a "vaccinate-to- kill" strategy and may be justified by the persistence of infected carrier animals. An alternative approach would be to simply monitor the vaccinated animals closely and kill only those that show evidence of infection, a vaccinate-to-live strategy. This strategy requires the use of effective DIVA vaccines.

LUMPY SKIN DISEASE

Lumpy skin disease (LSD) is a poxvirus-mediated disease of cattle, sheep, and goats. It is characterized by fever, nodules on the skin mucosa and internal organs, emaciation, lymphadenopathy, and death. LSD is endemic in Africa, the Middle East, and also southeast Europe. Attenuated strains may be used as live vaccines. Strains of capripox virus cross-react with LSDV and have been used as vaccines but they may produce severe local reactions.

RIFT VALLEY FEVER

Rift Valley fever (RVF) is a disease of humans in addition to sheep, cattle, and goats, and is restricted to Africa and the Arabian Peninsula. It is caused by a mosquito-borne Phlebovirus of the *Bunyaviridae* family. Rift Valley fever virus causes mass abortion and high neonatal mortality when it infects pregnant animals. Both live attenuated and inactivated vaccines are available for use in regions where RVF is endemic. The mouse-adapted Smithburn strain induces strong immunity within six to seven days. It should not be used in pregnant animals in which it may cause abortion or fetal malformations. Protection lasts for several years. These MLV vaccines should not be used in nonendemic countries. A formalin-inactivated vaccine is also available for use in pregnant cattle, sheep, and goats. It requires two doses, three to six months apart and annual revaccination.

BOVINE EPHEMERAL FEVER

This is an important arboviral disease affecting cattle, yaks, and water buffalo in East Asia and Northern Australia where it causes serious economic losses. It is caused by an Ephemerovirus. It causes a short (three-day) fever with profound depression, stiffness, and lameness. Cattle may be unable to rise. Vaccination is widely employed and both modified live and killed vaccines are available. They should be given in two doses, two to six weeks apart, well before the start of the mosquito and sand-fly season.

Mastitis Vaccines

Despite the fact that bovine mastitis is among the costliest animal diseases in much of the world, there are few successful vaccines against it. One reason for this is simply anatomical. The huge volume of milk produced by modern dairy cows effectively dilutes antibodies, lymphocytes, and neutrophils. Milk immunoglobulins are poor opsonins and complement does not work well in milk. Complement will not enhance the killing of *Staphylococcus aureus* by milk neutrophils. The neutrophil respiratory burst requires a relatively high oxygen tension while the inflamed udder has a low oxygen tension. Milk macrophages, although abundant, are loaded with fat droplets and are less able to phagocytose bacterial pathogens than those in blood. Additionally, milk is an excellent bacterial growth medium.

The main reason, however, for this apparent vaccine failure is that mastitis itself is an expression of a cow's innate immune response to invading pathogens. It is insufficient for any mastitis vaccine to simply promote innate and adaptive immune responses. They must in essence, be so effective that innate immune responses and inflammation are either not required or are somehow downregulated—a very difficult task indeed. Thus any vaccine that enhances a cow's innate immune responses to a mastitis pathogen will effectively promote the disease.

Many different parameters have been used to test vaccine efficacy. These include somatic cell counts; bacterial culture; milk yield; the incidence and severity of mastitis cases; and even milk immunoglobulin (Ig)G content. Unfortunately, these parameters do not correlate well and a vaccine that shows a benefit when measured by one parameter may be totally ineffective when measured by another.

The major causal agents of bovine mastitis are either contagious, e.g., *Staphylococcus aureus, Streptococcus agalactiae,* and *Streptococcus dysgalactiae,* or they are environmental contaminants such as *Streptococcus uberis* or coliform bacteria.

Staphlyococcus aureus causes subclinical intramammary infections that often become chronic. The goal of any *S. aureus* vaccine would be to prevent new intramammary infections, facilitate bacterial clearance and recovery, and minimize cow-to-cow transmission. In other words, enhance herd immunity. Several different *S. aureus* bacterins have been investigated as mastitis vaccines but most have yielded disappointing results. A bacterin that stimulates the production of antibodies against the pseudocapsule appears to be somewhat effective. This pseudocapsule interferes with the ability of milk leukocytes to phagocytose *S. aureus.* Antibodies induced by the vaccine thus promote opsonization and destruction of the bacteria. *S. aureus* vaccines designed to stimulate antibody production against its α toxin and the pseudocapsule, are also effective in some but not in all herds. Vaccines containing modified live bacteria may be more effective than killed ones.

Lysigin (Boehringer Ingelheim Vetmedica) is a vaccine consisting of a lysate of five strains of *S. aureus.* These are common mastitis-causing strains including phage types I, II, III, IV, and miscellaneous other groups. Preliminary experimental studies gave encouraging results because it reduced the incidence of intramammary infections, disease severity, somatic cell counts, and the development of chronic infections. The vaccine is given to heifers at six months of age, boosted two weeks later, and then boosted every six months until calving. The vaccinated cows had a 45% reduction in new *S. aureus* infections during the next lactation. Subsequent studies in experimentally challenged animals resulted in a milder shorter disease but cell counts remained unaffected. Other field studies have failed to show these effects. A second vaccine consists of an oil-adjuvanted *S. aureus* bacterin plus toxoid. Three subcutaneous doses are administered one month apart and it is only available in California. It is reported to reduce bacterial shedding, reduce California Mastitis Test scores, and reduce culling.

Other mastitis vaccines are marketed elsewhere. For example, Mastivac (Laboratorios Ovejero), is a complex combined bacterin available in Europe. It contains *S. aureus,* multiple streptococcal species, *Escherichia coli,* and *Trueperella pyogenes.* Little success has been reported using vaccines against *Streptococcus agalactiae* or *S. dysgalactiae.*

S. uberis vaccines containing the bacterial plasminogen activator (PauA) have shown good results in experimental studies. However, mutant strains of *S. uberis* lacking PauA still cause mastitis. This organism is also encapsulated and resists phagocytosis. Neutrophil influx does not correlate with protection. *S. uberis* is also highly variable, therefore complex strain mixtures may be required to induce immunity in different dairies. An oil-adjuvanted, *S. uberis* bacterin is available in the United States (Hygieia Laboratories).

Many different vaccines are available for the prevention of coliform mastitis. The J5 strain of *E. coli* is a mutant that expresses a lipopolysaccharide with portions of lipid A and core antigens exposed (Chapter 3). Encouraging results have been obtained by the use of a J5 mutant vaccine against coliform bacteria and against Re-17, a rough mutant of *Salmonella typhimurium.* Bacterins are available with different adjuvants and various methods of application. As in so many mastitis vaccine studies, successful experimental studies have not always been followed by successful field studies. However, these core antigen vaccines do provide some protection when administered during the drying-off period. They may reduce disease duration and decrease its transmissibility and also minimizing culling.

There are at least five licensed vaccines available against coliform mastitis in the United States. In general, these are given in multiple subcutaneous doses. One that is available in Europe and Canada, contains both *E. coli* J5 and *S. aureus* SP140 strain (Startvac, Hipra). As in so many cases it reduces the prevalence of *S. aureus* mastitis, but milk yield was reduced and it did not appear to affect the duration of disease. In other studies, the incidence of mastitis was unaffected but its severity was much reduced. One study suggested that the cost-effectiveness of using this vaccine was about 2.5:1. Other studies have failed to show this effect.

As described in Chapter 3, vaccines directed against a bacterial outer membrane siderophore receptor protein and porin proteins (SRP) block iron uptake by gram-negative enterobacteria. A vaccine containing a Klebsiella SRP appears to be very effective in reducing the prevalence and incidence of Klebsiella mastitis.

Herd-specific autogenous vaccines also been widely employed to control mastitis. Reported results are mixed, with some reporting excellent responses and protection whereas others are seemingly ineffective. Vaccination is no substitute for excellent hygiene, teat health, proper milking procedures, dry cow antibiotic therapy, and a well-considered mastitis control program.

Maternal Antibodies

Prebreeding vaccinations should be completed at least four weeks before the start of breeding to ensure that maximal antibody titers coincide with the onset of pregnancy. Vaccines given to prevent losses from abortions include those directed against bacterial diseases such as vibriosis, and leptospirosis; virus diseases such as IBR and bovine viral diarrhea (BVD); and protozoa such as Neospora and Trichomoniasis. It is often also appropriate to vaccinate cows at a time when they are undergoing pregnancy testing so that antibody titers will peak at a time of greatest susceptibility.

Precalving vaccines are intended to provide colostral immunity to the newborn calf. Vaccines are given to cows to protect their newborn calves from diseases caused by rotavirus, coronavirus, E. coli, Cl. chauvoei and Cl. perfringens types C and D. As a general rule, such vaccines should be given two to four weeks before calving to ensure maximal colostral antibody titers. Vaccination against diarrheal diseases is especially important at this stage.

Preweaning vaccinations help calves handle infections associated with weaning stress. These may include Clostridial vaccines and those directed against the components of the BRD complex.

Preconditioning is the preparation of feeder calves for marketing, shipping, and admission to the feedlot. It relies on vaccination of calves two to three weeks before shipping to give time for immunity to develop. Common vaccines given to these calves include those against clostridial diseases and the viral respiratory pathogens PI3, BRSV, BHV-1, and BVD. Vaccines against Mannheimia haemolytica, Pasteurella multocida, and Histophilus somni, may also be administered. Vaccination against respiratory pathogens is standard practice in many feedlots and occurs 24 hours after arrival. It makes sense to only use vaccines against agents known to cause problems in that feedlot. A basic minimum at this stage should be a respiratory disease vaccine plus a Clostridial vaccine. Any additional vaccines should be based on known risks.

Bulls should receive the same vaccines as the cow/calf herd, excluding brucellosis and trichomoniasis. Cows and bulls should receive respiratory viral vaccines including BHV-1, BVD, PI3, and BRSV. MLV-BHV-1 may be shed in semen so this is a concern especially if the semen is to be exported. They should also get reproductive disease vaccines, including vibrio and leptospirosis, and also a 7-way clostridial vaccine. Replacement heifers under one year of age should get the same vaccines and possibly brucellosis as well.

Adverse Events

Anaphylaxis (Type 1 hypersensitivity) is a potential vaccination hazard. In cattle the major shock organs are the lungs. It is characterized by profound systemic hypotension and pulmonary hypertension. The pulmonary hypertension results from constriction of the pulmonary vein and leads to pulmonary edema and severe dyspnea. The smooth muscle of the bladder and intestine contract, causing urination, defecation, and bloating. The main mediators of anaphylaxis in cattle are serotonin, kinins, and the leukotrienes. Histamine is of lesser importance.

Inadvertent intravenous administration of respiratory and clostridial vaccines in calves has been recorded as causing acute interstitial pneumonia, with multifocal pulmonary hemorrhages leading to fatal respiratory failure.

Attenuated BVD vaccines may cause problems because some are immunosuppressive. Thus they cause a reduction in lymphocyte and neutrophil numbers, neutrophil functions, and lymphocyte responses to mitogens. Some cattle are tolerant to and persistently infected with BVD. If these animals are then superinfected with another strain of BVD they may develop fatal mucosal disease. Administration of a BVD-MLV vaccine to these persistently infected animals may induce mucosal disease. Mucosal disease generally develops 7 to 20 days after vaccination in about 0.2% in vaccinated cattle.

Cattle vaccinated with a temperature-sensitive strain of BHV-1 intranasally develop latent infections. Administration of dexamethasone to these vaccinated cattle may result in shedding of the vaccine virus for up to eight days. These may be transmitted to in-contact animals. Even parenterally vaccinated calves may shed this virus transiently. It has also been reported that calves receiving MLV-BHV-1 within 48 hours after arrival at a feedlot have a higher mortality than unvaccinated calves.

Multiple vaccines administered at the same time may cause neck soreness. Gram-negative bacterins may contain sufficient endotoxins to cause a fever, anorexia, a drop in milk yield, and perhaps even abortion. Holsteins appear to be predisposed to these reactions. In general, therefore, no more than two gram-negative vaccines should be administered to an animal on the same day.

Two important vaccine-related adverse events that occur in cattle include hemolytic disease of the newborn and neonatal pancytopenia of calves. These are discussed in Chapter 10.

Sources of Additional Information

Angelos, J.A., Lane, V.M., Ball, L.M., Hess, J.F. (2010). Recombinant *Moraxella bovoculi* cytotoxin-ISCOM matrix adjuvanted vaccine to prevent naturally occurring infectious bovine keratoconjunctivitis. *Vet Res Commun,* 34, 229–239.

Benedictus, L., Otten, H.G., van Schaik, G., et al. (2014). Bovine Neonatal Pancytopenia is a heritable trait of the dam rather than the calf and correlates with the magnitude of vaccine induced maternal alloantibodies not the MHC haplotype. *Vet Res,* 45, 129.

Benedictus, L., Luteijn, R.D., Otten, H., et al. (2015). Pathogenicity of Bovine Neonatal Pancytopenia-associated vaccine-induced alloantibodies correlates with Major Histocompatibility Complex class I expression. *Sci Rep,* 5, 12748.

Chase, C.C.L., Fulton, R.W., O'Toole, D., et al. (2017). Bovine herpesvirus 1 modified live virus vaccines for cattle reproduction: Balancing protection with undesired effects. *Vet Microbiol,* 206, 69–77.

Diaz-San Segundo, F., Medina, G.N., Stenfeldt, C., Arzt, J., de Los Santos, T. (2017). Foot-and-mouth disease vaccines. *Vet Microbiol,* 20, 102–112.

Ellis, J.A. (2017). How efficacious are vaccines against bovine respiratory syncytial virus in cattle? *Vet Microbiol,* 206, 59–68.

Gershwin, L.J., Behrens, N.E., McEligot, H.A., et al. (2017). A recombinant subunit vaccine for bovine RSV and *Histophilus somni* protects calves against dual pathogen challenge. *Vaccine,* 35, 1954–1963.

Lalsiamthara, J., Lee, J.H. (2017). Development and trial of vaccines against Brucella. *J Vet Sci,* 18, 281–290.

Lee, R.W., Cornelisse, M., Ziauddin, A., et al. (2008). Expression of a modified *Mannheimia haemolytica* GS60 outer membrane lipoprotein in transgenic alfalfa for the development of an edible vaccine against bovine pneumonic pasteurellosis. *J Biotechnol,* 135, 224–231.

Leitner, G., Pinchasov, Y., Morag, E., et al. (2013). Immunotherapy of mastitis. *Vet Immunol Immunopathol,* 153, 209–216.

Madampage, C.A., Rawlyk, N., Crockford, G., et al. (2015). Reverse vaccinology as an approach for developing *Histophilus somni* vaccine candidates. *Biologicals,* 43, 444–541.

Marchart, J., Dropmann, G., Lechleitner, S., et al. (2003). *Pasteurella multocida-* and *Pasteurella haemolytica-*ghosts: New vaccine candidates. *Vaccine,* 21, 3988–3997.

Newcomer, B.W., Chamorro, M.F., Walz, P.H. (2017). Vaccination of cattle against bovine viral diarrhea virus. *Vet Microbiol,* 206, 78–83.

O'Neill, R.G., Fitzpatrick, J.L., Glass, E.J., et al. (2007) Optimization of the response to respiratory vaccines in cattle. *Vet Rec,* 161, 269–270.

Park, H.T., Yoo, H.S. (2016) Development of vaccines to *Mycobacterium avium* subsp. paratuberculosis infection. *Clin Exp Vaccine Res,* 5, 108–116.

Perez-Casal, J., Prysliak, T., Maina, T., Suleman, M., Jimbo, S. (2017). Status of the development of a vaccine against *Mycoplasma bovis. Vaccine,* 35, 2902–2907.

CHAPTER 17

Sheep and Goat Vaccines

Although vaccines are available against many infectious diseases of small ruminants, they labor under the difficulty that individual animals may be of low value, and consequently, the cost of vaccines must also be very low to make economic sense. This severely limits vaccine choices for these species. Additionally, many small ruminant operations are traditionally managed and function at a low technological level. Nevertheless, small ruminants are the most significant livestock species in many countries, especially in less developed or arid regions. Conversely, some sheep and goat products such as wool and mohair are of significant value, and the highly efficient sheep producing systems in countries such as Australia and New Zealand are important contributors to their economies. Therefore it is not surprising that these countries are the sources of some of the most innovative and effective small ruminant vaccines.

Vaccine Administration

As in other food animals, the veterinarian should be aware of the potential of injected vaccines to induce injection site lesions including blemishes in show animals. Reaction sites that require trimming at slaughter may result in a significant financial penalty. In general, subcutaneous injection in the caudolateral neck region is preferred, with an injection behind the elbow over the ribs as a possible alternative. Do not administer vaccines over the loin or hindquarters where the valuable meat cuts are located. As always, animals must be properly restrained to minimize struggling and to ensure proper delivery of the full dose of vaccine. The use of excessively long needles over 0.5 inches long should be avoided and they should be changed often. Remember, the needle used to withdraw vaccine from the bottle should not be used for injection.

Antibacterial Vaccines

CLOSTRIDIAL DISEASES

The most important vaccines given routinely to sheep and lambs in North America are those used to protect against Clostridial diseases. Specifically, the preferred vaccine is CD-T toxoid. This protects against enterotoxemia caused by *Clostridium perfringens* types C and D and also tetanus caused by *Clostridium tetani*. These Clostridial organisms can grow rapidly in an animal and secrete a complex mixture of toxins and enzymes. Seven toxinotypes (A–E) have been identified. *Cl. perfringens* type C causes a hemorrhagic enteritis ("bloody scours") in suckling lambs during the first few weeks of life. It may be triggered by changes in feed or receiving too much

215

milk. Vaccination of the ewe in late pregnancy, four weeks before lambing, offers protection. *Cl. perfringens* type D causes enterotoxemia (overeating disease) and pulpy kidney disease. It usually affects lambs over one month of age and is often precipitated by a change of feed. This results in abrupt changes in the intestinal microbiota and clostridial proliferation. This leads to sudden death in weaned lambs on a high carbohydrate diet. Like type C, the type D *Cl. perfringens* vaccine should be administered to pregnant ewes in late pregnancy to ensure adequate levels of antibodies in colostrum and protection of lambs for four to six weeks.

Polyvalent clostridial vaccines contain a complex mixture of toxoids and bacterins from up to eight different species. They are normally administered in two doses and elicit responses that are protective for at least a year. Studies however suggest that antibody levels peak about 36 days after vaccination and are maintained up to 90 days before declining rapidly. They may be undetectable by 6 months. Factors other than antibodies must be responsible for the prolonged immunity seen in practice. As might be expected, large individual variations in response occur between animals. Additionally, some antigenic competition occurs in these complex mixtures. *Cl. tetani* and *Clostridium novyi* type B are immunodominant and induce the highest antibody levels whereas *Clostridium septicum* the lowest.

Clostridial vaccines are available in 3-, 7-, and 8-way combinations, each containing a mixture of toxoids and bacterins. In addition to *Cl. perfringens* types -B, -C and -D, they may contain *Clostridium sordellii*, *Cl. septicum*, *Cl. novyi*, *Clostridium haemolyticum*, and *Cl. tetani* (Table 17.1). The 7- and 8-way vaccines are combination vaccines used to protect against other clostridial diseases such as malignant edema, "big head", and blackleg caused by wound infections. These should only be used if these other clostridia are known to be present in a flock.

Tetanus is a potential risk at docking and castration time. If their ewes were vaccinated when pregnant then revaccination of lambs is unnecessary. Vaccination at the time of docking or castration of lambs may not be protective because it takes about 7 to 10 days for antitoxic immunity to develop. Tetanus antitoxin should be used to provide immediate protection in such cases. Maternal antibodies will probably protect lambs and kids for about two months depending on their titer.

FOOTROT

Footrot is a common, complex, and important disease in the sheep industry. It is a painful and debilitating infection of the interdigital skin and is the most important cause of lameness in sheep. Footrot is primarily caused by a complex mixture of bacteria of which the most important is an anaerobic gram-negative bacterium, *Dichelobacter nodosus*. Infection by *D. nodosus* is preceded and accompanied by maceration and colonization of the interdigital skin by *Fusobacterium necrophorum*. Footrot causes significant losses because animals must be treated and/or culled. Based on the antigenicity of their fimbriae there are 10 major serogroups of *D. nodosus* (A-I and M), and within these serogroups there are additional serotypes. (Other classification systems have identified as many as 21 serotypes). Immunity is serogroup specific and multiple different serogroups may be found within a single sheep flock.

Sheep and goats can be immunized against footrot using vaccines against *D. nodosus* containing either whole cell antigens or fimbrial antigens. Whole cell vaccines are rarely protective against heterologous subgroups. The fimbriae provide the major antigenic determinants (also called epitopes) and as such are the major protective antigens. These fimbriae are composed of repeating protein subunits called pilins. Pilin monomers, although antigenic are not protective. Denatured fimbriae are not protective either. However, fimbriae containing pilin polymers are as effective as whole cell vaccines. These fimbrial antigens may be derived by physicochemical methods or produced in recombinant organisms.

Ideally footrot vaccines should contain antigens representing all the serogroups. A multivalent recombinant fimbrial vaccine containing ten serogroups (A, B1, B2, and C to M) is currently used in Australia and other countries. It is not ideal, and protection lasts for less than 10 weeks. Specific monovalent or bivalent vaccines, in contrast, can provide protection for up to 16 weeks

TABLE 17.1 ▪ A Suggested Vaccination Schedule for Lambs and Kids

Disease/Vaccine	Vaccine Timing	Comments
Bacterial Diseases		
Clostridial diseases—C, D, and T (CORE)	Vaccinate at 6–8 weeks, and revaccinate 3–4 weeks later. If ewes were not vaccinated for *Cl. perfringens*, their lambs may be vaccinated at 2–3 days of age and revaccinated 2–3 weeks later. Feeder lambs should be vaccinated at time of purchase, and 2–4 weeks later.	If not previously vaccinated, ewes must be vaccinated twice at 6–4 weeks before lambing, with the last dose 4 weeks before lambing. If previously vaccinated a single dose is sufficient. Revaccinate annually. Withdrawal time 21 days.
Footrot *Dichelobacter nodosus*	Vaccinate before the anticipated problem. Revaccinate between 6 weeks and 6 months later,	Revaccinate every 6 months. Withdrawal time 60 days.
Caseous lymphadenitis *Corynebacterium pseudotuberculosis*	Vaccinate sheep and goats over 3 months of age. Revaccinate 4 weeks later on the opposite side of the animal.	May be combined with clostridia. Annual revaccination. Withdrawal time 21 days. Do not use in known infected animals because a severe reaction may result.
Campylobacter fetus-jejuni bacterin	Vaccinate before breeding and revaccinate in 60–90 days.	Annual revaccination. Withdrawal time 21 days.
Bacterial pneumonia (*M. haemolytica* and *P. multocida*)	Vaccinate breeding ewes and revaccinate 2–4 weeks apart. Revaccinate again 2–4 weeks before lambing. Lambs vaccinated under 3 months should be vaccinated at 4–6 months.	Revaccinate ewes annually before breeding or during pregnancy according to the label recommendations. May be combined with clostridia. Withdrawal time 21 days.
Chlamydia	Vaccinate 60 days before breeding and revaccinate 30 days later.	Administered with Campylobacter bacterins. Annual revaccination. Withdrawal time 60 days.
Anthrax	In known problem areas vaccinate twice at a 2–3 week interval.	Withdrawal time 42 days. Annual revaccination.
Viral Diseases		
Soremouth	Vaccinate lambs at 1 month. Revaccinate 2–3 months later. Range lambs entering a feedlot should be vaccinated at least 10 days previously.	Use this vaccine well ahead of lambing or showing. Do not use within 24 hours of dipping or spraying. Withdrawal time 21 days.
Bluetongue	Vaccinate lambs over 3 months of age and revaccinate 3 weeks before the breeding season or after lambing.	Do not vaccinate pregnant animals. Vaccine is strain specific so select it carefully. Withdrawal time 21 days.
Rabies	Vaccinate lambs over 3 months of age.	Revaccinate annually or 3 yearly depending on the vaccine. Withdrawal time 21 days.

This table is an example of a consensus vaccination program. Individual programs are variable and will reflect animal health, local environmental and housing conditions, severity of challenge, and disease prevalence in addition to professional judgment. Be sure to follow the manufacturer's recommendations on the label.

or longer against homologous challenge. The reduced immunogenicity of multivalent vaccines appears to be caused by competition between their antigens. Attempts to produce a universal footrot vaccine have been unsuccessful.

Autogenous, outbreak-specific footrot vaccines have also been used successfully. In flocks infected with just one or two serogroups, serogroup-specific fimbrial or whole cell vaccines may be effective and permit eradication of the disease. If flocks are infected by more than one serogroup then sequential vaccination cycles using monovalent vaccines given at three-monthly intervals over several years may also prove effective.

Footrot is a seasonal disease because it results from animals standing in water and mud for prolonged periods. The vaccine should be given four months before the start of the "wet" season. Because duration of immunity is so short, sheep may require boosting every three to six months.

Vaccination for footrot is simply another tool that should be used in conjunction with other procedures, such as regular foot trimming and foot soaking in disinfectant baths in an effort to eliminate the infection.

CASEOUS LYMPHADENITIS

This disease of sheep is caused by *Corynebacterium pseudotuberculosis*. It causes abscess formation in lymph nodes. If the organism becomes systemic it can cause a chronic wasting disease. *C. pseudotuberculosis* also causes an acute disease of buffalo called edematous skin disease. Caseous lymphadenitis results from wound infections and may be associated with poor hygiene during shearing. It is a robust organism and can persist in the environment for up to a year. A formalin-inactivated bacterin using biovar 1 is used in healthy sheep and goats over three months of age. Adverse reactions have occurred in goats given the sheep vaccine. Once the prevalence of infection is reduced to a low level then infected animals should be culled rather than vaccinated.

CAMPYLOBACTER FETUS

Campylobacter fetus is one of the most common causes of abortion, late fetal loss in ewes, and the birth of dead or weak lambs. It is rarely a problem in goats. It may be prevented by vaccination given shortly before breeding. Two inactivated vaccines are available in the United States. They contain both *C. fetus* and *Campylobacter jejuni*. A third vaccine is available in Australia and New Zealand. This may contain multiple *C. fetus* strains (DL42, 6/1, 134) in addition to *C. jejuni*. Immunity develops in about 21 days. Do not use the vaccine licensed for cattle in sheep.

BACTERIAL PNEUMONIA

Bronchopneumonia caused by *Pasteurella multocida*, *Bibersteinia trehalosi*, and *Mannheimia haemolytica* is common in sheep and goats of all ages. It may be especially important in young lambs that have received insufficient colostrum. These organisms are normal inhabitants of the sheep nasopharynx. In times of stress caused by shipping, weather extremes, or overcrowding they can invade the lungs and cause pneumonia. Several types of vaccine are available to control these infections. These include whole cell bacterins, leukotoxin-toxoids, and cell surface iron binding proteins. The whole cell bacterins rely on outer membrane protein antigens specific for each serotype. *M. haemolytica* has 12 serotypes of which A2 is the most prevalent. Unfortunately, A2 is poorly immunogenic in sheep. As expected, these bacterins work reasonably well against homologous serotypes, but are less effective in protecting against unrelated serotypes.

Leukotoxins are critical virulence factors for *M. haemolytica* because they kill white blood cells. Addition of a leukotoxoid to these vaccines thus increases their efficacy. Like the outer membrane proteins, however, there is a great diversity in leukotoxin types.

M. haemolytica needs iron for growth. It expresses iron-binding proteins (siderophores) on its surface. Antibodies against these siderophores will effectively reduce its growth. Like the outer membrane proteins and leukotoxoids these proteins differ between different bacterial strains. However, when used in a vaccine against the appropriate strain they can be very effective.

The prevalence of respiratory disease in lambs increases beginning around three weeks of age. Maternal antibodies to these organisms appear to interfere minimally with vaccination of lambs so they can be vaccinated as early as 10 days of age. They should then be boosted three to four weeks later. A third booster may be needed around 12 to 14 weeks of age. If sheep are intensively housed and at high risk of respiratory disease then they may be revaccinated semiannually or annually.

OVINE ENZOOTIC ABORTION

The gram-negative intracellular bacterium, *Chlamydia abortus,* causes enzootic abortion in sheep and goats worldwide. Infected animals shed large amounts of the agent in the diseased placenta and uterine fluids. Killed vaccines are widely available. A temperature-sensitive mutant (strain 1B) has been generated by inducing mutations in a wild type strain (AB7) using the mutagen, N-methyl-N'-nitro-N-nitrosoguanidine. This organism has a reduced growth rate at 39.5°C. It is used in some European countries. Unfortunately, strain 1B has been implicated in cases of vaccine breakdown. Genomic sequencing has indicated that its genomic sequence is identical to its parent strain. As a result, it is not attenuated and can cause serious disease outbreaks. Vaccine-identical strains have been isolated from cases of disease.

Antiviral Vaccines

SOREMOUTH

Contagious ecthyma (orf, soremouth, or scabby mouth) is a skin disease of sheep and goats. The virus infects wounds around the mouth (often caused by abrasions or thorns such as from prickly pear cactus). As a result of these large painful lesions, the lamb or kid is unable to suckle. The infection may then spread to the ewe and cause mastitis.

Soremouth vaccine is unique because it contains virulent virus obtained from the scabs of affected animals. Lambs should be vaccinated when around one month of age. A booster may be administered two to three months later. The vaccine is brushed on to scarified, woolless skin at a time and place chosen by the sheep producer. It is commonly administered by a scratch to the inner thigh or foreleg of a lamb. The vaccine may be available in a container with the needle attached and a dye to ensure a successful take. Otherwise the vaccine may simply be brushed over the scratches. Ewes are vaccinated inside the ear or under the tail. The site should be checked 7 to 10 days after vaccination to ensure vaccine "take." If positive, the scratch will be raised and inflamed (Fig. 17.1). It produces an uncomfortable lesion, but after 12 to 14 days the scab falls off, the lesions heal, and the young animal is immune. They should be revaccinated annually. Ewes and does should be vaccinated well ahead of lambing. Animals should not be vaccinated immediately before a show. Vaccinated animals should be segregated from unprotected animals until the scabs have fallen off.

Soremouth is a zoonosis and will cause disease in humans. Vaccinators must therefore wear appropriate protection, including gloves and goggles. Flocks that are free of soremouth must not use this vaccine because it introduces the virus into a flock.

BLUETONGUE

Bluetongue virus (BTV) is a member of the Orbivirus genus in the *Reoviridae* family. Currently the BTV species contains 26 recognized serotypes, including Toggenburg virus (BTV 25) and

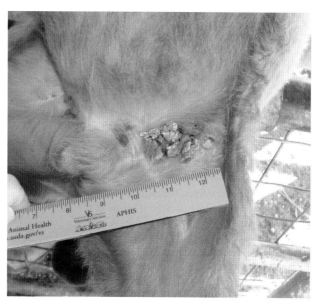

Fig. 17.1   A lesion produced on the inner thigh of a kid as a result of vaccination against soremouth (orf). (Courtesy of Dr. Jeffrey Musser.)

serotype 26 found in Kuwait. Serotypes 1, 2, 11, 13, and 17 are present in the United States. Serotype 8 is present in Northern Europe. It is transmitted by the bite of infected midges (*Culicoides*) and as a result it has a seasonal occurrence.

BTV can infect wild and domestic ruminants including sheep, goats, cattle, buffalo, deer, and antelope. Bluetongue infection is inapparent in most infected animals. Nevertheless, it can result in lethal disease in infected sheep and wild ruminants. BTV usually does not cause clinical disease in cattle except for serotype 8 in Europe.

Vaccination is used to minimize virus spread and allow the safe movement of animals. Both live attenuated and inactivated BTV vaccines are available for use in sheep or sheep and cattle. Studies suggest that they both provide protection for at least a year. Recombinant BTV vaccines have been investigated but none have been licensed.

Viruses for inactivated vaccines are grown in large-scale suspension cell systems under controlled conditions. When the culture reaches its maximum titer the cells are disrupted, the supernatant clarified and filtered. The virus is then inactivated by the addition of binary ethyleneimine or other inactivants. The inactivated virus is then concentrated and stored. Antibodies appear in response to vaccination by seven days but the duration of immunity is unclear.

Live attenuated vaccines have been produced by adapting field isolates to growth in tissue culture or embryonated chicken eggs. These modified live virus-bluetongue virus (MLV-BTV) strains retain the ability to replicate in the vaccinated animal and as a result can stimulate a strong antibody response after a single dose of vaccine. Antibodies appear by 10 days postvaccination, reach a maximum 4 weeks later, and persist for over a year. However, these vaccines, if underattenuated, may also depress milk production in lactating ewes. They also cause abortions and nervous system malformations in lambs especially if ewes were vaccinated during the first half of gestation. MLV-BTVs also cause a viremia and, as a result, may be spread by their vectors to other unvaccinated animals. Transmission of vaccine strains by the *Culicoides* vector midge has been documented in Europe and the United States.

A monovalent tissue culture derived, MLV-BTV type 10 vaccine, is available in the United States. It may be used in goats. A monovalent inactivated BTV-8 vaccine is available in the

United Kingdom and Northern Europe to fight an outbreak of BTV that began in 2006. The vaccine is given to sheep and cattle over 2.5 months of age. Animals require two doses of vaccine, 20 days (sheep) and 31 days (cattle) after the second dose, to develop protective immunity and prevent viremia. Nevertheless, blanket vaccination of cattle, sheep, and goats has brought the disease largely under control although occasional outbreaks continue to occur in France and Germany. Interestingly, cattle still had antibodies six years after receiving the BTV-8 vaccine.

Because many BTV serotypes may be circulating within a geographic area, polyvalent vaccines are often required. Thus in South Africa, 15 serotypes are administered sequentially in three formulations each containing five different serotypes attenuated by passage in embryonated chicken eggs and baby hamster kidney cells. Not all these serotypes induce a strong response so the animals are revaccinated annually.

RABIES

In rabies endemic areas, sheep and goats may be required to be vaccinated against rabies. This should be administered to lambs and kids over three months of age and repeated annually. Sheep grazing public lands and attending livestock shows may also be required to be vaccinated.

Other Vaccines

Q FEVER

Coxiella burnetii causes Q (query) fever in humans and coxiellosis in animals. It is a significant zoonosis. In small ruminants and cattle, it is associated with sporadic abortions, and dead or weak lambs and kids. It may cause infertility in cattle. An inactivated vaccine that contains phase 1 *C. burnetii* (Coxevac vaccine; Ceva) is available in parts of Europe. It is used in goats to prevent abortions and minimize bacterial shedding. The vaccine is given in two doses at least three weeks before breeding. Annual revaccination is required in affected areas.

In 2007, a massive Q fever outbreak occurred in the Netherlands. Many goat farmers used the inactivated *C. burnetii* vaccine. The Dutch government tested bulk milk from these dairy farms for the presence of Coxiella DNA. In 2010, several goat farmers claimed that their milk had tested positive for this DNA despite using the killed vaccine. Analysis showed however that the DNA did indeed originate in the killed vaccine. Thus the vaccine-derived DNA appeared in goat's milk two hours after vaccination and could persist for as long as nine days. It represented more than a million-fold dilution of the vaccine dose—an example of the extreme sensitivity of polymerase chain reaction (PCR) assays. The problem was "solved" by requiring a two-week interval between vaccination and bulk milk testing.

SHEEP AND GOAT POX

These two infections are endemic to northern Africa, the Middle East, and Asia. Some European countries have also experienced outbreaks. They cause skin and lung lesions leading to death in small ruminants. They are related to the poxvirus that causes lumpy skin disease and are collectively designated as capripox viruses. Both live and inactivated vaccines have been developed for these diseases. All strains of capripox, irrespective of their species of origin, share a major neutralizing epitope so that there is cross-protection among all three species. Inactivated vaccines generally give short-term protection. They contain only antigens from the intracellular virus and lack the major antigenic components from the virus envelope. It is important to determine virus strain identity and their degree of attenuation before a product is licensed because the protective dose required for prevention varies between strains. These capripox vaccines provide protection for 12 to 30 months depending on the strain employed.

BRUCELLOSIS

Brucellosis is a significant cause of abortion in sheep and goats. As in cattle, killed vaccines cannot prevent brucellosis in these species. As a result, the attenuated strain of *Brucella melitensis*, Rev.1 is widely used for the prevention of brucellosis in sheep and goats. Rev.1 was generated by the use of streptomycin as a selective agent from a virulent field strain of *B. melitensis*. It is injected subcutaneously or dropped into the conjunctiva of lambs and kids between three and five months of age. Conjunctival vaccination is considered safer than subcutaneous injection. Generally, the entire flock should be vaccinated at one time during the late lambing season or lactation, especially when they are managed under extensive conditions. Attempts to control the disease by vaccinating only young replacement females have been unsuccessful. The immunizing dose is from 0.5 to 2×10^9 viable organisms (cfu). *Brucella melitensis* strain Rev.1 vaccine like *B. abortus* S19, can infect humans so appropriate precautions should be taken against needlestick injury (Chapter 10). It should not be given to pregnant animals because a full standard dose may cause abortion. Reducing the vaccine dose may minimize abortions, but result in unsatisfactory immunity. Also, like S19, it has a smooth lipopolysaccharide that is detected by serologic assays and is thus incompatible with conventional test-and-slaughter programs.

Brucella ovis is a significant cause of epididymitis and infertility in rams. It is associated with abortions and perinatal mortality but its main impact is on males. There is no current vaccine specific for *B. ovis* but vaccination with *B. melitensis* Rev.1 is protective. Unfortunately, this also interferes with surveillance and eradication programs.

In China, *Brucella suis* strain 2 is the preferred attenuated vaccine to prevent ovine and caprine brucellosis. It is administered orally. It retains some virulence when injected parenterally and should not be used in pregnant animals.

CONTAGIOUS AGALACTIA

Caused by *Mycoplasma agalactiae,* this is a significant disease in Africa, Asia, and in the Mediterranean region. In addition to agalactia and mammary lesions, affected animals develop arthritis, conjunctivitis, respiratory disease, and abortion. Both inactivated and modified live vaccines are widely employed to prevent the disease. The major limitation is however strain specificity. Immunity is short so animals must be revaccinated every six months. The inactivated vaccines do not prevent infection but simply reduce disease severity.

LEPTOSPIROSIS

Leptospirosis may be a significant disease affecting some sheep and goat flocks where it can cause abortions, renal damage, and lamb deaths. The primary causes are *Leptospira interrogans* serovar Pomona and *Leptospira borgpetersenii* serovar Hardjo. Currently available combined bacterins provide protection for several months but the duration of immunity is unclear.

PESTE DES PETITS RUMINANTS

Peste des petits ruminants (PPR) is one of the most important and dangerous diseases affecting small ruminants in Africa, the Middle East, and in Central and Southeast Asia. PPR is caused by small ruminant morbillivirus (PPRV) closely related to rinderpest and distemper. (It is also called ovine rinderpest.) PPRVs have been grouped into four genetic lineages. All four lineages occur in Africa while lineage 4 also occurs in Asia. Cross-protection occurs among viruses of all four lineages. In December 2016, the disease reached Mongolia and in June 2018 it reached Bulgaria.

PPRV is highly lethal for goats with up to 100% mortality. It is less lethal for sheep who may be subclinically infected. Not only does PPRV infect sheep and goats, but occasionally also camels, cattle, and buffalo. It has caused massive mortalities in wild ungulates such as saiga antelope (*Saiga tatarica*). The animals develop a fever with the development of vesicular lesions on the oral mucosa, ocular and nasal discharge, leukopenia, diarrhea, and dyspnea. Death occurs as a result of bronchopneumonia, diarrhea, and dehydration. PPRV causes profound immunosuppression so affected animals may also die as a result of secondary bacterial and mycoplasma infections.

In 1989, an attenuated PPRV vaccine was developed by serial passage of a Nigerian strain in Vero cells. This vaccine was highly successful. Vaccinated sheep and goats were protected and the vaccine virus was not transmitted to contact animals. Subsequently attenuated vaccines against Indian goat and sheep strains have been developed using a similar technique and have also proved highly effective. These vaccines protect animals for at least four years.

One problem with live attenuated vaccines used in the tropics is maintaining the cold chain. Live attenuated PPRV strains are thermolabile, but have a shelf life of around one year at 4°C. Many efforts have been made to improve freeze-drying techniques and develop new stabilizers. Likewise, extensive efforts have been made to develop recombinant vectored vaccines involving capripox, fowlpox, or adenoviruses as vectors (Chapter 5). Some recombinant PPRV vaccines may therefore also protect against goat and sheep pox.

The major limitation of currently available vaccines is the absence of a DIVA capability that would enable vaccinated animals to be differentiated from naturally infected animals.

The global eradication of the related morbillivirus, rinderpest has had an interesting consequence in that PPR is spreading throughout Africa south of the Sahara and also the Middle East, Morocco, China, and Bhutan. Likewise, the Asian genotype 4 has now become established in the Sudan. A plan to globally eradicate PPR by 2030 was initiated by the World Organization for Animal Health (OIE) and Food and Agriculture Organization (FAO) in 2015. The virus has an estimated R_0 of 4.0 to 6.9 and the herd immunity threshold is 75% to 86%. Mass vaccination campaigns seek a minimum of 70% coverage.

PRODUCTION ENHANCING VACCINES

Sheep immunized with polyandroalbumin (androstenedione-7-carboxyethyl thioester linked to human serum albumin) produce about 23% more lambs than untreated sheep. These vaccines are marketed under the names Androvax, Fecundin, and Ovastim. Ewes are given two doses of this vaccine before mating. It is believed that the vaccine induces autoantibodies that reduce serum androstenedione levels. This temporarily blocks ovulation so that when the effect wears off, the ewe responds by producing more mature ova. Therefore if bred at this time the number of multiple births will be increased. The vaccine is used in young healthy ewes of breeds that can feed the increased number of lambs. Ewes that are in poor condition may not benefit from this vaccine. Adequate nutrition, parasite control, and shelter must be provided to take advantage of this increased productivity. The priming dose is given six to nine weeks before mating and the booster three to four weeks before breeding. A minimum of three weeks should elapse between boosting and breeding. Vaccinated ewes may be revaccinated annually three to four weeks before mating.

Adverse Events

In sheep, pulmonary signs predominate in anaphylaxis as a result of constriction of the bronchi and pulmonary vessels. Smooth muscle contraction also occurs in the bladder and intestine with predictable results. The major mediators of type I hypersensitivity in sheep are histamine, serotonin, leukotrienes, and kinins. Clostridial vaccines do tend to induce adverse reactions ranging from local swelling and stiffness to fever, pulmonary edema, abortion, and bloating. Aluminum adjuvants may cause injection site granulomas.

Related Species

GOATS

The most important "core" vaccine that should be used in goats is CD-T, the combined vaccine for *Clostridium perfringens* types C and D, plus tetanus. Pregnant does should receive the vaccine 30 days before birth. Kids should be vaccinated at five to six weeks of age, given a booster three to four weeks later, and boosted annually. It has been suggested that the duration of immunity against clostridia in goats is shorter than that in sheep so allowance may have to be made for this. Rabies vaccination should be considered in rabies endemic areas. Optional goat vaccines may include, caseous lymphadenitis, soremouth, rabies, footrot, Chlamydia, Leptospirosis, *Mannheimia haemolytica*, and *Pasteurella multocida*. As always, it is essential to keep a record of vaccinations given.

LLAMAS AND OTHER CAMELIDS

All vaccines used in llamas and related species have to be used in an extra-label fashion having been specifically developed primarily in cattle and small ruminants. Thus if a veterinarian uses a vaccine in a species not specified on the label or on the insert, then they assume full responsibility for product failure or any adverse consequences. A product licensed for use in another species may be used if there is a demonstrated need for it and if there is reasonable evidence that it can be expected to be efficacious.

As with sheep and goats, the most important llama vaccine is the triple clostridial vaccine CD-T. Although developed for small ruminants it would almost certainly be effective in llamas and alpacas. A typical vaccination schedule for llamas is similar to that described in goats above. Other optional llama vaccines may include other Clostridial vaccines, West Nile Virus, leptospirosis, rabies, and coronavirus.

Sources of Additional Information

Akan, M., Oncel, T., Sasreyyupoglu, B., Haziroglu, R., et al. (2006). Vaccination studies of lambs against experimental *Mannheimia (Pasteurella) haemolytica* infection. *Small Ruminant Research*, 65, 44–50.

Baetza, H.J. (2014). Eradication of bluetongue disease in Germany by vaccination. *Vet Immunol Immunopathol*, 158, 116–119.

Blasco, J.M. (1997). A review of the use of *B. melitensis* Rev 1 vaccine in adult sheep and goats. *Prev Vet Med*, 31, 275–283.

Council Report. (1994). Vaccination guidelines for small ruminants (sheep, goats, llamas, domestic deer, and wapiti). *JAVMA*, 205, 1539–1544.

Dhungyel, O., Hunter, J., Whittington, R. (2014). Footrot vaccines and vaccination. *Vaccine*, 32, 3139–3146.

Kumar, N., Barua, S., Riyesh, T., Tripathi, B.N. (2017). Advances in peste des petits ruminants vaccines. *Vet Microbiol*, 206, 91–101.

Kyriakis, C.S. (2015). Tomorrow's vector vaccines for small ruminants. *Vet Microbiol*, 181, 47–52.

Lacasta, D., Ferrer, L.M., Ramos, J.J., Gonzalez, J.M., Ortin, A., Fthenakis, G.C. (2015). Vaccination schedules in small ruminant farms. 181, 34–48.

Raadsma, H.W., Egerton, J.R. (2013). A review of footrot in sheep: Aetiology, risk factors and control methods. *Livestock Sci*, 156, 106–114.

Rossi, A., Monaco, A., Guarnaschelli, J., Silveira, F. et al. (2018). Temporal evaluation of anti-*Clostridium* antibody responses in sheep after vaccination with polyvalent clostridial vaccines. *Vet Immunol Immunopathol*, 202, 46–51.

van Rijn, P.A., Daus, F.J., Maris-Veldhuis, M.A., Feenstra, F., van Gennip, R.G.P. (2017). Bluetomgue disabled infectious single animal (DISA) vaccine: Studies on the optomal dose and route in sheep. *Vaccine*, 35, 231–237.

Porcine Vaccines

The basic principles of vaccinating pigs are the same as in other species. Thus for diseases that are threats to growing piglets, injectable vaccines should be administered as soon as maternal antibody titers have waned. This is generally considered to be around three to six weeks of age. These piglets may then need to be boosted two to four weeks later depending on the manufacturer's recommendations. Because maternal antibodies do not interfere with mucosal immunity, oral or intranasal vaccines may be administered much earlier. There are many infections that pose a significant threat to newborn piglets. These are controlled by vaccinating pregnant sows and thus promoting the production of colostral antibodies. It is noticeable that many pig vaccines appear to take a long time to induce protective immunity. Examples include the vaccines against foot-and-mouth disease, *Lawsonia intracellularis*, and porcine respiratory and reproductive syndrome (PRRS) (Tables 18.1 and 18.2).

Vaccine Administration

INJECTION

As always, it is essential to follow the manufacturer's recommendations regarding administration route, dose, and any withdrawal period. Vaccines given in an inappropriate manner or in the wrong place can trigger injection site reactions and carcass blemishes. As a result, subcutaneous vaccines should be administered, preferably behind the ear, using a short 12-mm, 18-gauge needle. Pigs must be restrained firmly to prevent needle breakage. If an intramuscular injection is required, a 38-mm, 18-gauge needle will be required for sows and gilts. For suckling pigs, a short 12-mm needle is adequate for injecting into muscle. The neck is the preferred site for intramuscular injections. It is important to ensure that the intramuscular vaccine is injected into the muscle, not into the subcutaneous fat. Multiple vaccines may be given on the same day but the injections should be given at different sites. When using a bottled multidose vaccine, a sterile needle should be used to withdraw the vaccine into the syringe, whereas another needle is used to inject the pig. Only healthy pigs should be vaccinated.

NEEDLE-FREE INJECTION

Swine producers are increasingly using needle-free injection devices, such as high-pressure jet injectors to improve vaccination speed and safety, and to minimize carcass quality issues arising from injection site lesions (Fig. 18.1). Use of these transdermal devices has many advantages

TABLE 18.1 ■ Vaccination of Piglets Under 6 Months of Age

Vaccine	Vaccine Timing	Comments
Antibacterial Vaccines		
Swine erysipelas	Vaccinate with 2 doses, 3–4 weeks apart beginning at 6–8 weeks of age.	An oral vaccine can be given to piglets over 8 weeks of age. Withdrawal time 21 days.
Colibacillosis	An oral vaccine may be given in the drinking water before weaning to prevent postweaning scours. To prevent edema disease, vaccines are administered in drinking water to piglets over 18 days.	Most vaccines against colibacillosis are given to sows before farrowing. Withdrawal time 21 days.
Mycoplasmal pneumonia	Vaccinate healthy piglets over 3 weeks of age. Revaccinate 2–3 weeks later.	There is also a single dose vaccine available given at 3 weeks of age. Semiannual revaccination is recommended for some vaccines. Withdrawal time 21 days.
Atrophic rhinitis (Bordetella)	Vaccinate intranasally within 1–3 days of age. The precise timing depends on the vaccine.	Withdrawal time 21 days.
Pleuropneumonia *Actinobacillus pleuropneumoniae*	Vaccinate at weaning (4–5 weeks) and 3–4 weeks later.	A third dose may be administered in the case of an outbreak or an imminent threat. Withdrawal time 21 days.
Porcine proliferative enteritis	Vaccinate piglets over 3 weeks of age with a single intramuscular dose. Oral vaccines are administered in drinking water to piglets over 3 weeks of age.	Withdrawal time 21 days.
Glasser's disease *Haemophilus parasuis*	Vaccinate piglets over 5 weeks of age and boosted 2–3 weeks later.	Some vaccines may be given at 7–10 days. Withdrawal time 21 days.
Salmonellosis	Drinking water vaccine given to piglets over 2–3 weeks of age. Injectable, given to piglets over 3–5 weeks of age. Intranasal may be given to piglets over 1 day of age.	Withdrawal time 21 days.
Streptococcus suis	Vaccinate piglets at 3 and 5 weeks of age if the sow has not been vaccinated.	Withdrawal time 21 days.
Antiviral Vaccines		
Porcine parvovirus	Vaccinate with 2 doses, 3–5 weeks apart with the second dose 2–4 weeks before breeding.	Revaccinate annually before breeding. Revaccinate boars semiannually. Withdrawal time 21 days.
Pseudorabies	Vaccinate piglets 1–7 days old intranasally, followed by intramuscular vaccination of all the other pigs on the farm.	Revaccinate breeding animals semiannually. Withdrawal time 21 days.
Porcine circovirus	Vaccinate at 3 weeks of age, revaccinate at 6 weeks. Some producers prefer 1 and 3 weeks of age or even at 2 and 4 weeks.	Withdrawal time 21 days.

TABLE 18.1 ■ Vaccination of Piglets Under 6 Months of Age (Continued)

Vaccine	Vaccine Timing	Comments
Porcine respiratory and reproductive syndrome virus	Vaccinate piglets over 3 weeks of age with a single dose. Another such vaccine may be given at 1 day of age. The autogenous intranasal vaccine may be administered at 7–10 days and at weaning (3 weeks).	Boosted semiannually. Withdrawal time 21 days.
Porcine epidemic diarrhea	Vaccinate piglets over 3 weeks of age and revaccinate 3 weeks later.	Withdrawal time 21 days.
Influenza	Vaccinate piglets over 3–5 weeks intramuscularly, followed by a second dose 2–3 weeks later. Vaccinate piglets over 1 day of age. intranasally.	Revaccinate semiannually. Withdrawal time 21 days.
Rotavirus	Vaccinate with the oral or injectable vaccine at 7–10 days preweaning.	If using the oral vaccine do not return the piglet to the sow for at least 30 minutes. Withdrawal time 21 days.

These tables are examples of consensus vaccination programs. Individual programs are variable and will reflect animal health, local environmental and housing conditions, severity of challenge, and disease prevalence, in addition to professional judgment. Be sure to follow the manufacturer's recommendations on the label.

TABLE 18.2 ■ Vaccination of Adult Pigs

Vaccine	Vaccine Timing	Comments
Antibacterial Vaccines		
Swine erysipelas	Vaccinate gilts and boars at 6.5 months or older and boosted 3–4 weeks later. Sows should be boosted on the day of weaning before rebreeding. Alternatively, pigs should receive 2 doses 3–5 weeks apart, with the second dose 2–4 weeks before breeding.	Withdrawal time 21 days.
Colibacillosis	Vaccinate gilts and sows 5 and 2 weeks before farrowing. Timing depends upon the brand of vaccine; two doses are given 4–8 weeks and 2–3 weeks before farrowing. In second or subsequent pregnancies a single dose may be given 2–3 weeks before farrowing.	Withdrawal time 21 days.
Leptospirosis	Vaccinate breeding pigs including boars, twice 4–6 weeks apart. Revaccinate every 6 months. Any new boars and gilts entering the breeding herd also need to be vaccinated. Do not vaccinate periparturient sows.	Withdrawal time 21 days.
Atrophic rhinitis (Bordetella)	Vaccinate sows about 2–5 weeks before farrowing.	Withdrawal time 21 days.

Continued on following page

TABLE 18.2 ▨ **Vaccination of Adult Pigs** (Continued)

Vaccine	Vaccine Timing	Comments
Clostridial dysentery	Vaccinate sows 2–6 weeks before farrowing. Revaccinate sows before each subsequent farrowing.	Withdrawal time 21 days.
Pleuropneumonia	Revaccinate annually or semiannually.	Withdrawal time 21–60 days.
Glasser's disease	Vaccinate feeder pigs on arrival and boost 2 weeks later.	Withdrawal time 21 days.
Streptococcus suis	Vaccinate gilts and sows 5 and 2 weeks before farrowing.	Withdrawal time 21 days.
Antiviral Vaccines		
Porcine parvovirus	Vaccinate breeding sows and boars 3–4 weeks apart. Sows should be boosted at each weaning. Boars should receive 6 monthly boosting.	Withdrawal time 21 days.
Pseudorabies	Vaccinate sows and piglets intranasally when 1–7 days old, followed by intramuscular vaccination of all the other pigs on the farm.	Withdrawal time 21 days.
Porcine respiratory and reproductive syndrome virus	Vaccinate sows and gilts 3–4 weeks before breeding or during pregnancy to prevent the reproductive form of the disease.	Withdrawal time 21 days.
Porcine epidemic diarrhea	Vaccinate pregnant sows, 5 and 3 weeks before farrowing.	In subsequent pregnancies give a single dose 2 weeks before farrowing.
Influenza	Vaccinate healthy breeding pigs in 2 doses 3–5 weeks apart. Revaccinate 2–4 weeks before breeding.	Revaccinate boars semiannually and sows annually before breeding. Withdrawal time 21 days.
Transmissible gastroenteritis	Vaccinate sows and gilts orally with two doses 3–5 weeks before farrowing and boost with the intramuscular (IM) vaccine one week before farrowing. Otherwise give the IM vaccine 5 and 2 weeks before each farrowing.	Prime with the oral vaccine and boost with an intramuscular vaccine. Withdrawal time 21 days.
Rotavirus	Used with transmissible gastroenteritis. Vaccinate sows 2–5 weeks before farrowing.	Prime with the oral vaccine and boost with an intramuscular vaccine. Withdrawal time 21 days.

These tables are examples of consensus vaccination programs. Individual programs are variable and will reflect animal health, local environmental and housing conditions, severity of challenge and disease prevalence in addition to professional judgment. Be sure to follow the manufacturer's recommendations on the label.

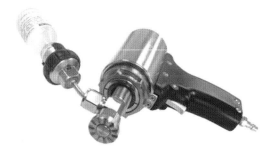

Fig. 18.1 A high-pressure jet injector used to vaccinate pigs. This instrument is powered by either compressed air or liquid CO_2. It delivers a vaccine dose of 0.1ml to 0.5ml. (Courtesy of Pulse NeedleFree Systems, Inc.)

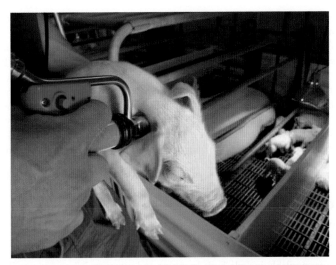

Fig. 18.2   The use of a high pressure jet injector in piglets is less traumatic, less painful, and reduces injection site lesions when compared with syringe and needle injections. (Courtesy of Pulse NeedleFree Systems, Inc.)

including improved safety as a result of the following: elimination of broken needles and accidental needle sticks; required needle disposal and consistent vaccine delivery; reduced vaccine volume, greater antigen dispersion, faster administration, and reduced pain and distress. As described in Chapter 8, these high-pressure jet injectors permit the vaccine antigen to penetrate the epidermis and dermis. They require one-half to one-tenth of a conventional dose of vaccine administered by syringe because of the widespread antigen dispersion and its subdermal location. Disadvantages include the start-up cost of equipment, its infrastructure (especially if using a high-pressure CO_2 gas supply), its maintenance, the required operator training, and some uncertainty as to the dose of antigen delivered. Newer devices have disposable nozzle faces that can be changed when necessary and when used in different farms. These devices therefore have the advantage of preventing the spread of infection that results from needle use. Transdermal jet injectors are best used at sites where the skin is thin, soft, and hairless. They should not be administered over bone or thick fat. In piglets the best site is the neck (Fig. 18.2).

PRRSV, porcine circovirus type 2 (PCV2), and *Mycoplasma hyopneumoniae* vaccines designed specifically for transdermal administration have been licensed in Europe.

ORAL VACCINATION

Although vaccines have traditionally been administered by subcutaneous or intramuscular injection, the growth of large pig growing enterprises has stimulated a switch to other methods of mass vaccination. Oral vaccination is increasingly used in swine operations. Individual animals may be drenched, but delivery through the watering system is preferred. The vaccine is added to the water delivery system to deliver the correct antigen dose to each pig. Generally, water is withheld from the pigs for one to two hours before vaccination depending on environmental conditions. All medications, sanitizers, and disinfectants must be removed from the drinking water first. Likewise, the system must be flushed with nonchlorinated water beforehand. Antibiotics or other antimicrobials should not be used from three days before to three days after vaccination (total seven days). However, a nonmedicated week is ideal after vaccination. The lines from the vaccine container to the furthest spigot or pen drinker must be precharged with vaccine solution. The amount should be such that the pigs receive the correct vaccine dose within four hours.

To accurately add the correct dose of vaccine to the water supply, a proportioner is used. This is a device that accurately feeds a measured amount of vaccine solution into the water supply. Before administering the vaccine, it is essential to calibrate the proportioner by measuring the flow-rate of water through the device for the same period and with the same pigs to be vaccinated to ensure that each pig receives an appropriate dose of vaccine. Alternatively, the vaccine solution can be added to the water line using a peristaltic pump, which will also require calibration. If these are not available, the vaccine may be added to a measured amount of water in a trough.

To ensure that the vaccine remains stable in the drinking water, it is common to add a stabilizer. In most cases thiosulfate blue is used to neutralize any chlorine. Skimmed milk may be used if thiosulfate blue is not available. The blue dye or the milk also indicates the presence of the vaccine in the water.

Antibacterial Vaccines

SWINE ERYSIPELAS

Erysipelothrix rhusiopathiae causes diamond skin disease in addition to arthritis, heart disease, and abortion. Vaccines available include both bacterins and attenuated live products. The immunity produced by these bacterins is relatively short lived, usually lasting no longer than one year and sometimes considerably less. For instance, a formalin-inactivated erysipelas bacterin protects for only four to five months, and breeding stock should therefore be revaccinated every six months. Modified live vaccines are available for use in breeding herds. Some brands may be given orally. However, the modified live strains may spread to other, unvaccinated pigs and reversion to virulence is a concern. It is also essential that piglets not be vaccinated before maternal antibody titers have waned. This is generally assumed to be around three to six weeks. Any earlier and maternal antibodies may block their responses. Vaccination failures are multifactorial and may occur in response to improper handling of vaccine, management stress, and occasionally as a result of strain specific antigenic differences. There is usually good cross-protection between different bacterial serotypes.

COLIBACILLOSIS

Escherichia coli is probably the commonest cause of severe scouring in newborn, suckling, and weaned piglets. The currently available vaccines in the United States are either bacterins or bacterin-toxoids (inactivated *E. coli* enterotoxins). The vaccines are given to gilts and sows before farrowing to ensure that newborn piglets receive high-titered colostral antibodies. Timing depends upon the specific vaccine used. Because this type of procedure depends upon the piglets receiving colostrum, it will not work if a piglet does not suckle or the sow lactates poorly. Failure of passive transfer is always a risk in these situations.

ATROPHIC RHINITIS

Atrophic rhinitis is characterized by nasal discharge, shortening and twisting of the snout, and atrophy of the turbinate bones. Two forms of the disease are recognized. A severe form is caused by toxigenic strains of *Pasteurella multocida*, either alone or in combination with *Bordetella bronchiseptica*. A milder form is caused by *B. bronchiseptica* alone. Several adjuvanted whole cell *B. bronchiseptica* bacterins together with toxigenic or nontoxigenic strains of killed *P. multocida* or a *P. multocida* toxoid are available. The *P. multocida* bacterins are usually of capsular type D, but some also contain capsular type A. Live attenuated vaccines containing *B. bronchiseptica* are also available. Bacterins containing *B. bronchiseptica* alone are not effective in preventing the severe form of the disease but may be of use in controlling the milder form. These vaccines do not prevent nasal colonization by these bacteria. The most important *P. multocida* antigen is a toxin. As a result, *P. multocida* toxoids are highly protective. However, the level of toxoid present in some bacterins may be insufficient to produce an effective antitoxin response. Unfortunately, toxoid purification also adds to the cost of product. Recombinant toxoids have been shown to be very effective and a DNA-plasmid vaccine containing the toxoid gene also works well.

LEPTOSPIROSIS

Leptospira infections in pigs give rise to a chronic carrier state and pigs then shed the organisms in their urine. The predominant species include *Leptospira interrogans* serovars Pomona, Icterohemorrhagiae, Canicola, Hardjo, and Bratislava; *L. borgpetersenii* serovar Hardjo-bovis and *L. kirschneri* serovar Grippotyphosa. The two most common serovars in swine leptospirosis are Pomona and Bratislava. Pigs are also the maintenance hosts for serovar Bratislava. Leptospirosis rarely causes acute disease but results in infertility, sporadic abortions, stillbirths, weak piglets, and increased piglet mortality. All available Leptospira vaccines are therefore combined bacterins containing multiple serovars. These bacterins may be combined with erysipelas in a single dose vaccine (Farrowsure B, Zoetis). Vaccination will not eliminate the carrier state. As discussed in other species, immunity to Leptospira is short lasting and requires frequent re-boosting.

CLOSTRIDIAL DYSENTERY

Clostridium perfringens type C causes fatal necrohemorrhagic enteritis in piglets under three weeks of age. A type C specific toxoid may therefore be given to sows three to six weeks before farrowing to provide maternal immunity to piglets. An antitoxin is effective if given to piglets within two hours of birth.

MYCOPLASMAL DISEASES

Mycoplasma hyopneumoniae causes porcine enzootic pneumonia, a highly contagious chronic respiratory disease that causes enormous economic losses worldwide. It damages the respiratory tract so that animals develop secondary bacterial and viral infections such as porcine pleuropneumonia. This infection is especially harmful when it occurs in association with immunosuppressive viruses such as porcine respiratory and reproductive system virus or porcine circovirus-2. The control of enzootic pneumonia is mainly based on management and vaccine-induced protection. Inactivated whole bacterial vaccines are most widely employed. These bacterins may be given to piglets and to introduced growers and breeders. They prevent or reduce the severity of lung lesions while improving daily weight gain. A modified live vaccine (*Mhp*-168 strain) attenuated by more than 300 serial passages *in vitro* is used in China and may provide superior protection. A bacterin is also available against *Mycoplasma hyorhinis* a cause of arthritis, pericarditis, and peritonitis in pigs.

PORCINE PLEUROPNEUMONIA

Actinobacillus pleuropneumoniae is a major pig pathogen that causes a highly contagious severe necrotizing hemorrhagic pneumonia with high mortality. Animals that survive, fail to thrive and become asymptomatic carriers. It causes significant losses to the pig industry. Effective vaccination is difficult because of the existence of two different biotypes and 16 different serotypes based on their capsular antigen structure. The predominant serotypes vary internationally. Killed, whole cell bacterins have been widely employed, but the protection afforded is inconsistent and is generally serotype specific. These bacterins, at best, reduce mortality but do not prevent infection or even the development of lesions.

Studies on the pathogenesis of porcine pleuropneumonia show that the organism releases soluble exotoxins called Apx toxins that play a central role in disease pathogenesis. Bacterins do not contain these Apx toxins, a factor that might partially explain their lack of efficacy. Vaccines are available in some countries that incorporate three inactivated exotoxins, Apx I, II, and III. These vaccines reduce pleuritis, mortality, and lung lesions while improving daily weight gain. They do not prevent clinical disease. Other important antigens include the outer membrane proteins and pilus proteins. A 42 kDa outer membrane protein is used in combination with the Apx toxins in some vaccines (Porcilis APP, Merck and Pleurostar APP, Novartis).

Currently only bacterins containing serotypes 1, 5, and 7 are available in the United States. Because of strain specificity, the serotype present on a farm should first be identified by culture and serology before deciding on vaccination. This situation is thus one in which the use of autogenous vaccines should be considered.

SALMONELLOSIS

Salmonellae are facultative intracellular bacteria. As a result, cell-mediated immunity is more important than humoral immunity. Nevertheless, many Salmonella bacterins have been developed. Some may contain more than one serovar. The organisms are killed with formaldehyde and then adjuvanted with aluminum hydroxide or mineral oil. Attenuated live vaccines are available in some countries. A live attenuated strain of *Salmonella choleraesuis* is available that can be administered intranasally or in drinking water.

LAWSONIA ENTEROPATHY

Lawsonia intracellularis is an obligate intracellular bacterium that causes either acute disease (proliferative hemorrhagic enteritis) or a chronic disease (porcine proliferative enteropathy). It occurs in grower and finisher pigs 3 to 12 months of age and can cause significant losses. The organism causes an increase in the thickness of the intestinal wall because of hyperplasia of infected enterocytes. The acute disease results in "ileitis" that results in enterocyte necrosis, bloody diarrhea, and sudden death. In the chronic form, disease symptoms such as lethargy, chronic enteritis, and weight loss develop progressively in weaner and grower pigs. Natural infection with *L. intracellularis* stimulates effective immunity.

Two types of vaccines are currently available. An inactivated intramuscular vaccine may be given to piglets over three weeks of age. Alternatively, modified-live oral vaccines may be administered in drinking water, drenched, or in liquid feed. These should not be administered before three weeks of age because of maternal antibodies. As with all live bacterial vaccines, antibiotics should be withheld before and after vaccination. These vaccines are reconstituted in an appropriate volume of drinking water. They should be consumed within four to six hours of thawing the vaccine. There is little or no fecal shedding of the vaccine strain. This live vaccine does not appear to induce strong immunity, nevertheless antibodies to the *Lawsonia* autotransporter A (LatA) protein in addition to the flagellae and the bacterial hemolysin have been found in the serum of vaccinated pigs. It is believed that immunoglobulin A (IgA) mediates most protection, but cell-mediated responses also contribute. It takes three to four weeks before immunity develops. The vaccine does not prevent infection and additional management interventions need to be employed to control the infection on a farm. Fecal shedding and clinical disease severity are reduced, although weight gain is improved in vaccinated pigs.

GLASSER'S DISEASE

Haemophilus parasuis causes systemic disease characterized by polyserositis, polyarthritis, and meningitis. Infection is controlled by a bacterin directed against serovars 4, 5, and 13. Thus the serovar present on a farm should be identified before using the vaccine. This vaccine may be combined with *Mycoplasma pneumoniae* vaccine.

STREPTOCOCCUS SUIS

Streptococcus suis is a zoonotic pathogen that causes septicemia, pneumonia, meningitis, arthritis, and acute death. There are multiple serotypes of this organism, but serotype 2 is the most virulent and significant. Bacterins are available but do not induce protection against heterologous strains. Subunit vaccines may also contain a virulence factor, suilysin, plus a muramidase-released protein and an extracellular protein factor. They are effective against most homologous and heterologous strains. However, these antigens are not conserved in all strains. Reverse vaccinology analysis has identified other conserved extracellular proteins that may serve as protective antigens.

Antiviral Vaccines

PORCINE PARVOVIRUS

Porcine parvovirus is common in pigs and is a major cause of reproductive failure in sows resulting in early death, mummified piglets, and infertility. It was initially called SMEDI (Swine Mummification, Embryonic Death, and Infertility). Because the infection is so common the main method of control is early vaccination. An inactivated vaccine may be given to breeding pigs before first breeding. Parvovirus vaccine is also available in combination with erysipelas and leptospirosis bacterins.

PSEUDORABIES

Also called Aujesky's disease, pseudorabies is a severe neurologic disease of pigs caused by Suid herpesvirus-1 (SuHV-1). Pigs are its natural hosts, and the virus can survive latently in them. It can also cause lethal disease in ruminants, carnivores, and rodents. Vaccination must be used as part of a comprehensive disease control program. The use of continuous large-scale vaccination using DIVA vaccines has permitted the detection and removal of pigs infected with a wild-type virus. As a result, the disease has been eradicated from Canada, the United States, Mexico, many countries in Western Europe, and New Zealand. This remarkable success can serve as a model for the eradication of other diseases through the use of genetically engineered marker vaccines employing a DIVA diagnostic strategy.

The earliest pseudorabies vaccines consisted of inactivated or modified live products. As expected, the attenuated live vaccines were more effective than the killed products and they were well attenuated. Hence, they were considered very safe for application but were not DIVA compatible making eradication challenging. They protected pigs from clinical disease and decreased viral shedding, but they did not induce sterile immunity nor prevent latent infections.

These early attenuated strains, designated the Bartha or K-61 strain and the BUK (Norden) strain were used in many vaccines. Genetic sequencing revealed that both were missing a large gene segment the gene for viral glycoprotein (g)E and the Bartha strain was also missing an additional gene encoding gI. Passage of a field strain in cell culture in the presence of the mutagen bromodeoxyuridine, also resulted in loss of virulence as a result of a deletion in the virus's thymidine kinase (TK) gene.

With this knowledge, a genetically engineered TK-negative mutant became the first licensed genetically modified vaccine. Other deletion mutants soon followed. These deletions usually involved gE and gI, but gG- and gC-deleted strains have also been produced. Because these major antigens are missing, it was soon recognized that these could form the basis of a DIVA strategy.

Antibodies to gE present in wild viral strains are relatively easy to detect. Countries seeking to eradicate pseudorabies employ gE-deleted vaccines. Commercial ELISA kits are available to test for antibodies to gE. Currently in the United States there is a single modified live vaccine available with gI and gX deletions. It can be given intramuscularly or intranasally. The modified live vaccine (MLV) multiplies at the site of inoculation and in regional lymph nodes. The lack of thymidine kinase ensures that the virus will not survive in nervous tissue. It is administered after maternal immunity has waned followed by semiannual revaccination. Breeding herds should be vaccinated quarterly. Some current vaccines appear to be ineffective against variant SuHV-1 viruses that have recently emerged in China.

PORCINE RESPIRATORY AND REPRODUCTIVE SYNDROME

Porcine respiratory and reproductive syndrome (PRRS) is the most significant cause of pig infectious disease losses worldwide and the most economically significant disease affecting US pig production. It has been estimated that it causes economic losses in the United States alone of about US$664 million per year or up to US$156 per litter. It has been especially devastating in China and Southeast Asia.

PRRS viruses (PRRSV) are small, enveloped, single-stranded, positive-sense RNA viruses belonging to the family *Arteriviridae*. There are two distinct genotypes, the European (type 1), and the North American (type 2) with about 60% genetic identity between them. These two genotypes have been classified as two different species in the genus *Porartevirus*, PRRSV-1, and PRRSV-2. They cause clinically identical diseases. However, because these RNA viruses do not replicate faithfully, they generate a "mutant swarm" of diverse variants within each genotype. As a result, it has proven very difficult to produce effective broad-spectrum vaccines. For example, four distinct lineages are associated with PRRSV-1, and ten lineages have been identified within PRRSV-2. Recombination can occur between these lineages. Most isolates from North and South America, and Asia belong to PRRSV-2.

PRRSV infection is restricted to cells of the monocyte-macrophage lineage including dendritic cells. As their name implies, the PRRSVs cause a syndrome characterized by reproductive failure, infertility, abortions, anorexia, and secondary pneumonia. When they invade the respiratory tract, they kill alveolar macrophages, and as a result are immunosuppressive. This suppression of the immune defenses within the lungs results in an increase in secondary bacterial pneumonia. It takes about 32 weeks for T cells to produce interferon in PRRSV-infected pigs. This is exceedingly slow and is attributed to virus-mediated immunosuppression and excessive regulatory T cell activity. T cell memory is also very poor after revaccination. Conversely, when PRRSVs infect neonatal piglets, they develop polyclonal B cell activation, autoimmunity, enlarged lymph nodes, and hypergammaglobulinemia (a 100- to 1000-fold increase in immunoglobin G). Cell-mediated responses and virus-neutralizing antibodies to PRRSV do not develop for several weeks after challenge as a result of loss of CD4$^+$ helper T cells. Because of this, PRRSV can cause persistent infections lasting for up to six months. The ongoing mutations and constant emergence of new PRRSV variants as they adapt to existing immunity ensures that vaccines are of limited usefulness.

Inactivated PRRS vaccines have been licensed worldwide. They do not induce detectable antibodies and stimulate a very weak cell-mediated responses. When used in growing pigs and boars, these vaccines fail to reduce the duration of viremia, virus shedding in semen, and respiratory signs after virulent challenge. The benefits of inactivated vaccines are more obvious when given to infected animals where they improved reproductive performance, for example, increased farrowing rate, number of weaned pigs, and the health status of piglets born to vaccinated sows. Thus they act as therapeutic vaccines rather than preventative ones. More recently, an intranasal vaccine (Barricade PRRSV, Aptimmune), containing poly (lactic)-co-glycolic acid nanoparticle-entrapped inactivated autogenous PRRSV vaccine, together with a whole cell *Mycobacterium tuberculosis* lysate as the adjuvant, has been shown to induce cross-protective immunity against heterogeneous strains.

Modified live PRRSV vaccines have been licensed in several countries. Those in the USA have been developed from the North American, PRRSV-2, whereas the European vaccines contain PRRSV-1. These MLV-PRRSV vaccines elicit relatively weak innate, humoral, and cell-mediated responses. PRRSV-specific antibodies appear at about two weeks, and peak around four weeks after vaccination. Most of these antibodies, however, are directed against the viral N (nucleocapsid) proteins and have no neutralizing activity. Neutralizing antibodies appear about four weeks after vaccination and demonstrate relatively low titers.

The MLV-PRRS vaccines reduce deaths, and piglets born to vaccinated gilts had a higher body weight and improved survival at weaning than those born to nonvaccinated gilts. In PRRSV-infected sows, MLV vaccines reduce abortions and hasten the rate of return to estrus and increase the farrowing rate and the number of weaned pigs. In growing pigs, the MLV-PRRSV vaccines reduce viremia, respiratory signs, and improve growth performance.

Protection conferred by PRRSV-1 vaccine does not protect against PRRSV-2 challenge and vice versa.

One major concern regarding the use of MLV-PRRSV vaccines is their potential for shedding and the development of persistent infections. Vaccinated pigs may develop a viremia for up to four weeks after immunization. As a result, reversion to virulence may possibly occur. This may occur through mutations of the vaccine virus and/or recombination with wild-type virulent PRRSV strains. The reverted vaccine virus may cause both reproductive and respiratory disease and affect growth performance. Piglets born to these infected sows may become carriers and shed the virus. In addition, MLV-PRRS vaccinated boars can spread the virus in semen to naïve animals.

Another cause for concern is the potential for antibody-mediated enhancement. Nonneutralizing antibodies can enhance macrophage uptake of either the vaccine virus or a circulating heterogeneous virus. This probably accounts for the polyclonal B cell activation.

In an effort to control PRRS in Denmark in late 1996, pigs were vaccinated against PRRSV-2. Unfortunately, the virus in this introduced vaccine reverted and as a result both PRRSV species now circulate within Danish pigs. Because of the immunosuppressive effects of the vaccine virus, it may also reduce the efficacy of other pig vaccines.

DNA, subunit, and virus-vectored PRRSV vaccines are under development. All appear to suffer from the problem of the great antigenic heterogeneity of PRRSV so it will be important to identify broad neutralizing epitopes. Alternatively, chimeric vaccines containing multiple epitopes may broaden cross-protection.

PORCINE EPIDEMIC DIARRHEA

Porcine epidemic diarrhea virus (PEDV) is a positive sense single-stranded RNA alphacoronavirus that causes acute watery diarrhea, vomiting, anorexia, dehydration, and death in neonatal piglets. It first appeared in the United States in 2013. It has since spread to Canada. Mortality may reach as high as 80% to 100%, and it has been estimated that it has caused a 10% loss in the US pig population. PEDV can also cause diarrhea, agalactia, and infertility in sows. Multiple mutant strains are continuing to emerge, a feature that is causing problems with currently available vaccines in addition to creating a constant demand for new vaccines. Because of the early onset of this disease, maternal immunity is critically important. Vaccination of sows is the most widely employed protective procedure. The virus spike (S) protein is required for the virus to bind to host cell receptors. This highly variable virus protein is the most antigenic and the target of neutralizing antibodies. Variations in the S gene and thus the epitopes on the S protein have significant effects on its virulence and antigenicity. PEDV is a type I enteropathogenic virus that infects villous enterocytes and can be suppressed by local mucosal immune responses.

Multiple commercial PED vaccines have been developed, especially in Asia. They include inactivated and modified live products. They may be combined with transmissible gastroenteritis virus (TGE) and rotavirus vaccines. Two inactivated PED vaccines are available in the United States. One is an adjuvanted inactivated whole virus vaccine containing both the S- and M-proteins for prefarrowing vaccination of pregnant gilts and sows. The other inactivated vaccine contains the S-protein only and is not adjuvanted. It is also given to sows before farrowing. Studies have shown that administering the vaccine to sows in the early stages of pregnancy works equally well.

Modified live PED vaccines that have been attenuated in tissue culture have been widely used in Asia. For example, a trivalent, PEDV, TGEV and porcine rotavirus vaccine is used in China. They may reduce mortality but the most highly attenuated vaccines do not appear to prevent virus shedding after challenge. In an effort to improve vaccine efficacy multiple different vaccines may be used. Both live and killed vaccines can be administered in series such as live-killed-killed or live-live-killed-killed. The difficulty is compounded by the continual emergence of new virus strains. Oral attenuated vaccines are available in South Korea and the Philippines for use in sows. This makes good sense because one is seeking to induce high colostral and milk antibody levels. The MLV-PED vaccines reduce mortality in piglets born to orally vaccinated sows, but do not prevent infection or viral shedding.

An alphavirus replicon RNA vaccine against PED has been provisionally licensed by US Department of Agriculture (USDA) (Chapter 6). It is derived from a Venezuelan equine encephalitis replicon expressing the PEDV spike gene.

TRANSMISSIBLE GASTROENTERITIS

Transmissible gastroenteritis (TGE) is an enteric disease of pigs caused by an alphacoronavirus related to PEDV. A respiratory variant, porcine respiratory coronavirus is not a primary pathogen but is associated with the pig respiratory disease complex. TGEV multiplies in the intestinal enterocytes and causes villous atrophy and enteritis. Unlike PEDV, the prevalence of TGE is declining, as is the market for TGE vaccines. Both modified live and inactivated vaccines have been licensed in the United States. The inactivated vaccines are given to nursing or weaned piglets by intramuscular injection. They do not induce a strong protective response against acute disease but are useful in controlling low-level enzootic infections.

Modified live vaccines may be used in pregnant sows to induce maternal immunity or in nursing or weaned piglets to induce active immunity. Unfortunately, these vaccines do not stimulate a strong IgA response because they do not replicate sufficiently within enterocytes.

Other Important Vaccines
SWINE INFLUENZA

Influenza in pigs is a highly contagious disease characterized by fever, coughing, sneezing, nasal discharge, lethargy, and depressed appetite—just like humans. It is caused by an influenza A virus of the *Orthomyxoviridae* family (IAV-S). Morbidity is very high but mortality is low. It causes a significant reduction in the growth rate of affected pigs and contributes to the porcine respiratory disease complex. It is potentially zoonotic. Currently H1 and H3 subtypes are circulating associating with N1 and N2 neuraminidases (H1N1, H1N2, and H3N2). However, within each virus strain are diverse antigenic subtypes. The hemagglutinin (HA) is the major target of neutralizing antibodies and hence a key vaccine component. Only inactivated adjuvanted IAV-S vaccines are currently available in North America. Some may contain a single viral strain whereas others may contain two or three strains. An intranasal nanoparticle adjuvanted autologous vaccine is now available in some US states. There is also an alphavirus replicon RNA vaccine available (Chapter 6). Many of these vaccines are available in combination with other antigens. They generally prevent clinical disease but may not be able to prevent viral shedding.

A complicating factor to be considered in influenza vaccination is vaccine-associated enhanced respiratory disease. Thus when pigs are vaccinated using an oil-adjuvanted whole inactivated virus vaccine, and subsequently challenged with a homotypic but antigenically mismatched influenza virus, they may develop greater lung damage. In these cases, the vaccine induced antibody binds to, but fails to neutralize, the challenge virus. Thus immune-complex mediated damage occurs in addition to the virus-induced damage.

CLASSICAL SWINE FEVER (HOG CHOLERA)

Classical swine fever (CSF) is a highly contagious disease caused by a pestivirus in the family *Flaviviridae,* which is closely related to the bovine diarrhea viruses and sheep border disease virus. In acute outbreaks clinical signs are nonspecific with high fever and depression, diarrhea, or constipation, ataxia, paralysis, or convulsions. Most affected pigs die within 3 weeks.

CSF was eradicated from the United States in 1976. It currently exists in Central and South America, Asia, and sporadic outbreaks continue to occur in Eastern Europe. Vaccination is not permitted in CSF-free countries. Conversely, it may be mandatory in countries where the disease is endemic. Normal practice is to vaccinate all pigs over two weeks of age except for piglets born to vaccinated sows. These piglets should be vaccinated at eight weeks.

The immunodominant protective antigen is the envelope glycoprotein, E2. Inactivated vaccines have largely been replaced by safe and effective modified live attenuated vaccines. These vaccine viruses have been attenuated either by passage in rabbits (C strain), or in tissue culture passage at low temperatures (ALD-strain and the Thiverval strain). Although very effective, these vaccines do not yet have DIVA capability. As a result, there are severe movement restrictions placed on vaccinated animals and their products. Oral C-strain CSF vaccines are used in Europe and Japan to control the infection in wild boars (Chapter 20).

Subunit vaccines based on the expression of the E2 protein, and generated in a baculovirus system have also been developed. These permit a DIVA strategy but they are not as effective as the modified live products. Pigs develop immunity within 10 days and it lasts for 2 to 3 years. Maternal immunity lasts for six to eight weeks.

A pestivirus chimera vaccine, CP7_E2alf, (Suvaxyn CSF Marker, Zoetis), using BVDV as its scaffold has been licensed by the European Medicines Agency. The BVDV E2 gene has been replaced by the CSF E2 gene. This vaccine combines DIVA capability with efficacy and protects against multiple CSF genotypes.

In 1936, a vaccine was developed against CSF that involved adding the dye crystal violet to pooled blood from viremic pigs. It was then incubated at 37° C for 14 days to kill the virus. It appeared to work well. However, because it contained pig blood, it sensitized recipients to other pig blood group antigens. As a result, vaccinated sows produced antibodies against these blood groups. If these sows were mated to boars of a different blood group, their piglets were at risk of developing hemolytic disease of the newborn. The sensitized sows concentrated these antibodies in their colostrum. Piglets suckling this colostrum ingested antibodies against their red blood cells. Affected piglets did not necessarily show clinical disease, although their red cells were sensitized by antibody. Other piglets showed rapidly progressive weakness and pallor of mucous membranes preceding death, and those animals that survived longest developed hemoglobinuria and jaundice. The disease ceased to be a problem when the crystal violet vaccine was withdrawn.

AFRICAN SWINE FEVER

Caused by the only member of the *Asfarviridae* family, a very large and complex DNA virus, African swine fever virus (ASFV) causes an acute viral hemorrhagic fever with very high mortality in domestic pigs. It is a robust virus that persists in the environment and is also spread by some soft ticks as well as by contaminated pork products. Endemic in much of sub-Saharan Africa, since 2007, ASF has spread through Georgia and Russia to reach China, Vietnam, Mongolia, North Korea, Cambodia, and Laos. The virus has also spread to Eastern Europe and is making inroads into Western Europe transported by contraband pork products and spread by wild boar. It is an enormous threat to the swine industry worldwide especially because there are no effective vaccines against ASF. Animals that recover from the disease, although apparently healthy, are persistent carriers and shedders of the virus.

Attempts to make a vaccine against ASFV have so far yielded disappointing results. The double-stranded viral genome varies in length, ranging from 170 to 190 kilobases depending on the isolate. It encodes 68 structural proteins and more than 100 infection-related proteins. Few of these proteins have known functions and many are immunosuppressive. The current pandemic is caused by the highly pathogenic, genotype II strain.

Conventional inactivated vaccines have been totally ineffective even when modern adjuvants are used. Subunit, DNA-plasmid, and virus-vectored vaccines have been developed but have also had very limited success. One cause of this is the difficulty in determining which of the numerous viral proteins to use in the vaccine. Several different ASFV proteins appear to be immunogenic and associated with protection but none are sufficient to induce solid protective immunity in pigs. Likewise, the major protective immunity mechanisms are not well understood. Neutralizing antibodies are important but not sufficient and cell-mediated responses are also required for protective immunity.

Modified live vaccines using traditionally attenuated virus may induce long-term immunity to homologous strains with the same genotype but not against heterologous strains. Studies on ASFV strain diversity suggest that this is caused, in part, by variations in capsid genes. Some 24 distinct genotypes of the major capsid protein have been described. Variations occur in multiple other viral proteins as well and their role in immunity needs to be resolved.

The vaccine problem is exacerbated by the observation that, under some circumstances, the immune response may enhance the disease. Attempts in Spain and Portugal in the 1960s to vaccinate pigs with a live attenuated vaccine resulted in both high antibody levels and the development of persistent viral infection and a chronic debilitating disease, with joint swelling, skin lesions, fever, viremia, and hypergammaglobulinemia. The control of ASF is an urgent necessity if the global swine industry is to survive and prosper.

FOOT-AND-MOUTH DISEASE

Commercially available foot-and-mouth disease virus (FMDV) vaccines have traditionally contained inactivated virus either in an aqueous suspension with aluminum hydroxide, saponin, or oil emulsion adjuvants. The conventional aqueous vaccines, however, stimulate low titer, short-lived immunity in pigs. As a result, the pig vaccines must be adjuvanted with oil based emulsion adjuvants. Double oil emulsion (Water/Oil/Water) adjuvants have significantly improved vaccine performance. They are generally created using Montanide ISA206 (Seppic, Paris, France). They have a longer duration of immunity although a slower onset of protection than aqueous vaccines in pigs. It can take as long as six weeks before a satisfactory level of immunity is reached. Pigs require a priming dose, then a boosting dose at 10 to 14 days to achieve the same level of protection that cattle acquire after a single dose of high potency foot-and-mouth disease vaccine. These vaccines decrease viral shedding by pigs, an important consideration for such a contagious infection. They may also cause significant local injection site reactions. The duration of immunity is generally six months, but in areas where there is high virus challenge, the re-vaccination interval may need to be reduced.

PORCINE CIRCOVIRUS DISEASE

Several genotypes of porcine circovirus 2 (PCV2), a small DNA virus, are associated with multiple swine diseases such a postweaning multisystemic wasting syndrome, porcine respiratory disease complex, reproductive failure, granulomatous enteritis, necrotizing lymphadenitis, exudative epidermitis, and congenital tremors. Porcine circovirus (PCV) usually causes disease in pigs 6 to 12 weeks of age. These diseases may be classified as either systemic disease (PCV2-SD), or as reproductive disease (PCV2-RD). There are four genotypes of PCV2 circulating in the United States: PCV2a, 2b, 2d, and 2e, but the prevalence of these is shifting. Until 2005, 2a was the only known PCV genotype, but shortly thereafter 2b became predominant. In 2012, a mutant 2b was discovered. It differed from the nominate 2b by only one additional amino acid in the open reading frame 2 (ORF2). This mutant PCV2b with high virulence spread rapidly. It quickly displaced the nominate 2b as the predominant genotype and is estimated to be present in a third of US herds. It has now been reclassified as PCV2d. Especially severe disease occurs when PCV is combined with PRRSV, swine influenza, or *Mycoplasma hyopneumoniae.*

Twelve commercial vaccines are currently available in the United States. These include inactivated whole virus vaccines licensed for use in sows and gilts. Other vaccines have been developed for use in piglets. Two subunit vaccines contain the PCV2 capsid protein expressed in a baculovirus system. Also available is an inactivated chimeric vaccine in which the capsid gene from nonpathogenic PCV1 has replaced the same gene in PCV2. Another chimeric vaccine contains both PCV 2a and 2b antigens. All these vaccines stimulate both neutralizing antibodies and cell-mediated immunity against PCV2a and offer cross-protection against PCV2b and -d. PCV2 vaccines are also available in combination with *Mycoplasma* and PRRS vaccines. These vaccines reduce viremia and disease pathology and increase average daily weight gain.

AUTOGENOUS VACCINES

Autogenous vaccines are killed vaccines made from a specific bacterium or virus isolated from infected farms. They are usually made by a veterinarian or by a licensed producer under a special USDA license for use only in a client's flock or herd. In order for a producer to acquire and use an autogenous vaccine, there must be a valid veterinarian-client relationship. The selected organism is cultured, killed, usually with formalin and standardized for bacterial content. They are not usually tested for safety or efficacy. One example is that against *Actinobacillus pleuropneumoniae* where there are multiple different strains, few of which are present in commercial vaccines. These can be very effective if carefully prepared because the vaccine will contain all the bacterial antigens required for protection in that specific location. Another example is the use of autogenous bacterins against exudative epidermitis caused by *Staphylococcus hyicus*. Studies have shown that its use significantly reduced antibiotic use as well as morbidity and mortality in weaned pigs. Autogenous bacterins can be made against many pathogens including, *E. coli, Haemophilus parasuis, S. suis,* Pasteurella, and Salmonella. Autogenous swine influenza vaccines are also widely employed.

BOAR TAINT VACCINE

Adult boars accumulate androstenone and skatole in their adipose tissues that are responsible for the offensive odor in boar pork. The development of this odor is mediated by gonadotropin-releasing hormone (GnRH), which stimulates the production of follicle stimulating hormone

(FSH) and luteinizing hormone (LH). These stimulate testosterone production that induces the boar taint. Blocking of GnRH will effectively castrate the animals and consequently prevent the development of these odors. One way this can be done is to immunize boars with a vaccine consisting of an adjuvanted GnRH-protein conjugate. This induces short-lived antiGnRH antibodies that decline seven to eight weeks after the second injection. These antibodies neutralize endogenous GnRH and block its biological activity so that boar taint drops to undetectable levels. Vaccinated boars also show altered behavior that may improve weight gain, feed conversion, and carcass quality. It is obviously much less stressful for the pigs than physical castration. The vaccine, available in Europe, is administered in two doses subcutaneously with a four-week interval and four to five weeks before slaughter. It is potentially hazardous to the vaccinator should they inadvertently inoculate themselves.

Vaccination Timing and Protocols

Piglets should be vaccinated at weaning with circovirus and *Mycoplasma* and maybe with PRRSV vaccines (see Table 18.1). Weaning generally occurs at three to six weeks. Maternal immunity lasts for six weeks. Swine influenza vaccine should be administered at seven to eight weeks.

Prebreeding vaccines are given to sows to protect from reproductive failure. These may include Leptospirosis, Erysipelothrix, and parvovirus vaccines. Gilts should get two doses of lepto/parvo/erysipelas vaccine before breeding and perhaps also a PED vaccine. Many farms vaccinate pregnant sows against enterotoxigenic *E. coli* to provide colostral immunity against scours in piglets. Other vaccines that may be considered include those directed against PRRSV, swine influenza, and *Lawsonia intracellularis*.

Adverse Events

Allergic reactions are always a possibility. In pigs, anaphylaxis is largely the result of systemic and pulmonary hypertension, leading to dyspnea, and death. In some pigs the intestine is involved, whereas in others no gross intestinal lesions are observed. The most significant mediator identified in this species is histamine. Leptospira bacterins may induce a significant febrile response.

Sources of Additional Information

Afgah, Z., Webb, B., Meng, X.J., Ramamoorthy, S. (2017). Ten years of PCV2 vaccines and vaccination: Is eradication a possibility? *Vet Microbiol, 206,* 21–28.

Brar, M.S., Shi, M., Murtaugh, M.P., Leung, F.C. (2015). Evolutionary diversification of type 2 porcine reproductive and respiratory syndrome virus. *J Gen Virol,* 96, 1570–1580.

Blome, S., Moss, C., Reimann, I., Konig, P., Beer, M. (2017). Classical swine fever vaccines—State-of-the-art. *Vet Microbiol, 206,* 10–20.

Chase, C.C., Daniels, C., Garcia, R., Milward, F., Nation, T. (2008). Needle-free technology in swine, Progress toward vaccine efficacy and pork quality. *J Swine Hlth Prodn,* 16, 254–261.

Chen, Q., Madson, D., Miller, C.L., Harris, D.L.H. (2012). Vaccine development in protecting swine against influenza virus. *Anim Health Res Rev,* 13,181–195.

Freuling, C.M., Muller, T.F., Mettenleiter, T.C. (2017). Vaccines against pseudorabies virus (PrV). *Vet Microbiol,* 206, 3–9.

Gerdts, V., Zakhartchouk, A. (2017). Vaccines for porcine epidemic diarrhea virus and other swine coronaviruses. *Vet Microbiol,* 206, 4551.

Karuppannan, A.K., Opriessnig, T. (2018). *Lawsonia intracellularis*: Revisiting the disease ecology and control of this fastidious pathogen in pigs. *Front Vet Sci,* 5, 1–11.

Koera-Muro, A., Angulo, C. (2018). New trends in innovative vaccine development against *Actinobacillus pleuropneumoniae. Vet Microbiol,* 217, 66–75.

Lyons, N.A., Lyoo, Y.S., King, D.P., Paton, D.J. (2016). Challenges in generating and maintaining protective vaccine-induced immune responses for foot-and-mouth disease virus in pigs. *Front Vet Sci,* 3, 1–12,

Mengeling, W.L., Vorwald, A.C., Lager, K.M., et al. (1999). Identification and clinical assessment of suspected vaccine-related field strains of porcine reproductive and respiratory syndrome virus. *Am J Vet Res,* 60, 334–340.

Nautrup, B.P., Van Vlaenderen, I., Aldaz, A., Mah, C.K. (2018). The effect of immunization against gonadotrophin-releasing factor on growth performance, carcass characteristics, and boar taint relevant to pig producers and the pork packing industry: A meta-analysis. *Res Vet Sci,* 119, 182–195.

Park, J.E., Shin, H.J. (2018). Porcine epidemic diarrhea vaccine efficacy evaluation by vaccination timing and frequencies. *Vaccine,* 36, 2760–2763.

Song, D., Moon, H., Kang, B. (2015). Porcine epidemic diarrhea: a review of current epidemiology and available vaccines. *Clin Exp Vacc Res,* 4, 166–176.

Renukaradhya, G.J., Meng, X.J., Calvert, J.G., Roof, M. (2015). Inactivated and subunit vaccines against porcine reproductive and respiratory syndrome: Current status and future direction. *Vaccine,* 33, 3065–3072.

Rock, D.L. (2017). Challenges for African swine fever vaccine development–"perhaps the end of the beginning". *Vet Microbiol,* 206, 52–58.

Rose, N., Andraud, M. (2017). The use of vaccines to control pathogen spread in pig populations. *Porcine Hlth Management,* 3, 8–16.

Vincent, A.L., Perez, D.R., Rajao, D., Anderson, D.K., et al. (2017). Influenza A vaccines for swine. *Vet Microbiol,* 206, 35–44.

Poultry Vaccines

Chickens are the most common bird in the world, with about 23 billion living at any given time. These birds are primarily grown for industrial meat production. Their survival depends on human management, and, as a result, they are most intensively vaccinated livestock species. In intensive management systems, each bird may undergo an average of 12 to 20 vaccination procedures within its short life span. Immunization of poultry, although necessary for economic production and insurance, is no substitute for proper hygiene and appropriate biosecurity. Lack of hygiene and other stressors may result in less than satisfactory vaccine performance. Clearly, the role of vaccines is to protect birds against specific infectious diseases. In layers they are also needed to ensure that maternal immunity is passed to the chicks and to prevent vertical transmission of infections. Given the large size of many poultry operations and the small unit cost of individual birds, vaccines must be very inexpensive. For example, in early 2018, a vial of 10,000 doses of Newcastle-bronchitis vaccine cost US$23.99, 1000 doses of Marek's disease vaccine cost US$29.99, and 1000 doses of Fowlpox vaccine cost US$6.99. Vaccines are commodities in the poultry industry and an unavoidable part of doing business.

Vaccine Administration

The most convenient time to vaccinate chicks is before they leave the hatchery (Tables 19.1, 19.2, and 19.3). As in many intensive animal industries, the cost of labor is critical. Vaccination procedures are therefore directed toward effectively vaccinating the largest number of birds in the shortest time, by the fewest workers, without causing any loss in productivity. The methods employed will also depend, in part, on the way in which the birds are housed and the nature of their watering systems.

As with all vaccines, proper storage is essential. They should be stored carefully according to the manufacturer's instructions and under no circumstances should they be allowed to get hot. Ideally the refrigerator should have an alarm installed in case of failure. They should be allowed to warm to room temperature and reconstituted with the appropriate diluent immediately before beginning the vaccination procedure. Automatic syringes must be carefully sterilized, properly calibrated, and checked for accuracy before use. Needles should be changed regularly (at least after every 1000 chicks). The reconstituted vaccine should be used completely within 45 minutes.

TABLE 19.1 ■ Vaccination Programs for Broilers

Disease/Vaccine	Vaccination Schedule	Comments
Antiviral		
Marek's disease	Modified live viruses administered either in ovo or day 1.	Withdrawal time 21 days.
Newcastle disease	Given in ovo or at day one or days 9–14, either in the drinking water or by coarse sprayers.	Usually the B1 or LaSota strain. Withdrawal time 21 or 42 days.
Infectious bronchitis	Day 1 or 14–21 days administered in drinking water or by coarse spray. With Newcastle disease vaccine.	Use Massachusetts strain. Withdrawal time 42 days.
Infectious bursal disease	Given in ovo or on day 1 and boost at 8–12 days.	Withdrawal time 21 or 42 days.

TABLE 19.2 ■ Vaccination Programs for Broiler Breeders

Disease/Vaccine	Vaccination Schedule	Comments
Antibacterial		
Fowl cholera	Vaccinate all chickens in the flock at 10–12 weeks. Revaccinate at 18–20 weeks.	Leave at least a 6 week gap between vaccine doses. Withdrawal time 21 or 42 days.
Mycoplasmosis	Only where permitted. Vaccinate at 12–16 weeks of age. Two doses are administered.	
Infectious coryza	Vaccinate at 5–9 weeks of age. Revaccinate in 4 weeks.	No later than 3–4 weeks before onset of lay. Withdrawal time 42 days.
Colibacillosis	Given in drinking water or coarse spray. Vaccinate at 1 day of age and repeat in 3 weeks. Long lived birds may be revaccinated at 12–14 weeks of age.	Do not use antibiotics when using these vaccines. Withdrawal time 21 days.
Salmonellosis	*Salmonella enteritidis*. Vaccinate at 12–16 weeks and 4 weeks later. May revaccinate during molt. Other vaccines may be given by coarse spray or in the drinking water to 1 day of age chicks. A second dose should be administered 2 weeks later.	Withdrawal time 42 days.
Antiviral		
Newcastle disease	Vaccinate with bronchitis at 9–14 days. Revaccinate at 4, 6, and 8–10 weeks. Alternatively, vaccinate with a MLV and then revaccinate at 4 and 16–20 weeks. Every 3–4 months thereafter revaccinate by water or aerosol.	Use B1 or LaSota strains. Withdrawal time 21 or 42 days.
Infectious bronchitis	Vaccinate at 9–14 days combined with NDV. Revaccinate at 4 and 8 weeks in water or coarse spray. Repeat every 3–4 months.	Withdrawal time 21 or 42 days.

TABLE 19.2 ▪ Vaccination Programs for Broiler Breeders—cont'd

Disease/Vaccine	Vaccination Schedule	Comments
Infectious bursal disease	Vaccinate at 10–20 days and revaccinate at 8–10 weeks and 16–18 weeks.	Usually administered by intramuscular injection, spray, or in the drinking water. Intermediate or invasive vaccines are used to vaccinate broilers and commercial layer replacements. They are sometimes delivered to 1-day chicks as a coarse spray to protect chicks lacking maternal antibodies. Second and third applications may be administered if there is a high risk of virulent disease. Withdrawal time 21 or 42 days.
Tenosynovitis (Reovirus)	Spray vaccines can be given to 1-day chicks or in drinking water to birds over 12 weeks of age. Boost at 6–8 weeks, 10–12 weeks, and 16–18 weeks. 1 day chicks may receive live vaccine.	Withdrawal time 21 or 42 days.
Encephalomyelitis	Vaccinate at 10–12 weeks In the wing web.	Withdrawal time 21 days.
Fowlpox	Vaccinate 10–12 weeks In the wing web. In ovo and 1 day of age vaccines are available.	Do not vaccinate during lay. Examine the injection site at 7–10 days to ensure "take". Withdrawal time 21 days.
Chicken infectious anemia	Vaccinate birds over 12 weeks in the wing web. Do not vaccinate laying breeders.	Examine the injection site at 7–10 days to ensure "take." Withdrawal time 21 days.
Laryngotracheitis	Vaccinate in ovo or birds 5–8 weeks by eye drop, spray, or drinking water. Revaccinate at 16–20 weeks.	Withdrawal time 21 days.

These tables are examples of consensus vaccination programs. Individual programs are variable and will reflect animal health, local environmental and housing conditions, severity of challenge, and disease prevalence, in addition to professional judgment. It is essential that the instructions on the individual vaccine label be followed.

Withdrawal times are for meat unless otherwise stated. When a range is stated it means that some products have a longer withdrawal time than others. Check the label directions for the specific withdrawal time for each vaccine.

IN OVO VACCINATION

Embryonic chickens have a functioning immune system by 16 to 18 days incubation. Vaccination of embryonic chicks in ovo is therefore a highly effective method of vaccinating large numbers of birds in a very short time. Automatic egg injection machines have been widely adopted. Injection through the eggshell is performed at 18.5 days when eggs are routinely transferred to hatching trays to avoid turning in the setter compartment of the incubator. The window for in ovo vaccination is considered to be 17.5 to 19.2 days when the chick is in the ideal position for vaccination. The chick should be in the hatching position with its head under the right wing and no visible intestines in the yolk sac stalk. Once internal pipping starts and pulmonary respiration begins it is too late to vaccinate. Automatic systems can inoculate up

TABLE 19.3 ■ **Vaccination Programs for Layers**

Disease/Vaccine	Vaccination Schedule	Comments
Antibacterial		
Mycoplasma gallisepticum	Vaccinate at 10–14 weeks by spray or 18 weeks parenterally.	
Antiviral		
Newcastle disease	Vaccinate together with infectious bronchitis by water or coarse spray. At 14–21 days, 5 weeks, and every 5–6 weeks thereafter. B1 can be administered by eye drop or spray at 1 day. B1 or LaSota at 18–21 days, drinking water, LaSota at 10 weeks, and an inactivated adjuvanted vaccine at point of lay.	Withdrawal time 21 or 42 days.
Infectious bronchitis	Vaccinate on day 1, and then revaccinate at 14–21 days, 5 weeks, 8–10, 12–14, and 16–18 weeks. Revaccinate layers and breeders at 13–18 weeks of age.	Withdrawal time 21 or 42 days.
Infectious bursal disease	Vaccinate at 10–17 days. Revaccinate at 7 weeks and 6 months	Withdrawal time 21 or 42 days.
Encephalomyelitis	Vaccinate birds over 8 weeks but at least 4–6 weeks before start of lay.	Withdrawal time 21 days. Do not vaccinate during egg production.
Fowlpox	Vaccinate at 10–12 weeks in the wing web. They should be over 8 weeks, but at least 4 weeks before start of lay.	Examine the wing site to ensure that the vaccine has taken. Withdrawal time 21 days. Do not vaccinate during egg production.
Laryngotracheitis	Vaccinate at 8–12 weeks by eye drop. Revaccinate at 4 months.	Withdrawal time 21 days.

These tables are examples of consensus vaccination programs. Individual programs are variable and will reflect animal health, local environmental and housing conditions, severity of challenge and disease prevalence in addition to professional judgment. It is essential that the instructions on the individual vaccine label be followed.

Withdrawal times are for meat unless otherwise stated. When a range is stated it means that some products have a longer withdrawal time than others. Check the label directions for the specific withdrawal time for each vaccine.

to 60,000 eggs per hour and eliminate the need for posthatching vaccination (Fig. 19.1). The machines can deliver precise amounts of vaccine without causing significant trauma to the developing chick. The machines work by gently lowering an injection head onto the top of the egg. A small diameter hollow punch makes an opening and the needle then descends through this hole to a controlled depth—1 inch. A specified volume of vaccine is injected, the needle withdrawn and cleaned in a sterilization wash.

Correct placement of the vaccine is critical. Vaccine deposited in the air sac confers no protection; vaccine in the allantoic fluid protects about a quarter of the birds; vaccine delivered to the amniotic fluid or the body of the embryo results in over 90% protection. Success also depends on timing. If given slightly earlier (around 17 days) the vaccine will mainly enter the amniotic fluid

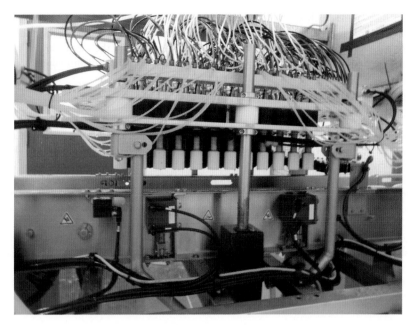

Fig. 19.1 An in ovo vaccination machine. This photograph shows the injection section of the machine. A tray of eggs is conveyed into this section. The white components descend to hold the eggs in position and then the drill and needle are lowered through the eggshell and a measured dose of vaccine injected. (Courtesy Alberto Torres and Mike Bonner.)

and be swallowed by the embryo. If given slightly later (around 19 days), the needle will likely enter the embryo—ideally the right breast. When properly done this does not result in significant damage. It is also important that the eggs be correctly aligned in the injector. For example, the embryo should develop with its head toward the large end of the egg so that it can emerge through the air sac. If the egg is upside down it results in embryonic malpositions and decreased hatchability.

In ovo vaccination requires specialized equipment, great accuracy, and a very high degree of hygiene because once opened to the environment by a needle puncture, eggs are susceptible to bacterial or fungal invasion. With appropriate hygienic precautions, however, the method is highly satisfactory. It is predominantly used for Marek's disease vaccines containing the CVI 988/Rispens strain of virus. It may also be used for control of infectious bursal disease in addition to fowlpox, and avian influenza. More than half the broilers in the United States are vaccinated against Marek's disease using this system. Studies have shown that compared with vaccination at hatching, in ovo vaccination significantly reduces condemnations and early mortality.

Basic precautions must be taken to achieve the best results, especially good hatchery sanitation and proper disinfection of the hatching eggs. One special problem is aspergillosis. This fungus is often present in moldy litter and can give rise to "brooder pneumonia" in hatchlings. To minimize this risk, airflow patterns must be carefully regulated to ensure that it flows from clean to dirty areas. Moisture management, disinfection, and careful sanitation are all essential. The equipment must also be carefully and precisely maintained. Vaccines must be reconstituted in a clean room, preferably well away from any sources of feather dander. Vaccine vials are stored in liquid nitrogen. They must be thawed in a water bath; once thawed they are injected slowly into the diluent bag before use. All these steps must be performed aseptically. Generally, the diluent also contains a dye to confirm vaccination. It is important to ensure that the vaccine and diluent are thoroughly mixed. The work area should be sanitized before and after any procedure

SUBCUTANEOUS NECK INJECTION

Day-old chicks may be vaccinated with a subcutaneous injection of 0.2 to 0.5ml vaccine into the skin behind the neck or intramuscular injection into the thigh. Automatic vaccination machines (poultry service processors) are primarily designed for neck injection. Some robots can take day-old hatchlings, debeak them, and then inject them with one or two measured doses of vaccine subcutaneously in the neck region (Figs. 19.2 and 19.3). The vaccine dose is adjustable and delivered at low pressure, thus minimizing tissue damage. Needles are automatically sterilized between each chick using a disinfectant spray. The newest robots can vaccinate up to 3500 chicks/hour (20,000–30,000/day)! A colored dye may be mixed with the vaccine to permit quality assurance and the chicks are monitored for hemorrhage or vaccine leakage. This can identify any chicks accidentally missed. The presence of blood may indicate a blunt needle or that the machine needs to be readjusted.

When injecting the vaccine by hand, the neck skin should be lifted up and the vaccine injected subcutaneously along the mid-line with the needle pointing away from the head. Other possible

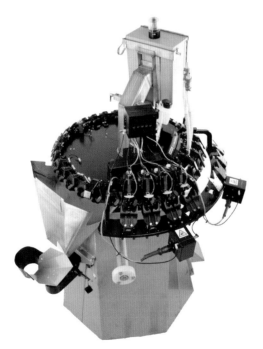

Fig. 19.2 A robotic poultry service processor. Operators pick up the chicks and place them in neck holders. These are then transported into a debeaking sector and then into an injection sector where they are injected with a measured amount of one or two vaccines in the correct subcutaneous location in the neck. After vaccination the chicks are removed from the holders and then placed on a discharge conveyer or manually boxed. These machines can accurately vaccinate up to 3500 chicks an hour. (Courtesy Mr. Andrew Gomer and NovaTech Inc.)

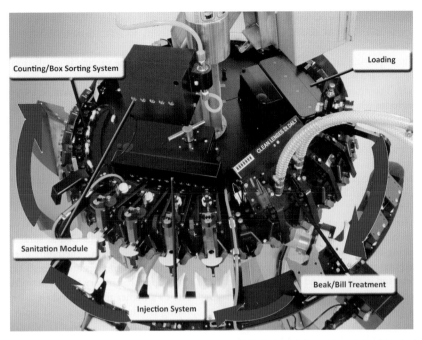

Fig. 19.3 Details of a poultry service processor. Chicks are carried around the track and are debeaked and vaccinated before being counted and placed in boxes for shipment. (Courtesy Mr. Andrew Gomer and NovaTech Inc.)

injection sites include the inguinal fold, the breast muscle, the biceps, or the tail head and the gastrocnemius muscle. It should always be borne in mind however that muscle lesions should be avoided in birds destined for human consumption.

SPRAY VACCINATION

Spray vaccination is a very effective method of immunizing large numbers of birds. It works especially well against respiratory diseases such as Newcastle disease and influenza. The type of sprayer used determines the vaccine droplet size. This in turn determines how far down the chicken's respiratory tract the droplets will penetrate. Large droplets will be trapped in the nasal cavity, smaller droplets will reach the pharynx and trachea, while the smallest will reach the lungs and air sacs. These small droplets are deposited at the bifurcations of the primary to secondary bronchi. Here they are taken up and processed by antigen presenting cells.

Spray vaccination can be performed with the birds enclosed in a spray cabinet or by spraying birds within an entire house. Droplets less than 50 μm are classified as aerosols, droplets 50 to 100 μm are considered fine spray, and 100 to 300 μm droplets are considered coarse spray. When using a spray cabinet, a measured amount of vaccine can be delivered to each batch of chicks. Each manufacturer will have recommendations for the volume of vaccine used per box. The sprayer should aim to generate "coarse" droplets. However, remember that droplet size depends not only on nozzle size, but also on the spray pressure. Higher pressure generates smaller droplets. The distilled water used should be cool but not cold. The delivery of the vaccine can be visualized either by means of a dye or simply by the amount of moisture present on the plumage. Factors such as air pressure and spray pattern and the volume delivered must be carefully monitored.

In a hot dry environment, droplet size will shrink as the water evaporates. The distance between the nozzle and the bird also affects droplet size. Avoid trying to reach distant birds by raising the nozzle.

When spraying an entire house, backpack sprayers are used. The vaccine is usually reconstituted in distilled water. The sprayers must not have been used for other purposes such as pesticide spraying. The droplet size should be 80 to 120 μm for young chicks. This size will be affected by the degree to which the backpack sprayer is pumped up. A team of sprayers dressed in appropriate protective clothing plus gloves, masks, and goggles, should walk slowly through the house spraying at least 1 gallon of vaccine per 100 feet. Each vaccinator should spray one side of the house and the nozzle should be directed about 3 feet above the heads of the birds. The objective of the process is to deliver droplets to the eyes, nares, and the respiratory tract. Vaccine deposited on litter and equipment is wasted. Fans and heater should be turned off. Curtains should be closed in open houses. Birds should be settled before spraying begins, perhaps by dimming the lights.

In hatcheries, live attenuated vaccines against infectious bronchitis virus (IBV) and Newcastle disease virus (NDV) are administered as a coarse spray on day of hatch. Coarse spraying, by generating droplets greater than 100 μm, prevents the vaccine virus from penetrating deep into the respiratory tract. This in turn, prevents vaccine virus from causing lesions there. The large droplets land in the eyes and nares and are confined to the upper respiratory tract. These droplets do not damage the virus particles so that they replicate to a higher titer and induce a stronger protective response. Despite precautions, vaccine spraying is often suboptimal and many birds may be missed. Once vaccination is completed, equipment must be cleansed thoroughly with hot water and the fans and heaters turned on again.

GEL VACCINATION

Gel diluents have been introduced to enhance coccidiosis vaccination. The vaccine is mixed with a thick gel diluent and then applied to chicks through a gel application bar. The gel remains on the feathers until preened off by the bird. It works well for coccidia where oocysts must be ingested. It may also work for infectious bronchitis and other viral diseases.

DRINKING WATER VACCINES

Another common method for the mass administration of vaccines to large numbers of poultry is through their drinking water. To ensure that poultry drink the water, it should be withdrawn for 1 to 4 hours before vaccine administration depending upon the ambient temperature to ensure that they are somewhat thirsty. All birds should have access to the vaccine water at the same time to ensure that vaccine uptake is evenly distributed across the flock. It is important to determine daily water consumption beforehand to estimate the appropriate vaccine dose. The amount of water to be used for vaccination should be about one-third of average daily consumption. There are, however, standard guidelines based on the temperature including the birds' age and type. The drinking water should not contain any chlorine or disinfectants. Likewise, sanitizer use should be discontinued 48 hours before vaccination. Lines should be flushed with a product that can remove litter, feed, and feces, in addition to detergents, minerals, and biofilms. The pH of the water supply should be between 7 and 6.5. Filters and oxygenators should be removed or disconnected. Waterers should be scrubbed with chlorine free water. Commercial products are available that may be added to the water to neutralize chlorine and other oxidants and optimize pH. Ideally the vaccine should be administered early in the morning and all birds should have easy access to it. Keep the waterers out of direct sunlight. Skim milk powder may be added as a stabilizer and also dye. The vaccine solution is placed in the drinkers or water tanks according to the manufacturer's recommendations, and the water system is primed. Unvaccinated water should be drawn off and discarded. Birds should drink all the vaccine solution in 1 to 2 hours. If water has been cut off for too long, some thirsty birds may drink it so fast that the others may not get a sufficient dose. The water should remain free of chlorine medications or disinfectants for at least 24 hours after vaccination. Unfortunately, field conditions are often such that not all birds receive the vaccine. Perhaps as few as 60% may be vaccinated successfully with drinking water.

EYE-DROP/INTRANASAL VACCINATION

Some commercial poultry vaccines are approved for administration by eye drops. The vaccines should be reconstituted with appropriate diluent and an eyedropper cap used. Allow one full drop to fall into the open eye of the bird and hold it until it swallows. Birds will usually get 0.03 ml of vaccine into the eye or nasal cavity where it is rapidly absorbed.

WING-WEB VACCINATION

Some vaccines may be administered into the plucked wing web using a two-pronged needle that has been dipped in the vaccine solution. It is given in the underside of the wing avoiding vulnerable structures such as veins, bone, or nerves.

Antibacterial Vaccines

Antibacterial vaccines are especially significant in the poultry industry where the short production cycle precludes the use of antibiotics. Although viral diseases are of greater overall significance, antibacterial vaccines are also essential.

PASTEURELLOSIS

Fowl cholera is caused by *Pasteurella multocida*, an acute fatal septicemia in chickens and turkeys. *P. multocida* vaccines include bacterins adjuvanted with aluminum hydroxide or oil emulsions, or they may contain attenuated live organisms. Multivalent Pasteurella vaccines usually contain the commonest serotypes 1, 3, and 4. The inactivated vaccines are usually given by injection. The attenuated live vaccines (M9 or PM-1 strains) may be given by the wing web or in drinking water. Protection develops in about two weeks.

MYCOPLASMOSIS

These diseases are caused by several pathogenic Mycoplasmas. The most important are *Mycoplasma gallisepticum* (MG) and *Mycoplasma synoviae* (MS). MG causes chronic respiratory disease, whereas MS causes respiratory disease or synovitis. It is generally best to maintain mycoplasma-free flocks, but inactivated, attenuated live and fowlpox-vectored vaccines are available for use in countries where vaccination is permitted. The use of these vaccines is prohibited in some states. Vaccines should only be used in flocks with birds of all ages and where infection is considered inevitable.

Bacterins consist of suspensions of MG in an oil emulsion. These can protect against respiratory disease or egg production losses but will not prevent infection with field strains of MG. Live MG vaccines contain the mild F strain, or the safer avirulent ts-11 or 6/85 strains. The F strain is administered by the intranasal or eye drop method; the ts-11 strain is given in eye drops; the 6/85 strain is given by fine spray. A fowlpox recombinant MG vaccine is also available. It is administered in the wing web. The use of the attenuated vaccines has been characterized as controlled exposure by giving a mild infection at an age when little damage occurs. Pullets are generally vaccinated between 12 to 16 weeks of age. One dose is sufficient to make the birds permanent carriers. A live MS vaccine containing the MS-H strain is administered by eye drop.

INFECTIOUS CORYZA

This is an acute respiratory disease of chickens caused by *Avibacterium paragallinarum*. It is characterized by nasal discharge, sneezing, conjunctivitis, diarrhea, and facial swelling. Affected hens show a significant drop in egg production. Coryza may be complicated by the simultaneous presence of many other bacteria in addition to infectious bronchitis virus. There are three serovars of *A. paragallinarum* (A, B, and C). These are not cross-protective so it is essential that any vaccines contain the appropriate serovar for that population of birds. Commercial bacterins are available in the United States and other countries. These generally contain all three serovars. Some vaccines produced by large manufacturers are marketed internationally and contain the most prevalent bacterial strains. However, there are concerns that these may not provide protection against more localized variants.

COLIBACILLOSIS

Colibacillosis is caused by avian pathogenic *Escherichia coli*. This commonly starts as a respiratory infection and eventually leads to colisepticemia, sickness, deaths, and carcass condemnation. Colibacillosis is a leading cause of economic loss in the poultry industry. Vaccination is an obvious solution to this problem and many different inactivated and live vaccines have been developed. However, at the present time there is only a live attenuated vaccine available in the United States. The vaccine contains an *aroA*-deleted mutant designed for coarse spray or drinking water administration.

SALMONELLOSIS

Salmonellae present the poultry farmer with two potential problems. One is the fact that they may kill large numbers of birds. The other is that they may cause human food poisoning caused by the contamination of eggs and poultry meat with *Salmonella enterica* serotype Enteritidis. This is of major concern to the poultry industry for both legal and financial reasons. In Europe, for example, 10% to 15% of poultry meat at the retail level may be Salmonella positive. Young chickens may be infected by both vertical and horizontal transfer and they probably acquire the infection soon after hatching. Once established in the intestine, the Salmonellae can prevent colonization by other serovars.

It is well established that cell-mediated immunity is essential for the control of Salmonellosis. If birds are vaccinated against one of the host-specific serovars such as *Salmonella gallinarum*, it induces a strong specific immunity. However, vaccination against the nonhost specific serovars is much less effective. The host-specific infections normally cause a septicemic disease involving macrophage colonization and minimal enteric infection. In contrast the nonspecific serovars tend to colonize the intestinal tract. These are the serovars that cause human food poisoning. Thus the greatest number of available vaccines are directed against serovar Enteritidis. These are all administered subcutaneously around 10 to 14 weeks of age and given in two doses 4 to 6 weeks apart. Many are combined with Newcastle and bronchitis vaccines. Some salmonella vaccines also contain other serovars such as Typhimurium, Kentucky, and Heidelberg. Spray and drinking water vaccines are also available for use in chickens and turkeys.

Antiviral Vaccines

MAREK'S DISEASE

Marek's disease virus (MDV) is a member of the genus *Mardivirus*, an alphaherpesvirus. It causes a lymphoproliferative and neuropathic disease that affects the nerves, viscera, muscle, and skin of chickens. It is also immunosuppressive. As with other herpesviruses, chickens may become persistently infected without showing any clinical signs. There are three species of MDV: Gallid herpes virus 2 (serotype 1), Gallid herpesvirus 3 (serotype 2), and Meleagrid herpesvirus 1 (serotype 3, also called herpesvirus of turkeys, HVT). Serotype 1 includes all the virulent poultry strains and some attenuated vaccine strains.

Marek's disease is primarily controlled by vaccination either in ovo at day 18, or by subcutaneous injection at day of hatch. The need for vaccination against MDV has a significant economic impact on the poultry industry.

Bivalent vaccines containing serotypes 1 and 3 or trivalent vaccines containing serotypes 1, 2, and 3 are used. These vaccines contain live virus and although they prevent tumor production they do not generate sterilizing immunity. Vaccinated chickens still get infected and can shed virulent field virus. It is suggested that this has resulted in the increased virulence of field strains of the virus.

Several different modified live virus vaccines are available to control Marek's disease. Turkey herpesvirus (HVT or MDV-3) is an avirulent virus that can effectively protect chickens against MDV. Strain FC126 of HVT is the most widely used MDV vaccine and commonly given to broilers as a monovalent vaccine and as a polyvalent vaccine in breeders and layers. Serotypes 1 and 2, and HVT are highly cell-associated and must be stored frozen in liquid nitrogen. Thus they must be carefully stored and thawed before use. This includes the use of safety glasses and gloves when removing the vaccine vials from the liquid nitrogen tank. The thawed vaccine is diluted appropriately and mixed well before use. Cell-free vaccines are available in some countries. These are less immunogenic but easier to store.

HVT has an excellent safety record and like other herpesviruses is persistent. Immunity to HTV is not inhibited by maternal antibodies if given on the day of hatch or in ovo. It can also be used as a vector virus for recombinant vaccines against infectious laryngotracheitis, Newcastle disease, infectious bronchitis, avian influenza, and bursal disease. These recombinants are very effective in protecting against systemic disease, but immunity to mucosal infections such as NDV is inconsistent.

MDV-2 strain is another naturally occurring avirulent strain of MDV used in vaccines. It only provides limited protection but it may be used in combination with other strains. There are situations in which HVT alone and MDV-2 alone cannot protect against very virulent strains. However, a combination vaccine containing both HVT and MDV-2 may show a synergistic effect.

Attenuated MDV-1 vaccines have also been generated by serial cell culture passage. Strain CVI988 or Rispens is considered the most efficacious current vaccine (Dr B.H. Rispens was the first to isolate strain CVI 988 in 1972). It was attenuated by serial passage in chicken kidney cells. This vaccine has some residual virulence in susceptible chickens and can spread between birds. It is predominantly used for in ovo vaccination. Higher passage variants are less virulent but also less immunogenic. CVI988 is the vaccine strain of choice against very virulent strains of MDV.

NEWCASTLE DISEASE

Newcastle Disease is a serious respiratory disease caused by virulent strains of avian paramyxovirus serotype 1 of the genus *Avulavirus*. All strains of the virus (NDV) are contained in a single serotype, but they are divided into two classes, class I and class II. Class II is then divided into 16 genotypes. Class 1 viruses are primarily found in wild birds because NDV can infect many different avian species.

The incubation period of NDV lasts from three to six days. Clinical signs are nonspecific, namely depression, ruffled feathers, anorexia, hypothermia, and death. Some birds may develop neurologic disease with torticollis, ataxia, and paralysis. Viscerotropic velogenic ND is the most severe form of the disease resulting in the development of diphtheritic and necrotic, or hemorrhagic lesions along the gastrointestinal tract.

Class II NDVs vary greatly in their virulence for chickens. They are classified as velogenic—rapidly lethal; mesogenic—intermediate; and lentogenic—relatively low virulence, based on their lethality for chick embryos. For example, class II, genotype II strains are so lentogenic that some, such as Hitchner B1 and LaSota, can be used in modified live vaccines.

Because all the strains of NDV belong to a single serotype, proper vaccination should protect against all of them. Immunity is mainly derived from neutralizing antibodies against their hemagglutinin (H) and the fusion (F) glycoproteins. However, cell-mediated immune responses also reduce viral shedding, presumably by killing virus-infected cells. Sterilizing immunity is not achieved with current NDV vaccines. Vaccines prevent clinical disease and mortality, and they may reduce virus shedding and increase the dose of virus needed to infect a bird. Flock immunity is another positive outcome of vaccination although it is estimated that this will only have an impact when greater than 85% of the flock have hemagglutination inhibition titers greater than 8 after two doses of vaccine.

Inactivated vaccines are given by the intramuscular or subcutaneous routes. They are often given to layers or breeders to provide persistent high antibody levels that can be transferred to their chicks. They are usually inactivated with formaldehyde or beta-propiolactone and adjuvanted by emulsification in mineral or vegetable oil. Because birds have to be handled individually, these vaccines are more expensive than the MLV vaccines. Permissible withdrawal times between vaccination and slaughter must also be taken into consideration because of the persistence of vaccine antigen. This may be 21 or 42 days depending upon the vaccine.

Modified live lentogenic or mesogenic strains are used in MLV-NDV vaccines. The live vaccines are usually grown in embryonated chicken eggs or in tissue culture. Lentogenic strains used in these vaccines include B1, C2, LaSota, V4, NDW I2, and mesogenic strains used include Roakin, Mukteswar, and Komarov. The mesogenic vaccines cause mild disease so they are generally used in countries where Newcastle disease is endemic. In countries largely free of ND only lentogenic strains are permitted. These live vaccines are given in drinking water, by coarse sprayer, or by intranasal or intraocular administration. A lentogenic strain is also available for in ovo use. Some mesogenic strains may be given by wing web inoculation.

The severity of vaccine reactions depends on the strain of the virus employed. For example, of the two major vaccine strains of Newcastle disease, the LaSota strain is a good immunogen but may provoke mild adverse reactions. In contrast, the B1 strain is considerably milder but is less immunogenic, especially if given in drinking water. Where disease risks are high, live LaSota vaccine can be given in the drinking water or as a spray at 5 to 6 weeks, followed by another dose at 10 weeks, and an inactivated vaccine at point of lay. It is also important to bleed and test samples of bird sera after vaccination to ensure that they develop protective antibodies.

Recombinant vectored NDV vaccines using turkey herpesvirus or fowlpox vectors incorporating the hemagglutinin gene or the F gene, or both, are also available. Some of these may be appropriate for in ovo vaccination. NDV itself may also be used as a vector for other vaccines such as those against IBD or avian influenza.

As with other poultry vaccines, maternal antibodies can interfere with early vaccination procedures. The significance of this varies between farms and between birds and two strategies have been employed to overcome this. One is to delay vaccination until two to four weeks when most birds can develop immunity. Alternatively, the birds are vaccinated at one day by coarse spraying or eye drop vaccination. This will infect the chicks until maternal immunity has gone and they can then respond to the infection themselves. However, these vaccines may cause respiratory problems in very young chicks. Reactions in spray-vaccinated birds may be significantly more severe than those receiving eye-nose drops, however, their antibody response is slightly but significantly greater. Although NDV vaccines can prevent clinical disease and mortality, a major impediment to prevent outbreaks is uneven vaccine application when using these mass administration techniques. It has proved difficult to attenuate live NDV strains sufficiently for in ovo use without affecting hatchability. Recombinant NDV vaccines expressing the fusion (F) gene may solve this problem. Layers may be vaccinated at frequent intervals to ensure adequate immunity. For example, they may be primed with an inactivated vaccine and then repeatedly boosted with more immunogenic live vaccines.

INFECTIOUS BURSAL DISEASE

Also called Gumboro disease, the causal agent of IBD is an *avibirnavirus*.

It infects multiple bird species, but causes clinical disease only in chickens less than 10 weeks of age. The virus destroys B cells within the Bursa of Fabricius resulting in bursal atrophy and subsequent suppression of the antibody responses. This immunodeficiency will result in a poor response to other vaccines and overwhelming secondary infections. There are two serotypes of IBDV but severe bursal disease is only associated with serotype 1. All commercial vaccines are directed against this serotype. There are no reports of clinical disease caused by serotype 2. As with all RNA viruses, IBDV is rapidly evolving and as a result there is much variation in antigenicity and virulence, features that complicate vaccine development.

Many different types of IBD vaccine are available, both monovalent and in combinations. These include live attenuated vaccines, inactivated oil-adjuvanted vaccines, live recombinant vaccines, or even immune-complex vaccines. Because this disease affects very young chicks it is important to exploit maternal immunity by vaccinating hens.

The inactivated vaccines are water-in-oil adjuvanted products. They are mainly used to induce long-term immunity in breeding stock. They are safe to use in young valuable birds with maternal antibodies. They are best used in birds at 16 to 20 weeks that have been primed by live vaccines at 8 weeks of age.

The viral structural protein 2 (VP2) is the major protective antigen in IBVD. This antigen can be expressed in different vector systems such as *E. coli*, yeast, fowlpox virus, baculovirus, and in plants. Commercially available VP2 recombinant vaccines include those from *E. coli*, the yeast *Pischia pastoris,* and baculovirus systems. They are not highly immunogenic and have to be boosted repeatedly. Given that these birds develop antibodies against only VP2, these have the potential to be DIVA vaccines.

Modified live vaccines have been attenuated by serial passage in tissue culture or eggs. Depending on their degree of attenuation, live attenuated IBDV vaccines may be classified as mild, intermediate, or invasive based on their ability to replicate and cause bursal lesions. This also reflects their ability to overcome maternal immunity. Mild vaccines are used to prime broiler breeders before boosting with an inactivated vaccine. If chicks have maternally-derived antibodies, then vaccination should be delayed until this has waned. The mild vaccines show poor efficacy in the presence of maternal antibodies or against very virulent strains of IBDV. The intermediate or hot strains are more immunogenic but may induce bursal lesions. The vaccine is usually given in a spray or in drinking water.

Immune-complex vaccines are made by mixing a live intermediate IBD virus with IBDV-specific hyperimmune chicken serum (IBDV-Icx vaccine, Cevac, Transmune). The advantage of this vaccine is that it can be used for in ovo vaccination. It can also be administered subcutaneously to one-day-old chicks. Studies on the fate of the immune-complex-bound virus indicate that it does reach the bursa, but five days later than uncomplexed virus. As a result, it causes much less bursal and splenic damage. It is likely that the immune-complexed virus localizes in areas within the spleen and bursa where it is more effectively processed and presented by follicular dendritic cells. Immune-complexes are much more immunogenic than vaccine antigen given alone. This is supported by the observation that chicks receiving the immune-complex vaccine develop many new germinal centers in their spleen. This vaccine is not available in the United States.

Recombinant vectored vaccines use the herpesvirus of turkeys to express the VP2 antigen of IBDV. As a result, they can be used in a DIVA strategy because they only induce antibodies against VP2 in contrast to whole virus vaccines that induce antibodies against all IBDV proteins. They are designed so that they can be injected either into 18-day eggs or into 1-day-old hatchlings, where they are not inhibited by maternal antibodies.

INFECTIOUS BRONCHITIS

Infectious bronchitis is an economically significant respiratory disease of chickens that also causes nephritis, decreased egg production, poor growth, and high morbidity. It is caused by a *gammacorona* virus, avian infectious bronchitis virus (IBV). The combination of high morbidity, and loss of performance, together with secondary bacterial infections can lead to unsustainable losses. As a result, almost all commercial poultry are vaccinated against this virus. However, the ability to control or prevent infectious bronchitis outbreaks is rendered very difficult by the continuous emergence of new IBV genotypes, serotypes, and variants as a result of mutation and recombination. Over 50 serotypes and hundreds of variants have been identified and more continue to emerge. These variants arise as a result of sequence changes in a hypervariable region of the viral spike (S) glycoprotein. There is also a lack of cross-protection among these genotypes. Thus as variants appear and disappear, they necessitate the continual development of new vaccines. Both inactivated and live attenuated IBV vaccines are available. Currently most of these vaccines contain the Massachusetts strain either alone or in combination with the Arkansas, Connecticut, Georgia, Huyben (Holland), or Delaware strains. They are usually given in combination with Newcastle disease vaccines.

Inactivated vaccines may be used alone or in combination with modified live virus (MLV) vaccines in layer/breeder flocks to induce maternal immunity and thus protect chicks from an early age. As we have seen with other diseases, the inactivated vaccines induce a relatively weak immune response without cell-mediated immunity, and thus require multiple doses and the use of adjuvants. These in turn increase handling costs and may cause significant injection site lesions.

Modified live IBV vaccines containing three common serotypes are administered in the drinking water, or by coarse spray, and given at day one or within the first week. Some short-lived broilers receive only this single dose. For longer-lived broilers, a second dose is generally given two to three weeks later. Long-lived broiler breeders and layers receive multiple vaccine doses at two, four, and six weeks. Revaccination after that depends upon the local threat assessment. There is great diversity among the MLV strains employed depending on geographic location. For example, in North America the major vaccine strains are M41 (Massachusetts), Arkansas, and Connecticut. In Europe strains 4/91 and D274 predominate. These may be ineffective in other countries or locations. The Chinese QX strain has caused outbreaks in Africa, the Middle East, Europe, and Asia. These modified live vaccines induce a potent protective response but reversion to virulence, recombination, or mutation are ever-present risks. There are currently no licensed recombinant vaccines available.

INFECTIOUS LARYNGOTRACHEITIS

An economically important respiratory disease caused by gallid herpesvirus 1, ILT affects chickens, peafowl, pheasants, and partridges. The principle lesion is tracheitis and the disease can vary in severity from lethal asphyxiation to very mild or subclinical infection. As with other herpesviruses, infected birds may become healthy carriers. The disease is usually prevented by the use of either live attenuated vaccines or recombinant vectored vaccines.

Modified live vaccine viruses have been attenuated either by prolonged passage in tissue culture or by passage in embryonated chicken eggs. The MLV vaccine may then be administered by spray, eye drops, or in the drinking water. Residual virulence may be an issue with some of these vaccines especially when delivered by spray vaccination. Reversion to virulence may also be an issue. Some recent ILT outbreaks have been attributed to egg adapted vaccines that have regained virulence. The chicken embryo passaged vaccine is the most widely used ILT vaccine. It induces rapid immunity and is easily administered through drinking water. In general, long-lived birds are routinely vaccinated against ILT, but short-lived birds such as broilers are only vaccinated if an outbreak is threatened

As a result of residual virulence in modified live vaccines, efforts have been made to generate safer vaccines by developing viral vectored vaccines. These recombinant ILT vaccines contain either herpesvirus of turkeys (Marek's serotype 3), or fowlpox virus expressing one or more of the ILT glycoproteins. The fowlpox-vectored vaccine expresses the glycoprotein B and UL32 genes. It may be given in ovo or by wing web puncture to one-day-old commercial layers. There are two HVT vectored vaccines, one expressing glycoproteins I and D, the other expressing glycoprotein B. They induce protective immunity against both ILT and Marek's disease. They are not transmitted between birds and do not revert to virulence. They are also administered by subcutaneous vaccination to one-day-old chicks or in ovo. They are not as protective as the attenuated vaccines and are less able to prevent shedding.

AVIAN REOVIRUSES

Avian reoviruses belong to the genus Orthoreoviruses in the *Reoviridae* family. They cause arthritis/tenosynovitis, proventriculitis, a runting-stunting syndrome, and "blue-wing disease" in broilers. Because these diseases affect very young birds, reovirus vaccines are often administered to breeding hens to stimulate maternal immunity and protect the newly hatched chicks. Both inactivated and modified live vaccines are available.

The inactivated oil-emulsion adjuvanted vaccines may contain multiple strains and different pathotypes. They are used in replacement and breeder hens and are often used in combination with NDV, Marek's or bronchitis vaccines.

Live vaccines may contain the avirulent 2177 or 1133 strains. Some are given subcutaneously to one-day-old chicks. Others are given in drinking water to birds between 10 and 17 weeks of age. Over the past six years there has been a gradual increase in the number of disease outbreaks in vaccinated flocks. This is a result of changes in the circulating strains of the viruses, and so new, updated vaccines are needed.

AVIAN INFLUENZA

According to the US Department of Agriculture (USDA), the outbreak of highly pathogenic avian influenza (HPAI) that occurred in 2015 was the worst animal disease outbreak in US history. More than 200 premises were affected in 15 states and more that 48 million birds were depopulated. These recent outbreaks have made mass slaughter prohibitively expensive. Consideration is therefore being given to use vaccination to block or slow the spread of the disease when this disease recurs. In most countries where the disease is not endemic, vaccination against HPAI is actively discouraged or banned because it interferes with the detection of infected flocks. Vaccination alone is not a solution to the problem of HPAI, or H5/H7, low pathogenic avian influenza (LPAI) viruses because it raises the possibility that these strains could become endemic in avian populations. Additionally, although vaccines may prevent sickness and death, they will not prevent infection or viral shedding.

In the United States, the USDA has established the National Veterinary Stockpile in case a decision has to be made regarding avian influenza vaccination. The stockpiled vaccines are primarily inactivated vaccines but a DNA-plasmid vaccine has also been conditionally licensed. If a decision to vaccinate is made, domestic distribution and use will be supervised and controlled by USDA veterinary services as part of an official USDA program. Vaccination may be used in control programs for both HPAI and LPAI. The recent emergence of pandemic influenza A strains such as H7N9 and H5N1, reveals the tremendous challenges to our current influenza control strategies. Better vaccines that provide protection against a wide spectrum of influenza viruses and long-lasting immunity are urgently needed.

Over 95% of all avian influenza virus (AIV) vaccines used in poultry are inactivated, adjuvanted products given by injection. Vaccines containing mineral or vegetable oil based adjuvants generally induce the highest antibody titers. These vaccines are prepared from infectious allantoic fluid that is inactivated with beta-propiolactone or formaldehyde.

Inactivated influenza A vaccines have been used in turkeys in the United States against LPAI and non-H5/H7 influenza A viruses. A vaccine against H1 and H3 swine influenza viruses has also been used in breeder turkeys. Vaccines against H9N2, H7N3, H5N2, H5N1, have been used extensively in Asia in response to specific disease outbreaks.

Advances in molecular biology have allowed Marek's disease (HVT) vectored vaccines, expressing the influenza virus hemagglutinin (HA), to be sold commercially. As a group, these vectored vaccines can stimulate both cellular and humoral immunity and are effective at preventing clinical disease and reducing virus shedding. All the licensed recombinant vaccines, because they only express the HA, may be used to differentiate vaccinated from infected birds. The vectored vaccines also work well with a prime-boost strategy where the vectored vaccine is given first and birds are revaccinated with a killed adjuvanted vaccine two or three weeks later. The use of a killed vaccine with a homologous hemagglutinin and a heterologous neuraminidase may allow the serologic differentiation of vaccinated and infected birds.

A recombinant fowlpox influenza vaccine (TROVAC-AIV H5) expressing the hemagglutinin of avian influenza H5 has been licensed for use in Mexico, Guatemala, and El Salvador where it is widely employed. It can be administered to one-day-old chicks and serologic tests can readily distinguish vaccinated from naturally infected birds.

FOWLPOX

Fowlpox is caused by an Avipoxvirus, a large, complex DNA virus. They are transmitted through aerosols or by biting insects. It is a slowly spreading infection characterized by proliferative skin lesions (dry pox) on unfeathered skin, or by diphtheritic lesions in the mucosa of the mouth, esophagus, larynx, or trachea (wet pox). The latter can result in asphyxiation of young chicks. In general mortality is low but may reach 50% in stressed flocks. Modified live fowlpox or pigeon poxvirus vaccines attenuated in cell culture or embryonated eggs are available. They may be given as monovalent vaccines or in combinations. Most are administered into the wing web after maternal immunity has waned. Some are administered subcutaneously to one-day-old chicks and there is also an in ovo recombinant vectored vaccine available that expresses ILT antigens. They may be used in situations where the disease is endemic because the infection spreads relatively slowly and may be administered in the face of an outbreak. They have also been used in pigeons, turkeys, and quail, in addition to chickens.

AVIAN ENCEPHALOMYELITIS

The cause of epidemic tremor, avian encephalomyelitis virus is a picornavirus that affects the central nervous system. In young chickens it induces paralysis, ataxia, and muscular dystrophy. In older chickens, infection is usually subclinical but causes a decline in egg production and hatchability. Several modified live vaccines are available. Some may be combined with fowlpox. Most are administered by wing web vaccination using a double needle applicator. Breeder chickens are vaccinated at 10 to 16 weeks of age, at least 4 weeks before start of lay. The site of inoculation should be examined for "take" at 7 to 10 days postvaccination. A positive take is indicated by a swelling or scab at the site of inoculation. If given to laying flocks this vaccine can cause a serious drop in egg production.

EGG DROP SYNDROME

Egg drop syndrome (EDS) is caused by an adenovirus infection in laying hens. It is characterized by production of soft-shelled and shell-less eggs and also a 10% to 40% drop in egg production. An inactivated vaccine containing EDS'76 virus strain BC14 in a water-in-oil emulsion may be available. It should be administered intramuscularly to layers and breeders no later than 4 weeks before the expected onset of lay.

ANTIPARASITE VACCINES

Coccidiosis

Infection with Eimeria coccidia induces a strong, species-specific protective immunity. As a result, several live coccidial vaccines are used in commercial poultry. These vaccines typically contain live sporulated oocysts from multiple Eimeria species and strains. Some consist of virulent, drug-sensitive organisms administered repeatedly in very low doses of oocysts (trickle infection). Some of these organisms have been attenuated by repeated passage through eggs, but this only works well for *Eimeria tenella*. Other Eimeria species have been selected for precocity. Precocious strains mature very rapidly (30 hours faster than the parent strain), and, as a result, have less time to replicate, produce fewer oocysts, are less virulent because they cause less tissue damage, yet are highly immunogenic. This precociousness is a stable trait and the parasites do not regain virulence. All of these vaccines provide solid immunity to coccidia when applied carefully under good conditions. Nevertheless, the dose of coccidia vaccine must be carefully controlled, and the vaccines must be harvested from the feces of infected birds. Vaccinated birds shed oocysts that are transmitted to other birds. Because of regional strain variation, vaccination may not be effective in protecting against field strains in all locations.

A transmission blocking subunit vaccine has been developed that contains two purified glycoproteins (Gam56 and Gam82) from the wall-forming bodies of macrogametocytes of *Eimeria maxima*. It is believed that the antibodies produced inhibit oocyst wall formation. This vaccine (CoxAbic, Netanya, Israel) is administered by injection with an oil-in-water adjuvant. It is given to breeder hens twice before the breeding season to provide maternal immunity to their chicks.

Conventional live coccidiosis vaccines are delivered to day-old chicks either at the hatchery or on the farm by coarse spray, gel, or feed vaccination. The vaccine containers should be shaken gently at intervals to ensure that the oocysts do not settle but stay in suspension. Spray application of these vaccines involves the use of a large droplet size and the vaccine is dyed to stimulate preening and consumption of the vaccine by the birds. Likewise, the sprayed chicks should be placed in well-lit areas to encourage them to preen. Administration on feed involves spraying the feed with the diluted vaccine to moisten it.

Maternal Immunity

Newly hatched birds emerge from the sterile environment of the egg, and like mammals, require temporary immunological assistance. Serum immunoglobulins are actively transported from the hen's serum to the yolk while the egg is still in the ovary (Fig. 19.4). During egg production about 30% of the hen's immunoglobulin (Ig)Y will transfer from her plasma to the yolk. IgY in the fluid phase of egg yolk is therefore found at levels equal to or greater than those in hen serum. As the fertilized ovum passes down the oviduct, IgM and IgA from oviduct secretions are acquired with the albumin. As the chick embryo develops in ovo, it absorbs the yolk IgY, which then appears in its circulation. At the same time, the IgM and IgA from the albumin diffuse into the amniotic fluid and are swallowed by the embryo. Thus when a chick hatches, it possesses IgY in its serum, and IgM and IgA in its intestine. The newly hatched chick does not absorb all its yolk sac antibodies until about 24 hours after hatching. These maternal antibodies effectively prevent successful vaccination until they disappear between 10 and 20 days after hatching. Newly hatched chicks begin to make their own IgA at day three in the bursa, and day seven in the gut and lung. Interestingly, maternal IgA persists for at least seven days because it appears to be

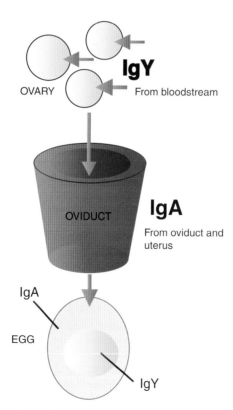

Fig. 19.4 The passive transfer of protective immunoglobulins from the hen to her eggs and hence to her chicks.

retained by the intestinal mucus. The presence of maternal antibodies may neutralize live vaccine strains and day of age vaccination is not therefore ideal. That is why in ovo vaccination is employed.

Assessment of Vaccination

The evaluation of serum antibody levels is an important tool for poultry flock management. The presence or absence of specific antibodies can be determined by serologic tests such as ELISAs, hemagglutination and agglutination tests. Serum samples are routinely and repeatedly obtained from poultry flocks. They are tested for the presence of antibodies against major poultry pathogens such as *Mycoplasma gallisepticum*, avian influenza, Newcastle disease, infectious bronchitis, salmonellosis, and infectious bursal disease. If antibody levels are deemed too low then the flock may be reimmunized until the birds generate a satisfactory titer. This procedure also permits an assessment of the comparative efficacy of different poultry vaccines. It serves as a diagnostic tool in disease outbreaks, either to prove freedom from a disease such as pullorum disease or fowl typhoid, or to confirm the presence of a new disease. It also permits evaluation of the level of maternal antibodies and thus the optimal time to vaccinate chicks. Bleeding schedules will depend upon the specific farm situation and their vaccination program.

HATCHERY VACCINATION

Hatchery vaccination can be performed in several different ways. These include in ovo vaccination before hatching in addition to spray or subcutaneous vaccinations administered at the day of hatch before the birds are moved out to barns. Although not an optimal time because of maternal antibodies, vaccination at one day can stimulate innate immunity such as interferon production that will provide early immunity (Chapter 4).

LAYER CHICKENS

Layers live for very much longer than broilers and accordingly need greater disease resistance. A typical protocol would be to administer Marek's disease vaccine at day 1; infectious bursal disease, Newcastle disease, and infectious bronchitis at weeks 2, 6, and 12; ILT and fowlpox at week 8 to 12; and *Mycoplasma gallisepticum* at week 12 to 16.

BROILER CHICKENS

These birds receive Marek's disease vaccine in ovo or on day 1; they get infectious bronchitis and Newcastle disease vaccines at day 1 and day 14; and they are vaccinated against infectious bursal disease in ovo, or on day 1, with a boost on day 8. Remember that these birds go to market at around 35 days so prolonged protection is not required.

SMALL FLOCKS

Although commercial poultry operations employ a great variety of vaccines, small flock owners use very few. This may be exacerbated by the cost of vaccines. Many are sold in 500 to 10,000 dose vials. Small flock owners generally only need to vaccinate if they have had problems in the past. Vaccination may also be recommended if they mix with other birds at poultry shows or if new birds from multiple sources are introduced into the flock. Marek's disease is ubiquitous and vaccination is strongly recommended. Birds purchased from hatcheries should be vaccinated before sale otherwise the owner should vaccinate their own chicks. Possible vaccines may also include, Newcastle disease, infectious bronchitis, laryngotracheitis, fowlpox, fowl cholera, and avian encephalomyelitis.

Adverse Events

Many of the problems associated with poultry vaccination relate to improper vaccination techniques. For example, in birds injected into the neck, accidental intradermal inoculation can result in swellings. These may rupture; bleed and other birds in the flock may cause secondary damage by pecking. Accidental intramuscular injection can cause muscle damage, scarring and possibly twisted necks. Injections that hit the spinal cord may be lethal. Birds injected close to the head may develop head swelling that can reduce performance and feed conversion.

Granulomas may form in the breast muscle of birds injected at this site and can cause issues when processing. Generally, vaccine volume should be minimized if injecting into small muscles such as the leg or wing.

Accidental human injection with oil emulsion vaccines is a serious potential problem. If these vaccines are injected into the hands or fingers, they can cause severe injury. Immediate treatment will involve removing the oil-emulsified product to improve healing in the affected area. This should be done by a qualified medical professional. Proper injection technique and bird handling will reduce the potential for this hazard. Bird handlers must present the birds for injection at the proper angle for the chosen site of injection. If the syringe operator has difficulty reaching the site of injection, the chance of accidental injection is significantly increased.

Ducks

Commercial duck production in the United States is largely restricted to parts of New York State. As a result, the source of duck vaccines in North America is the International Duck Research cooperative at Cornell University. Other countries such as China and India are major producers of duck vaccines (Table 19.4).

DUCK SEPTICEMIA

The cause of duck septicemia (also called infectious serositis or New Duck disease). *Reimerella anatipestifer* is a gram-negative bacterium. It causes the most economically important disease of farmed ducks and geese worldwide. The infection affects ducklings under eight weeks of age. It causes high mortality, and high condemnation rates as a result of weight loss. The bacterium is antigenically complex and 21 different serotypes have been described. There is much regional

TABLE 19.4 ■ **Vaccines for Ducks**

Vaccine/Disease	Vaccination Schedule	Comments
Antibacterial		
Reimerella anatipestifer	Vaccinate with the MLV at day 1 by spray and revaccinate at 10–14 days in drinking water. Vaccinate with the bacterin subcutaneously at 3 weeks.	From Cornell University Duck Laboratory.
Antiviral		
Duck viral hepatitis	A modified live vaccine injected into ducklings lacking maternal antibodies and also breeder birds.	
Duck viral enteritis	Vaccinate breeder birds at 4 weeks.	It may be administered to younger birds in the face of a developing outbreak.

variation in the prevalence of these serotypes. Bacterins generally provide short lasting protection. More recently, an avirulent live vaccine, which includes the three most common and virulent serotypes of *R. anatipestifer* (1, 2, and 5) found in North America, has been approved for use in ducks. Breeder ducks can be vaccinated with the live vaccine to provide maternal immunity that may last for up to two to three weeks of age in ducklings. A combined *E. coli-R. anatipestifer* formalin-killed bacterin is also available. It is given in two doses at two and three weeks of age. Autogenous bacterins may also be used in the case of outbreaks caused by less common serotypes.

DUCK VIRAL HEPATITIS

This is an acute highly contagious, rapidly fatal disease that affects ducklings and geese with sudden, high, and persistent mortality caused by an avihepatovirus, duck hepatitis A virus (DHAV) in the family *Picornaviridae*. The most pathogenic of the genotypes is DHAV type 1 (DHAV-1) that affects ducklings under four weeks of age. A live attenuated virus vaccine is available. It is generally given to breeder ducks to induce high levels of maternal antibodies and thus confer passive immunity on ducklings. The live attenuated vaccine may also be administered to one-day-old ducklings to control the disease in birds that lack maternal antibodies. It does not apparently spread from vaccinated birds. It is administered subcutaneously or intramuscularly. An inactivated vaccine can be used to boost breeder birds that have been primed by the modified live product.

Bacterial recombinants containing VP1 genes and expressing viral protein-1 from both DHAV-1 and DHAV-3 have been generated. Ducks that received a single dose of this recombinant vaccine were protected against challenge with both viruses, as early as three days after vaccination. Viral replication was blocked in vaccinated ducks by one week postvaccination. Tissue culture attenuated DHAV-1 also protected ducklings against challenge. Immunization of ducklings with yeast-derived recombinant VP1 induced a significant immune response and may also prove to be an effective vaccine.

DUCK VIRAL ENTERITIS

Duck plague is caused by Anatid herpesvirus 1. It is most commonly seen in mature ducks. In addition to malaise, bloodstained greenish diarrhea develops. Affected birds may show bloodstained feathers around the vent and nostrils, and sudden death is common. Attenuated live vaccines are available. They are given to broiler or breeder ducks over two weeks of age.

DUCK PARVOVIRUSES

These viruses can infect commercial Muscovy ducks and geese. Parvovirus disease occurs primarily in birds less than six weeks of age but older birds may act as carriers. The disease causes lethargy and wasting, and mortality can reach 100%. A variant, the Derzsy's parvovirus causes dwarfism and beak deformities in Mulard ducks (hybrid of Pekin and Muscovy ducks). Inactivated and modified live vaccines are available in Europe against these viruses.

Turkeys

In addition to turkey-specific infectious diseases, turkeys are also susceptible to many agents affecting chickens. For example, licensed turkey vaccines include those against the following: Pasteurella, Bordetella, *Mycoplasma gallisepticum*, Salmonellosis, Colibacillosis, fowlpox, viral encephalomyelitis, Newcastle disease, and paramyxovirus 3 (Table 19.5).

TABLE 19.5 ■ **Vaccines for Turkeys**

Vaccine/Disease	Vaccination Schedule	Comments
Antibacterial		
Fowl cholera	Vaccinate at 6 weeks revaccinate at 3–6 weeks and revaccinate layers or breeders at 3 month intervals. Other vaccines may be given at 15–18 weeks and revaccinated 8 weeks later.	Withdrawal time 21 or 42 days.
Erysipelas	Vaccinate at 8 weeks and revaccinate 2–3 weeks later. Revaccinate every 3 months.	Withdrawal time 21 days.
Mycoplasma gallisepticum	Vaccinate between 4 and 10 weeks of age.	Withdrawal time 21 or 42 days.
Colibacillosis	Vaccinate at 3 days and repeat at 3 weeks.	Withdrawal time 21 days.
Turkey Coryza *Bordetella avium*	Vaccinate at 1 day of age, revaccinate at 14 days, and revaccinate every 4–6 weeks as necessary. Another is given at 10 days and revaccinated at 24 days.	Withdrawal time 21 days.
Antiviral		
Newcastle disease	Either vaccinate birds over 3 weeks by eye drop or inject subcutaneously in birds between 16 and 24 weeks.	Withdrawal time 21or 42 days.
Hemorrhagic enteritis (Adenovirus 2)	Vaccinate in drinking water to birds 22–42 days of age.	Withdrawal time 21 or 42 days.
Turkey rhinotracheitis (Pneumovirus)	Vaccinate either in ovo or in drinking water at 1 week of age and revaccinate 4 weeks later.	Boost by eye drop or drinking water. Withdrawal time 21 days.
Encephalomyelitis	Vaccinate tween 10 weeks of age and 4 weeks before production.	Applied in the wing web. Withdrawal time 21 days.
Paramyxovirus 3	Vaccinate before laying at 20–24 weeks and revaccinate 4–6 weeks later.	Withdrawal time 42 days.
Fowlpox	Vaccinate turkeys over 4 weeks or older (8–18 weeks).	Withdrawal time 21 days. Do not vaccinate within 4 weeks of egg production.

TURKEY ERYSIPELAS

Two vaccines are available against *Erysipelothrix rhusiopathiae* in turkeys. One is a two-dose vaccine administered in drinking water given at 8 and 11 weeks of age. The other is an injectable bacterin. It confers limited immunity and requires multiple doses given every three months.

TURKEY CORYZA

Bordetella avium causes turkey coryza, an upper respiratory tract infection with high morbidity, seen between two and eight weeks of age. Live attenuated vaccines are available against this infection. They are administered by spray or drinking water. Some are given at 1 day of age, boosted at 14 days, and revaccinated every 4 to 6 weeks as necessary. Another is given at 10 days and revaccinated at 24 days.

TURKEY RHINOTRACHEITIS

Rhinotracheitis of turkeys is caused by an avian metapneumovirus that causes a severe upper respiratory tract infection. The agent is a single stranded, negative sense, RNA paramyxovirus. Four antigenic subtypes have been identified. Both an inactivated oil-emulsion adjuvanted vaccine and live attenuated vaccines are available. The live vaccines have been attenuated by passage in duck embryonated eggs, or in tissue culture, or by alternating between these two procedures. These live vaccines are used in young birds (one to seven days) to prevent disease onset. They can also be used for a primary dose before boosting with an inactivated vaccine. They are usually applied by coarse spray, eye drop, or in drinking water. The inactivated vaccines are used to produce strong consistent immunity in breeder turkeys primed with the live vaccine.

TURKEY HEMORRHAGIC ENTERITIS

Hemorrhagic enteritis virus is an adenovirus of the genus *Siadenovirus*, associated with acute hemorrhagic gastrointestinal disease in turkeys. This is a disease of young birds seven to nine weeks of age characterized by severe depression and bloody droppings. Surviving birds are profoundly immunosuppressed. This may predispose them to secondary bacterial infections such as colibacillosis. Avirulent strains of this virus can be effectively used as vaccines. They may be prepared using a crude spleen homogenate or attenuated *in vitro* by passage in RP19 cells, a turkey lymphoid cell line. The cell-cultured vaccine is commercially available. It is given via drinking water in four to six week old birds after maternal immunity has waned. If necessary, a booster may be given a week later to ensure maximal protection.

PARAMYXOVIRUS 3

There are 12 recognized serotypes of avian paramyxovirus (PMV). The most important of these is PMV-1, Newcastle disease. However other PMV serotypes may occasionally cause disease. PMV-3 causes respiratory disease, reduced egg production, and lower hatchability in turkeys. Secondary bacterial infections make the disease more severe. Inactivated oil emulsion vaccines are used in turkey breeder flocks.

Guinea Fowl

Guinea fowl housed with poultry are susceptible to Newcastle disease and fowlpox and so should receive these vaccines.

Sources of Additional Information

Abdul-Cader, M.S., Palomino-Tapia, V., Amarasinghe, A., et al. (2018). Hatchery vaccination against poultry viral diseases: Potential mechanisms and limitations. *Viral Immunol,* 31, 23–33.

Bande, F., Arshad, S.S., Bejo, M.H., Moieni, H., Omar, A.R. (2015). Progress and challenges towards the development of vaccines against avian infectious bronchitis. *J Immunol Res,* 2015, 424860.

Choi, K.S. (2017). Newcastle disease virus vectored vaccines as bivalent antigen delivery vaccines. *Clin Exp Vacc Res,* 6, 72–82.

Dimitrov, K.M., Afonso, C.L., Yu, Q., Miller, P.J. (2017). Newcastle disease vaccines *Vet Microbiol,* 206, 126–136.

Garcia, M. (2017). Current and future vaccines and vaccination strategies against infectious laryngotracheitis (ILT) respiratory disease in poultry. *Vet Microbiol,* 206, 157–162.

Higgins, D.A., Henry, R.R., Kounev, Z.V. (2000). Duck immune response to *Reimerella anatipestifer* vaccines. *Dev Comp Immunol,* 24, 153–167.

Jackwood, D.J. (2017). Advances in vaccine research against economically important viral diseases of food animals: Infectious bursal disease virus. *Vet Microbiol,* 206, 121–125.

Jones, R.C. (2000). Avian reovirus infections. *Rev Sci Tech,* 19, 614–625.

Jordan, B. (2017). Vaccination against infectious bronchitis virus: A continuous challenge. *Vet Microbiol*, 206, 137–143.

Kapczynski, D.R., Afonso, C.L., Miller, P.J. (2013). Immune responses of poultry to Newcastle disease virus. *Dev Comp Immunol*, 41, 447–453.

Muller, H., Mundt, E., Eterradossi, N., Islam, M.R. (2012). Current status of vaccines against infectious bursal disease. *Avian Pathol*, 41, 133–139.

Reddy, S.M., Izumiya, Y., Lupian, 1. B. (2017). Marek's disease vaccines: Current status and strategies for improvement and development of vector vaccines. *Vet Microbiol*, 206, 113–120.

Sharman, P.A., Smith, N.C., Wallach, M.G., Katrib, M. (2010). Chasing the golden egg: vaccination against poultry coccidiosis. *Parasite Immunol*, 32, 590–598.

Suarez, D.L., Pantin-Jackwood, M.J. (2017). Recombinant viral-vectored vaccines for the control of avian influenza in poultry. *Vet Microbiol*, 206, 144–151.

Singhe, R., Verma, P.C., Singh, S. (2010). Immunogenicity and protective efficacy of virosome based vaccines against Newcastle Disease. *Trop Anim Health Prod*, 42, 465–471.

Vaccination of Exotic and Wild Species

Although exotic mammals and birds are susceptible to many of the diseases that affect their domestic counterparts, they are rarely presented to veterinarians in sufficient numbers to justify the development of specific vaccines for each species. Mink, foxes, and rabbits raised commercially for their fur and meat respectively are exceptions. As a result, it is usual to vaccinate exotics "extra-label." Should a veterinarian use a vaccine in a species not specified on the label or on the package insert, they must assume full responsibility for product failure or any adverse consequences. Vaccines developed and considered safe for a specific domestic species may not be safe or efficacious in related wild species. However, captivity may expose animals to a greater risk of contact with pets or livestock, and exposure to pathogens, compared with their free-living counterparts. In many cases, there is a significant lack of information on diseases in exotic species. Before considering vaccination of exotic pets, the veterinarian must ensure that the owner is legally in possession of the animal because in many jurisdictions, ownership of certain species is restricted. As always, informed consent is critical considering the lack of hard data regarding the use of vaccines in these species.

Constraints on new vaccine production and marketing include the cost and complexity of production, in addition to the relatively small size of the market for exotic species. The relative complexity of many new vaccines, and expensive and complex licensing requirements are reflected in vaccine cost. A serious expense gap exists between our ability to make sophisticated vaccines in a laboratory setting and to manufacture and market these products at a reasonable price. Manufacturers are therefore reluctant to make a large investment in new vaccine production for less abundant species.

Vaccination of free-living species presents totally different considerations. Because wildlife vaccination is primarily undertaken by, and often restricted to, government agencies either for public health reasons such as rabies or plague control, for conservation reasons as in saving an endangered population, or for population control purposes, no commercial market for wildlife vaccination exists.

Mammals

Modified live vaccines pose a health risk to exotic mammals and may not be effective. Vaccines attenuated for domestic mammals such as dogs and cats may retain significant virulence for wild mammals.

ERYSIPELAS

The bacterium, *Erysipelothrix rhusiopathiae,* is pathogenic for peccaries, nondomestic pigs, cetaceans, and pinnipeds. An erysipelas bacterin can be administered by a standard protocol to nondomestic pigs (including pot-bellied pigs) and peccaries. Some dolphins may be healthy carriers of this organism. Erysipelas bacterins are not widely used in captive cetaceans because of the risks involved in immobilization, and the prevalence of adverse reactions, especially hypersensitivities leading to death. Vaccination is not recommended for pinnipeds.

LEPTOSPIROSIS

Leptospirosis occurs sporadically in many different mammals. Although vaccination with a Leptospira bacterin is considered noncore in dogs, vaccination should be considered when exotic species are housed in an endemic area, or if this disease is known to be a problem in the collection. Selection of serovars depends upon those known to be present in a region. However, serovars Canicola and Icterohaemorrhagiae should be included in any vaccine. Carnivores should be vaccinated at six to eight weeks of age, boosted two weeks later, and revaccinated every six months. Ruminants, pigs, and peccaries should receive the 5-way bacterins including Pomona, Hardjo, Icterohaemorrhagiae, Canicola, and Grippotyphosa. Because the available bacterins are poorly immunogenic, semiannual vaccination is probably necessary to maintain immunity.

CLOSTRIDIAL DISEASES

Many exotic species are susceptible to clostridial diseases, especially tetanus. These include equids, elephants, great apes, deer, camelids, and also sheep and goats. The equids and elephants should be vaccinated on the same schedule as domestic horses with primary immunization at three to four months, a second dose one month later and annual revaccination. Ruminants including deer, antelope, and camelids should receive 8-way combined clostridial bacterins. Other domestic hoof stock should receive tetanus toxoid according to the manufacturer's recommendations. Pot-bellied pigs should be vaccinated against tetanus.

Primates should receive human tetanus toxoid. Two intramuscular doses given at an interval of 4 to 5 weeks followed by revaccination 6 to 12 months later, and subsequent boosting every 3 to 5 years or after an injury.

Exotic sheep, goats, llamas, and alpacas should receive the core sheep vaccines, especially *Clostridium perfringens* toxoids C and D and other clostridial vaccines as required in addition to tetanus (Chapter 17) (Box 20.1). *Clostridium botulinum* has caused lethal disease in many different mammals especially mink. Botulism type C toxoids for mink have been available for many years.

BOVINE HERPESVIRUS 1

As described in Chapter 16, there are numerous vaccines available to protect domestic cattle against rhinotracheitis caused by bovine herpesvirus 1. It would be safer to use inactivated vaccines in exotic hoof stock in view of the known hazards of the modified live vaccines. The same applies to bovine virus diarrhea vaccines.

PARAINFLUENZA 3

Sheep and goats are susceptible to respiratory disease caused by *Mannheimia haemolytica* and parainfluenza 3. Modified live vaccines are available for domestic sheep and goats. Intranasal

---

BOX 20.1 ■ Camelpox Vaccines

Both species of old-world camels (*Camelus dromedaries* and *Camelus bactrianus*) constitute an economically important pair of species because they are used for milk, wool, and meat. However, they may suffer from camelpox caused by an orthomyxovirus very closely related to smallpox (variola) virus. This virus also causes disease in the introduced camels in Australia and the new-world camelids such as llamas. The infection is zoonotic and can affect humans. In camels it causes morbidity including weight loss and a decline in milk yield. Mortality may reach 100% in young camels. Nomadic camel herders used to vaccinate against the disease by scarifying animals with a mixture of camelpox scabs and milk.

Both inactivated and live attenuated camelpox vaccines are currently available. The formalin inactivated product adjuvanted with aluminum hydroxide provides protection for about a year and requires annual revaccination. The attenuated vaccines include a Saudi isolate (Al Jouf-78), and a South African isolate (Ducapox). These vaccines protect for at least 6 years although young camels require a booster at 6 months. The live vaccine may be combined with contagious ecthyma (soremouth) vaccine.

(Balamurugan, V., Venkatesan, G., Bhanuprakash, V., Kumar Singh, R. [2012]. Camel pox: an emerging orthopox viral disease. *Indian J Virol*, 24, 295–305.)

---

vaccines should be administered as directed on the label for domestic species with annual boosting.

CANINE DISTEMPER

Most of the Carnivora including canids, hyenas and aardwolves, procyonids, mustelids, especially mink and otters, viverrids, and both giant and red pandas are susceptible to distemper. Large felids such as lions, leopards, and tigers (*Panthera spp.*) are also susceptible to canine distemper virus (CDV) so that this should be considered a core vaccine in these species, although its efficacy is unclear. The risk of distemper in small felids appears to be low, but lethal distemper has been reported in lynx. Recent molecular evidence suggests that CDV isolates from large felids are distinctly different from current vaccine strains.

Xenarthra such as sloths are also susceptible to distemper. However, there is some debate as to the best canine distemper vaccine to use in these exotic species.

One of the major issues with vaccinating exotic species is a history of modified live virus (MLV) vaccines causing lethal distemper in nondomestic species. The newer canarypox-vectored subunit distemper vaccines appear to be safe and usually effective, although they may not stimulate as strong an antibody response as traditional MLVs. It is suggested that the first vaccine dose should be given to canid pups when maternal antibodies wane around 6 to 9 weeks, followed by boosters every 2 to 3 weeks until 16 to 20 weeks, followed by annual revaccination. The persistence of maternal antibodies also varies among species so current recommendations suggest that the final dose should be given at 18 to 20 weeks in raccoons, and after 10 weeks in ferrets. The duration of immunity following vaccination in these species is unclear. For some, such as red foxes, immunity lasts about 3 years, but data is lacking for others.

A common distemper virus strain used in modified live CDV vaccines is Snyder Hill. This strain retains significant virulence. Thus when this vaccine was administered to gray foxes it killed them. The infection was also transmitted from vaccinated to unvaccinated contacts. Subsequent analysis suggested that a single passage through foxes resulted in a measurable increase in viral virulence. Similar cases of distemper have been reported in young kinkajous (*Potos flavus*) and red pandas (*Ailurus fulgens*). The lethal effects of MLV CDV vaccine in black-footed ferrets are discussed below.

It is assumed that the primary reservoirs of CDV are unvaccinated domestic dogs. However, other species such as raccoons may also be reservoir hosts. Distemper-infected ferrets (*Mustela putorius faro*) develop severe lymphopenia and secondary diarrhea, cutaneous lesions, and neurologic signs. Ferrets die within two weeks as a result of sepsis and multiorgan failure, and the disease is nearly 100% fatal. The only vaccine currently licensed in the United States for use in ferrets is a live canarypox vectored recombinant. It is given to ferrets over eight weeks of age, boosted three and six weeks later, and then revaccinated annually. There are also several inactivated vaccines that may also be given after 12 weeks and boosted annually. As with all other species, the decision to vaccinate should be subjected to a careful risk assessment. This may also influence any decision as to when to revaccinate. It has been suggested that ferrets are more likely to develop adverse events following distemper vaccination and that veterinarians should obtain signed consent forms before vaccinating ferrets. Some recommend pretreating ferrets with diphenhydramine, an antihistamine, before vaccinating them. Do not forget that ferrets must also be vaccinated against rabies. In addition to residual virulence, there have been several reports of injection site-associated sarcomas occurring in ferrets. These have been associated with the use of rabies and distemper vaccines.

PARVOVIRUSES

Canine, feline, and mink parvoviruses are closely related. Canids, felids, mustelids, procyonids, and viverrids are susceptible to at least one of these. Thus canids and mustelids such as otters should get canine parvovirus vaccines; exotic felids, raccoons, and mink should get feline panleukopenia vaccine. Only inactivated vaccines should be used in these species. Vaccines should be administered according to the manufacturer's recommendations with annual revaccination. Some species such as lions may be less responsive to these vaccines than others such as tigers. Red wolves (*Canis rufus*) have positive antibody titers after three years, but otherwise the duration of immunity is unknown. Pigs of all species should also receive porcine parvovirus vaccination.

CANINE ADENOVIRUS

Canine adenoviruses 1 and 2 can cause disease in foxes, wolves, coyotes, wild dogs, mustelids, binturongs (*Arctictis binturong*), and bears (Fig. 10.5). Cross-protection occurs between the two viral species so a single vaccine protects against both. Although a killed vaccine is not commercially available, this should be considered to be a core vaccine for captive canids. Risk of vaccine-induced disease exists because an MLV- CA2 vaccine has induced hepatitis in a maned wolf (*Chrysocion brachyurus*). In general, the vaccination protocol should be the same as used in domestic dogs.

FELINE CALICIVIRUS

A core vaccine in exotic felids, the killed calicivirus vaccine may be administered in combination with feline rhinotracheitis vaccine. This is not a highly immunogenic vaccine and antibody responses are unpredictable. Annual revaccination is recommended.

FELINE HERPESVIRUS

This is a core vaccine in exotic felids. Combined vaccines with feline panleukopenia are available. Timing of vaccination should be the same as recommended in domestic cats.

EQUINE ENCEPHALITIDES

Nondomestic equids are susceptible to the viral encephalitides. They should therefore receive bivalent (EEE-WEE) or trivalent (EEE-WEE-VEE) vaccines, perhaps in combination with tetanus toxoid. They should be primed with two doses three to four weeks apart with annual revaccination. It would be prudent to vaccinate tapirs in the same manner.

EQUINE HERPESVIRUS

Equine herpesviruses 1 and 4 can cause abortion in exotic equids. They should therefore receive a killed vaccine. They should be vaccinated at four months and at four-month intervals up to one year. Pregnant mares should be vaccinated during pregnancy (Chapter 15).

HUMAN VACCINES

Primates are susceptible to many of the infectious diseases that affect humans. It is usual to vaccinate them, especially the Pongidae, with children's vaccines: mumps, measles and rubella, as well as diphtheria, pertussis, and tetanus (DPT). The great apes are also susceptible to poliomyelitis and they should therefore receive polio vaccine. The oral vaccine is easier to administer than the injectable one, but the modified live oral vaccine has the potential to cause disease. The oral vaccine may be administered on a sugar cube at six months, and then the animal should be isolated from unvaccinated primates for one month after vaccination. Should human polio vaccination be discontinued it would be no longer necessary to vaccinate captive primates.

RABIES

All mammals are susceptible to rabies. Therefore rabies vaccination should be considered essential in canids and felids and recommended for use in other mammals such as elephants where the potential for infection is high. Unfortunately, none of the currently available rabies vaccines are licensed for use in exotic captive mammals. The sole exception is for ferrets where killed vaccines are available for use in animals over 12 weeks of age. Ferrets must be vaccinated against rabies in an approved manner as prescribed in the compendium for rabies control.

Birds

Most avian vaccines are licensed for use in commercial species such as poultry, mallards, and turkeys, but can probably be used safely in exotic species. Some vaccines designed for use in non-avian species are also routinely used in an "extra-label" manner to prevent disease. Nevertheless, infectious diseases remain a constant threat to pet birds. Although these threats stem mainly from viral infections, clostridial and mycoplasmal infections are examples of bacterial diseases that are better prevented or avoided than treated.

AVIAN POLYOMA VIRUS

Avian polyoma viruses (APV) cause acute mortality in fledgling budgerigars, nestling macaws, and finches. Adjuvanted and nonadjuvanted vaccines are available and used to vaccinate birds before shipment for commercial sales. Seroconversion does not differ significantly between the two vaccines.

HERPESVIRUSES

Pacheco disease, caused by Psittacid herpesvirus 1 (PDV), is an acute fulminating hepatitis resulting in up to 100% mortality in new world parrots. Survivors may eventually develop cloacal papillomas or hepatomas. Several oil-adjuvanted, inactivated vaccines have been developed against this disease. However, none appear to be commercially available at present. The oil emulsion adjuvanted vaccines may cause injection site reactions including swelling, muscle necrosis, or granuloma formation. Cockatoos appear to be especially sensitive to these types of reactions.

WEST NILE VIRUS (WNV)

Since its introduction to North America in 1999, West Nile Virus (WNV) has spread across both American continents causing neurological disease in humans, horses, and many species of birds. WNV is maintained in the wild in a transmission cycle between birds and mosquitoes. Corvids are highly susceptible to WNV infection. Other susceptible North American birds include some endangered or threatened species. As in humans, juvenile and aged birds may be more susceptible to disease. Although a clear threat, no avian-specific WNV vaccine is available. Therefore valuable susceptible species, especially captive cranes, raptors, penguins, flamingos, and corvids may be vaccinated using equine vaccines.

The formalin inactivated, adjuvanted whole virus vaccine, West Nile Innovator, has been used extensively in birds, especially in emergency situations where it is considered essential to protect large valuable populations. For example, this vaccine has been tested in Sandhill cranes (*Antigone canadensis*). Other species that have received this vaccine include penguins, flamingos, and prairie chickens. All were vaccinated intramuscularly at least twice and no adverse effects were reported. WNV vaccination has also been undertaken in California condors (*Gymnogyps californianus*), both in captivity and in the wild.

AVIAN INFLUENZA

Influenza vaccines have been used in species other than poultry. For example, birds have been vaccinated against avian influenza virus using an inactivated H5N9 vaccine. Significant species variation in response was noted. Vaccination may provide protection from highly pathogenic avian influenza outbreaks in zoos and should be regarded as an important adjunct procedure in addition to increased biosecurity and monitoring.

NEWCASTLE DISEASE

Newcastle disease virus (NDV) vaccines are used in commercial ostrich flocks. Ostriches respond to vaccination with LaSota strain NDV vaccines. NDV causes neurologic disease and diarrhea in pigeons. As a result, racing pigeons are commonly vaccinated using the LaSota strain of NDV. Adult birds are given the chicken vaccine by eye drop seven weeks before breeding. Annual revaccination is recommended. Vaccination may be mandatory for racing pigeons in many countries. A single vaccination gave protection lasting one year.

Other Pigeon Vaccines

Paratyphoid caused by *Salmonella typhimurium* var. Copenhagen, is a problem in many pigeon lofts. A killed adjuvanted vaccine (KM-1) is given subcutaneously to pigeons over five weeks of age and boosted three to four weeks later. It contains a mixture of pigeon isolates. Annual revaccination is also recommended. Pigeons also suffer from pigeon pox and circovirus infections and some pigeon breeders may elect to use extra-label poultry vaccines in their birds despite the lack of evidence of efficacy.

POXVIRUSES

Avipoxvirus infections occur in many domestic, pet, and wild bird species. These viruses are spread either by mosquito bites or via aerosol. Many different vaccines are available to control fowlpox infections in poultry. A chicken fowlpox vaccine has been reported to protect zebra finches. A live pigeon pox vaccine has been tested in falcons. There is a commercially available live attenuated canarypox vaccine (Poximune C, Ceva Biomune) available for use in canaries. It is administered through the wing web and an obvious reaction occurs at the site 7 to 10 days later. Birds should be revaccinated at 6 to 12 month intervals. Birds should also be revaccinated four weeks before laying or the beginning of the mosquito season.

Commercial Exotic Vaccines

MINK VACCINES

Mink are intensively farmed for their fur. As a result of high stocking density, infectious diseases are a constant threat. It is important to remember that the pelt is the most valuable product from these animals. Injection site lesions thus present a special problem. Vaccine site infections with *Arcanobacterium phocae* are also an emerging issue. This bacterium causes a severe necropurulent dermatitis at the injection site in the hind leg and is believed to be the cause of a skin disease, fur animal epidemic necrotic pyoderma, in mink, foxes, and raccoons.

BOTULISM

The use of cheap, low-quality food has resulted in serious food poisoning episodes, especially botulism from rotting meat among mink. *Cl. botulinum* type C grows and produces its toxin when contaminated meat is stored at temperatures over 15°C and anaerobic growth can occur. When this meat is consumed, mink die within 24 to 72 hours with paralysis and dyspnea. Losses may reach 100%. *Cl. botulinum* type C toxoid is available for use in mink. It may be given to kits as early as six to seven weeks of age. Protection develops in three weeks. Annual revaccination is encouraged.

CANINE DISTEMPER

Mink are highly susceptible to canine distemper. Attenuated live CDV vaccines produce prolonged dependable immunity. Inactivated vaccines have given erratic results in mink. Historically, such vaccines were made by formalizing infected mink tissues. On occasion however, the formaldehyde failed to inactivate contaminating Aleutian disease parvovirus. As a result, outbreaks of Aleutian disease caused serious losses. Almost all young mink in North America receive a single dose of distemper vaccine during the summer after they reach 10 weeks of age and maternal antibodies have waned. Revaccination may not be necessary because of herd immunity and the fact that mink are generally pelted around three years of age. Mink distemper vaccine is commonly given as a 3- or 4-way vaccine with pseudomonas, enteritis, and botulism.

MINK VIRUS ENTERITIS

Mink virus enteritis is caused by a parvovirus that is closely related to the feline and canine parvoviruses. In kits, mortality may reach 75%. Only inactivated vaccines are available commercially. Kits may be vaccinated at 10 to 13 weeks of age. Breeding mink should be revaccinated annually. Parvovirus vaccines are commonly combined with vaccines against botulism, distemper, and Pseudomonas.

HEMORRHAGIC PNEUMONIA

Pseudomonas aeruginosa causes hemorrhagic pneumonia in mink. It is associated with the stress of the warm days in the fall. The mink show lethargy and anorexia progressing to respiratory disease and death. Successful vaccination requires immunization with all the pathogenic serotypes. Pseudomonas bacterins should contain serotypes 5, 6, 7, and 9. Like the other vaccines, it should be administered after maternal antibodies have waned. Adult mink should be revaccinated annually.

Rabbit Vaccines

RABBIT PASTEURELLOSIS

A killed bacterin against *Pasteurella multocida* for the prevention of rabbit "snuffles" is available in North America.

RABBIT HEMORRHAGIC DISEASE

Rabbit hemorrhagic disease is a highly contagious disease of European rabbits caused by small, single-stranded RNA caliciviruses. There are two such viruses: classical rabbit hemorrhagic disease virus-1 (RHDV-1) and a variant virus, (RHDV-2 or RHDVb). RHDVs cause a disease characterized by convulsions, paralysis, and respiratory signs, including depression and inappetence. Morbidity and mortality may reach up to 90% within 36 hours. In captivity, transmission is by the oral-fecal route. In the wild it is likely spread by mosquitos and fleas.

In countries where RHD is endemic, the disease is controlled by good biosecurity and variant-specific vaccination. If the virus type is unknown then vaccination should be directed against both variants because cross-protection between RHDV-1 and -2 vaccines is variable and unpredictable. Both monovalent and bivalent inactivated adjuvanted vaccines against RHDV are available. Most are directed against RHDV2 but a bivalent product is preferable.

The first injection is given subcutaneously between four weeks and two months depending upon the product. It is usual to vaccinate only breeding stock and they should be revaccinated at six months. Immunity develops in 7 to 10 days and persists for over a year. They do not protect rabbits against myxomatosis

MYXOMATOSIS

This disease is caused by the myxoma virus (MYXV), a member of the *Poxviridae* family. Its natural hosts are found in South America and California. Myxomatosis is characterized by the development of large skin lesions accompanied by immunosuppression or respiratory disease. Mortality varies from 20% to 100% in European rabbits. Two types of modified live vaccine have been developed. One has been prepared from the Shope fibroma virus (SFV), an avirulent Leporipoxvirus. The others are prepared from attenuated strains of MYXV. Both may be administered subcutaneously or intradermally. The SFV vaccines are somewhat less immunogenic and are no longer used in the meat rabbit industry. The live attenuated MYXV vaccines are more immunogenic and protection lasts for four to six months. They should be followed by annual revaccination. However, these vaccines are immunosuppressive. A recombinant live MYXV vectored vaccine expressing the rabbit hemorrhagic disease virus capsid protein and thus protecting against both of these important diseases is available in Europe.

Wildlife Vaccines

Many infections in humans and their animals come from wildlife reservoirs. These may include major public health zoonoses such as rabies and sylvatic plague, or threats to livestock such as brucellosis, anthrax, pseudorabies, classical swine fever, and tuberculosis. In many cases lethal control procedures may neither be feasible nor acceptable. An alternative control strategy is oral vaccination. This has been highly successful for rabies and encouraging results have been observed for sylvatic plague. For oral vaccination to work three factors must come together: an effective oral vaccine, a suitable way of delivering it, and a species-specific bait.

RABIES

Wild caught carnivores have a high risk of transmitting rabies and should not be kept as pets. Indeed, this is illegal in many areas. Do not assume that a baby animal is not infected. Foxes, raccoons, and skunks may acquire infection at an early age and may incubate the disease for more than a year. In the United States, wild mammals account for over 90% of human rabies exposures. If vaccination of pet wildlife is necessary then only killed vaccines should be used.

More importantly, wild animals must be vaccinated if rabies is to be controlled. This requires the oral administration of vaccines. It needs an economical and effective vaccine, a vaccine that is environmentally stable, and a vaccine that works extremely well by the oral route. Several different vaccines have been used in oral rabies vaccination programs. Most have used a live, attenuated rabies virus. More than 13 million doses of the attenuated rabies strain, ERA-BHK21 were distributed across Eastern Ontario to control the disease. In Europe, more than 650 million doses were distributed between 1978 and 2014 using attenuated SAD (Street-Alabama-Dufferin) Bern, its derivative strain SAD B19 or SAG2 (SAD Avirulent Gif). More recently, wildlife vaccinators have switched to recombinant vaccines using either vaccinia or adenovirus vectors.

For example, the gene for the rabies envelope glycoprotein, (G-protein), from the avirulent ERA strain has been inserted into a vaccinia vector (RABORAL V-RG, Boehringer Ingelheim). When this is ingested, the resulting infection induces neutralizing antibodies to the G-protein and the development of immunity within 10 to 14 days. This vaccine is distributed in a small plastic sachet and either surrounded by solid fishmeal polymer (FP bait), or coated with wax and fishmeal crumbs (CS bait) (Fig. 20.1). It may also contain tetracycline as a biomarker because this

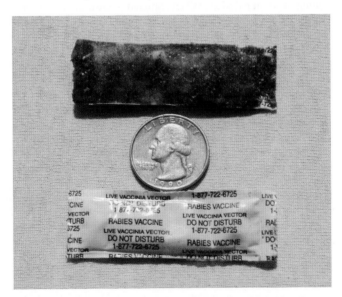

Fig. 20.1. Rabies vaccine fishmeal crumbs sachet baits. The upper sachet has been coated with a wax-based bait. The lower sachet is uncoated. (Courtesy Animal and Plant Health Inspection Service (APHIS), US Department of Agriculture.)

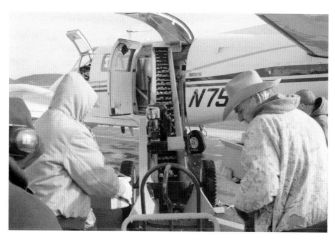

Fig. 20.2 Rabies vaccine fishmeal polymer bait being loaded onto a plane before dropping it over rural Texas. (Courtesy Dr. Ken Waldrup.)

will stain the recipient's teeth. RABORAL V-RG is licensed for use in the United States in coyotes, raccoons, and gray foxes.

An alternative adenovirus vectored vaccine (ONRAB, Artemis Technologies) is a live recombinant that also expresses the rabies glycoprotein gene. It is delivered in a blister pack coated with a wax and fat-based bait.

These baited vaccines can be distributed over a very wide area by dropping from aircraft (Fig. 20.2). Beginning in 1989 in Europe, live vaccines inserted into meat baits had immediate success in preventing rabies in red foxes. When scattered in areas known to contain red foxes it resulted in a dramatic reduction in fox rabies. They have also been used in Ontario to prevent the spread of raccoon and red fox rabies, in the eastern United States to establish a barrier along the Appalachian ridge to prevent the westward spread of raccoon rabies, and in Texas to block the northward spread of coyote rabies from Mexico and to eliminate rabies in gray foxes in west-central Texas.

A comparative study examined the effectiveness of both vectored rabies vaccines in New England and New Brunswick in an effort to prevent raccoon rabies entering New Brunswick. Both were equally immunogenic, but raccoons appeared to prefer the fat-based bait.

In Ontario, oral rabies virus baits were distributed by aircraft or hand. The baiting started near the center of the outbreak and was then extended during successive years. Within 5 years the reported cases of rabid foxes dropped from 203 cases/year to 4 cases. Spillover cases in skunks and livestock dropped from 36 and 42 cases/year to zero, 5 years later.

Oral baiting for rabies in south Texas was initiated in 1995 in the form of a northern barrier. In subsequent years the baited area was extended south toward the border with Mexico. Since 1995, 17.5 million doses of vaccinia-vectored rabies vaccine have been airdropped over 255,500 square miles (661,745 sq km) of Texas. The number of rabies cases dropped from 122 cases in 1995 to 0 in 2004. Currently Texas continues to drop the baits in a zone 30–65 km wide along the international border to provide a barrier of immune animals. These vaccines are effective against rabies in coyotes, raccoons, and red foxes.

Oral rabies vaccines have been extensively tested in several less developed countries in an effort to prevent the spread of rabies by pet and feral dogs. Pet dogs may simply be provided a vaccine sachet by the owner, "the hand-out model," Dogs that cannot be handled or dogs encountered in the street are simply offered a bait. Feral dogs may simply have access to scattered baited vaccine in suitable locations such as garbage dumps, public markets, or paths used by dogs. The vaccine strains employed must not be able to infect humans by licking or biting. Baits that have been used include chicken heads, minced meat with breadcrumbs, boiled chicken intestines, or dog biscuits. Interestingly dogs in different countries have different bait preferences. This strategy can complement traditional dog vaccination programs to achieve the desired level of herd immunity.

SYLVATIC PLAGUE

The blackfooted ferret (*Mustela nigripes*) is a specialized predator of prairie dogs (*Cynomys* Sp), once prevalent across the prairies of North America from Saskatchewan to Texas. As prairie dog populations have declined because of hunting, poisoning, and the plague, the numbers of blackfooted ferrets have declined as well. At one time it was believed that the species was extinct. In 1981 however, a small wild population was discovered in Wyoming. Unfortunately, at least four died as a result of being vaccinated with a modified live canine distemper vaccine. By 1987, the population was reduced to 18 individuals. These however provided sufficient animals to begin a very successful captive breeding program. Over 200 ferrets are now held in captive breeding facilities, and about 2600 animals have been reintroduced into the wild. Although successful so far, the ferrets suffer from two serious diseases, canine distemper and sylvatic plague caused by *Yersinia pestis*. Plague is endemic throughout the Western states. It was introduced to California around 1900 and spread eastward. Outbreaks can totally wipe out an infected prairie dog colony and their accompanying ferrets.

Yersinia pestis is transmitted by fleas or by eating infected prairie dogs. Ferrets may, however, be vaccinated against the plague using a purified subunit vaccine also developed for use in humans. Ferrets released from the captive breeding facility are given two doses of the injectable vaccine before release and this works very well. Unfortunately, this does not protect wild ferrets and more importantly does not protect their prey, the prairie dogs.

An experimental vaccine consisting of a recombinant raccoon poxvirus engineered to express two protective *Yersinia pestis* antigens, F1 and a truncated version of the V protein is being field-tested. It is delivered through the use of vaccine-loaded oral bait. Studies have shown that the vaccine remains viable for up to 7 days at 28°C. Trials are underway involving the use of drones incorporating a bait-spraying device that will shoot baits in 3 directions simultaneously at 30 ft intervals. Prairie dogs appear to like peanut butter very much so the baits consist of "candy" containing vaccine-laden peanut butter. A dye is added to the mix so that it will show up on the animal's whiskers (Fig. 20.3). Preliminary analysis indicates that the use of such vaccines has increased prairie dog numbers and survival.

CLASSICAL SWINE FEVER

Wild boars in Europe and Japan can carry classical swine fever (CSF) and thus present a significant threat to their domestic swine industries. As a result, considerable efforts have been made to develop appropriate oral vaccines. These vaccines currently consist of the modified live attenuated Chinese C strain in an aluminum foil blister package. This is wrapped in a bait consisting of corn meal and milk powder with an almond odorant in a wax base. The vaccine packets are hand-delivered by hunters on the boar's feeding grounds. Control is based on bait distribution in three double dose campaigns conducted in spring, summer, and fall with a 28-day interval between the two doses. Vaccine uptake by the boars is significantly affected by seasonality, reflecting the availability of other, more attractive, food sources. It is also an expensive approach because it requires

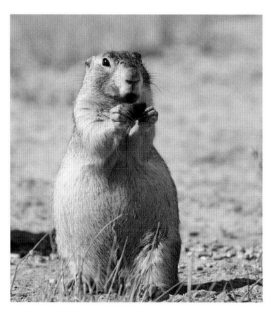

Fig. 20.3. A Gunnison prairie dog holding a piece of bait loaded with sylvatic plague vaccine. (Courtesy Dr. Tonie E. Rocke, US Geological Survey.)

a huge effort and much manpower. However, this is the only effective method of CSF control in wild boars in large forested areas.

BRUCELLOSIS

In the United States, Brucellosis has been eliminated in domestic cattle. However, the infection persists in bison and elk within and around Yellowstone National Park. Public sentiment and the need to maintain genetic diversity will not permit their slaughter. How can they be vaccinated? One method is to shoot it into them. Ballistic vaccination involving shooting calves in the hind leg with a methylcellulose pellet containing lyophilized S19 or RB51 vaccine has been investigated. This method is however relatively inefficient and is unlikely to vaccinate sufficient animals to generate herd immunity.

Ongoing studies are under way to investigate the feasibility of vaccinating white-footed mice for Lyme disease, vaccinating bighorn sheep for pneumonic Pasteurellosis, vaccinating koalas for Chlamydia, vaccinating dolphins against morbillivirus, and vaccinating cheetahs and rhinos against anthrax in Namibia. There is an ongoing debate in the UK regarding vaccinating badgers against tuberculosis. In all such cases little consideration seems to have been given to methods of vaccine delivery.

IMMUNOCONTRACEPTION

Under some circumstances it is desirable to reduce the size of wild animal populations without killing individuals. This may be accomplished by fertility control. Vaccination can do this. It is completely reversible, easily administered, cost effective, and efficacious in multiple species. Killing is irreversible whereas vaccination is not.

Although there are many different antigens that might be targets for contraceptive vaccines, two have proven successful. One consists of zona pellucida (ZP) glycoproteins. These are glycoproteins that form a matrix around the oocyte. The antiZP vaccine likely works by binding to these proteins in the ZP and either blocking sperm binding, or causing structural changes that block sperm penetration. This approach has the benefit that vaccination has no hormonal side effects and animal behavior is unaffected. The ZP proteins are conserved across different phyla and the vaccine can be used in multiple species although there are great variations in antibody levels, effectiveness, and duration. A vaccine directed against porcine zona pellucida (PZP) has been used successfully to reduce fertility in at least 85 mammalian species. Three PZP glycoproteins have been the antigens of choice. Adjuvants are critical to the success of these vaccines. Several different adjuvants have been tested including complete and incomplete Freund's adjuvant, and synthetic trehalose dimycolate (Chapter 7).

For free-roaming animal populations the PZP vaccine may be administered by darting or in baits. As might be expected, remote darting from a helicopter is somewhat less effective because it does not always deliver intramuscular injection. In captive situations such as zoos, these vaccines have also been very effective. Most ungulates follow a consistent response pattern. After receiving a booster at three to six weeks, antibody levels peak at one to three months, and maintain high levels for eight months to one year. Contraception lasts for at least 12 months, so annual revaccination is necessary. Some species such as Munjac deer (*Muntiacus* Sp.) require revaccination every six months, whereas zebras require revaccination every nine months. Other species such as Himalayan tahr (*Hemitragus jemlahicus*) and Dall sheep (*Ovis dalli*) may mount a prolonged response and remain infertile for up to three years.

The second type of successful contraceptive vaccine is designed to immunize animals against gonadotropin releasing hormone (GnRH). GnRH vaccines have an advantage over PZP vaccines in that by reducing sex hormone production they eliminate estrus and its associated misbehaviors. Multiple molecules of this small poorly immunogenic peptide are conjugated to a single large immunogenic protein such as mollusk hemocyanin. The GnRH-hemocyanin conjugate is adjuvanted with a water-in-mineral oil emulsion. This vaccine, GonaCon was developed as a reproductive inhibitor for wildlife by the National Wildlife Disease Center of the US Department of Agriculture. GonaCon induces antibodies that bind and neutralize GnRH. These block the release of gonadotropins such as FSH and LH from the pituitary. This in turn inhibits reproduction and its behaviors in both males and females. GonaCon has induced contraception with a single dose for up to five years in domestic cats, pigs, wild horses, bison, and white-tailed deer. It is currently registered by the Environmental Protection Agency as a contraceptive for white-tailed deer and wild horses, thus effectively managing overabundant wildlife populations. The vaccine is classified as a restricted use pesticide. Tests showed that a single dose reduced fertility in urban white-tailed deer by 88% in the first year and 47% in the second. In adult female wild horses and burros, it also inhibits sexual behavior. Although working well in domestic species, GnRH vaccines encounter the same difficulties as PZP vaccines when used in wild, free roaming wildlife. The product can be delivered by injection, jab stick, or darting.

GonaCon may also be used for the prevention of adrenocortical disease in domestic ferrets. The development of adrenal hyperplasia, adenomas, and adenocarcinomas in neutered ferrets is believed to be a result of continuous overproduction of luteinizing hormone (LH) caused by a lack of gonadal feedback. Subcutaneous vaccination with a single dose of the GnRH vaccine generates antibodies to endogenous GnRH and suppresses its production. This in turn suppresses production and release of LH. This causes clinical remission of adrenocortical disease in these ferrets and can prevent disease recurrence for up to three years.

Sources of Additional Information

Council Report. (1994). Vaccination guidelines for small ruminants (sheep, goats, llamas, domestic deer, and wapiti). *JAVMA*, 205, 1539–1544.

Cross, M.L., Buddle, B.M., Aldwell, F.E. (2007). The potential of oral vaccines for disease control in wildlife species. *Vet J*, 174, 472–480.

Faber, M., Dietzschold, B., Li, J. (2009). Immunogenicity and safety of recombinant rabies viruses used for oral vaccination of stray dogs and wildlife. *Zoonoses Publ Hlth*, 56, 262–269.

Fayrer-Hosken, R. (2008). Controlling animal populations using anti-fertility vaccines. *Reprod Dom Anim*, 43, 179–185.

Heatley, J.J., Payne, S., Tizard, I. (2018). Avian vaccination: Current options and strategies. *Vet Clin Exot Anim*, 21, 379–397.

Kirkpatrick, J.F., Lyda, R.O., Frank KM. (2011). Contraceptive vaccines for wildlife: A review. *Am J Reprod Immunol*, 66, 40–50.

Olsen, S.C., Kreeger, T.J., Schultz, W. (2002). Immune responses of bison to ballistic or hand vaccination with Brucella abortus strain RB51. *J Wildlife Dis*, 38, 738–745.

Risi, E., Agoulon, A., Allaire, F., Le Dréan-Quénec'hdu, S., Martin, V., Mahl, P. (2012). Antibody response to vaccines for rhinotracheitis, caliciviral disease, panleukopenia, feline leukemia, and rabies in tigers (*Panthera tigris*) and lions (*Panthera leo*). *J Zoo Wildl Med*, 43, 248–255.

Rocke, T.E., Kingstad-Bakke, B., Berlier, W., Osornio, J.E. (2014). A recombinant raccoon poxvirus vaccine expressing both Yersinia pastis F1 and truncated V antigens protects animals against lethal plague. *Vaccines*, 2, 772–784.

Rossi, S., Staubach, C., Blome, S., Guberti, V., et al. (2015). Controlling of CSFV in European wild boar using oral vaccination: A review. *Front Microbiol*, 6, 1141.

Salkeld, D.J. (2017). Vaccines for conservation: Plague, prairie dogs and black-footed ferrets as a case study. *Ecohealth*, 14, 432–437.

Sterner, R.T., Meltzer, M.L., Shwiff, S.A., Slate, D. (2009). Tactics and economics of wildlife oral rabies vaccination, Canada and the United States. *Emerg Inf Dis*, 15, 1176–1184.

Wade, L.L. (2018). Vaccination of ferrets for rabies and distemper. *Vet Clin Exot Anim*, 21, 105–114.

Fish Vaccines

Aquaculture is the most rapidly developing food industry. Many different fish species are farmed worldwide, but about 65% are extensively farmed carp. The remainder are high value species, such as salmon, farmed on an industrial scale. As a result, the global fish yield from aquaculture now exceeds that of wild-caught fisheries. In addition, wild caught fisheries are reaching their maximum output, and a quarter of wild fish populations are overfished or seriously depleted. As a result of this intensification, stocking densities in commercial aquaculture have risen. This has caused increased stress, and greatly increased the risk of infectious disease outbreaks in farmed fish. Infectious diseases are therefore a major issue for the industry and as a result, Intensive bacterial and viral vaccination is essential for its commercial success. Vaccine use has enabled the intensive industry to significantly reduce antibiotic consumption. In general, industrial scale vaccination is mainly limited to larger, high-value fish such as salmon and trout, and seeks to get the fish to market weight with only a single cycle of vaccination. As a result, there is a reliance on early vaccination followed by boosters to provide long-lasting disease protection. Killed bacterial vaccines predominate in the fish industry. It has proven to be much more difficult to produce effective viral vaccines, whereas the use of modified live vaccines is discouraged because of potential environmental risks. Vaccines are therefore used in 77 species of fish against more than 22 different bacterial diseases and 6 viral diseases.

Fish Immunity

A major consideration concerns the methods used to administer vaccines to fish. This includes not only their aquatic environment, but also the great variations in size and feeding behavior as fish grow. The first licensed vaccines against *Yersinia ruckeri* and *Vibrio anguillarum* for fish in the United States were introduced into commercial aquaculture in the early 1980s. Thereafter many killed bacterial vaccines have been used routinely. About 30 licensed fish vaccines are available worldwide. These differ between countries and some are specific for a single fish species. It should also be noted that, as in all animal vaccines, they must be cost-effective. Thus there are enormous differences in vaccination practices between the large commercial fisheries raising Atlantic salmon and the small-scale carp-production activities in villages in East Asia.

ADAPTIVE IMMUNITY

Bony fish (teleosts) have a complete set of lymphoid organs except for a bone marrow, and they can mount both innate and adaptive immune responses. Their lymphoid organs are very different from those in mammals. For example, their thymus may involute in response to hormones or season. Age involution is inconsistent, and a thymus may be found in old fish. Fish kidneys differentiate into two sections. The opisthonephros or posterior kidney is similar to the mammalian kidney. In contrast, the pronephros or anterior kidney is a lymphoid organ containing antibody-forming cells and phagocytes. Its function is analogous to mammalian bone marrow and lymph nodes. Fish have a spleen with a structure and function similar to that in mammals. Aggregates of lymphocytes are prominent in the fish intestinal tract. Fish also have clusters of macrophages containing melanin and hemosiderin. These melanomacrophage centers are found in the spleen, liver, and kidney. Antigens may persist in these centers for long periods, and they appear to be precursors of the germinal centers found in more evolved vertebrates. Teleosts also have dendritic-like cells that can present antigens to T cells.

Fish lymphocytes resemble those of mammals. B cells can be found in the thymus, anterior kidney, spleen, Leydig organ, and blood, and their surface immunoglobulins act as antigen receptors. These B cells can mature into plasma cells. Unlike mammalian B cells, however, teleost B cells can phagocytose particles, generate phagolysosomes, and kill ingested microbes. Both helper and cytotoxic T cells can be detected in fish.

Fish antibody responses are characterized by the predominance of IgM produced by plasma-like cells in the anterior kidney. In the presence of complement, fish antibodies can lyse target cells, but there is no evidence that they can act as opsonins. The blood vessel walls of fish are permeable to immunoglobulin (Ig)M. As a result, antibodies are found in most tissue fluids including plasma, lymph, and skin mucus.

Fish do not produce IgA, but they secrete a mucosal IgM together with IgD. One significant difference between fish and other vertebrates is that their antibodies do not undergo class switching or affinity maturation. IgT is the major mucosal and skin immunoglobulin in teleosts.

Not all antigens are effective immunogens in fish. Soluble protein antigens are poorly immunogenic, in contrast to particulate antigens such as bacteria that are very potent. Environmental temperatures have a significant influence on vaccine responses. Antibody production in vaccinated Atlantic salmon is significantly less in fish held at 2°C than in those held at 10°C. Social interactions can also influence their immune response; fish kept at a high population density are immunosuppressed, a matter of some concern in commercial aquaculture.

Methods of Vaccination

Administration of vaccines to large numbers of fish presents challenges. One major issue is the vulnerability to infection of very small larval or fry stages before immune system development and before they are large enough to vaccinate. Three routes are available for vaccination of larger fish: injection, immersion, and oral. Each has advantages and disadvantages.

INJECTION

The usual way to vaccinate fish on an industrial scale is by intraperitoneal or intramuscular injection (Fig. 21.1). The effectiveness of vaccines is greatest if injected, but the process does place significant stress on the fish. In addition, injected vaccines can only be used on larger fish. The best results are obtained with vaccines incorporating oil-emulsion based adjuvants such as mineral oil with an emulsifier or a vegetable/animal oil with pristane or squalene. When vaccinating very large numbers, the fish are carried through pipes from the rearing tanks to an anesthetic bath. Once lightly anesthetized, the fish are removed from the bath, placed on a table, and injected by the vaccination team using repeating injection guns connected to a vaccine bag or bottle. Each fish has to be handled individually and injected by hand. The fish is held ventral side

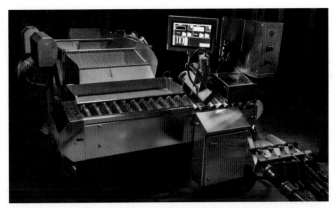

Fig. 21.1 A semiautomatic fish vaccination machine. Back left in the picture is the holding tank and anesthetic bath where the fish are brought in before vaccination. The sedated fish are then emptied on to the vaccination table where an operator places each fish, head down and belly to the left, in the trays of the transporter belt taking the fish to the vaccination station on the right. Every fish is photographed and a computer program tells the machine where to place the injection point. How far from the nose and how deep the injection is placed depends on the fish size. The fish data can be transferred to other computer units for later use and analysis. After vaccination the fish are sorted into three different sizes that have been set by the machine operator. Front right on the picture. One of the sorting stations is used for rejected fish, that is fish that are either too small or placed the wrong way onto the belt. The machine can vaccinate unsorted fish from 10 grams to 250 grams. Software that makes the machine suitable for specific species such as salmon, trout, sea bass, and tilapia has been developed. (Courtesy PHARMAQ Fishteq AS.)

up with its head facing away from the operator. The vaccine is injected into the abdominal area of each anesthetized fish. The needle is inserted about 5mm. Depending on the vaccine, 0.05 to 0.2mL of fluid is injected. The recommended volume is 0.1 mL per fish weighing a minimum of 39 g. Using automatic injection guns, four skilled operators can vaccinate 5000 salmon per hour. However high labor costs have led to the development of automated vaccination machines that can vaccinate up to 20,000 fish per hour (Fig. 21.2). Intraperitoneal vaccines are generally used to deliver water-in-oil emulsion vaccines whereas intramuscular injection is employed for DNA vaccines.

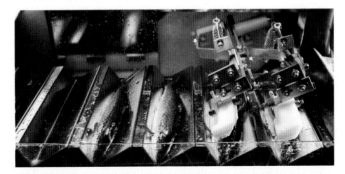

Fig. 21.2 Correctly placed salmon smolts in the fish trays of the transporter belt. A machine vision (photo technology) records their size and decides where to place the vaccine injection. Clamps gently hold the fish in place while the vaccine is injected, two fish are injected simultaneously in tray "one" and "two." (Courtesy PHARMAQ Fishteq AS.)

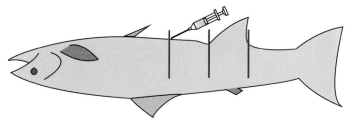

Fig. 21.3 Intraperitoneal vaccines should be administered on the midline, one fin length in front of the pelvic fin.

Before vaccination fish must be fasted for 12 to 24 hours, the fish tanks made ready, and the water aerated. This reduces stress and anesthesia complications. As with all vaccines, only healthy fish should be vaccinated and it is essential not to overstock them.

The most commonly used anesthetic in Europe and the United States is MS-222 (also called Tricaine methanesulfonate or Tricane-S). This is a sodium channel blocker with a wide safety margin approved for use in food fish. It does not affect their respiratory system and fish recover rapidly. The dose ranges from 20 to 50 mg/L depending on the species. MS-222 is light sensitive, and should be stored appropriately and prepared fresh each time. Although highly soluble, it will acidify the tank water so it should be buffered with sodium bicarbonate. This may not be necessary for seawater.

Fish should be vaccinated at water temperatures from 1°C to 18°C and preferably below 15°C. The vaccination equipment should be disinfected before use. The vaccine should be left to slowly reach 15°C to 20°C by keeping it at room temperature and should be well shaken before use. To reduce the risk of adverse reactions, it is important to deposit the entire dose in the abdominal cavity. The injection needle used should have appropriate diameter, and length to penetrate the abdominal wall by 1 to 2 mm. The entire needle should be inserted into the midline about 1 to 1.5 pelvic fin lengths anterior to the base of the pelvic fin (Fig. 21.3). When using automated methods, anesthetized fish are wedged into an enclosed space and auto-injected. This may be less satisfactory than the use of hand injectors because the number of injection site lesions is increased.

Inactivated vaccines must be administered by injection to induce protective immunity, but for some viral diseases, this may not be practical. Thus injection is not appropriate for small fish and so cannot be performed very early in life. This means that there may be a window of disease susceptibility as the fish are growing before reaching a size suitable for injection. Vaccine injection also needs complex machinery and a skilled staff so that the cost of labor is significant. Depending upon the adjuvant employed, complications such as postvaccinal fungal diseases, or severe local reactions with tissue damage may occur. For this reason fish farmers are reluctant to give fish more than one injection in the production cycle. There is also a desire to incorporate as many vaccines as possible into that injection. On the other hand, injection gives long lasting immunity, and each fish is assured of getting the correct dose of vaccine.

IMMERSION VACCINATION

Given the cost, complexity, and risks of injection, fish farmers have turned to immersion vaccination where fish are placed in a dip or bath containing the vaccine antigen. They remain for a suitable time period while the antigen is absorbed through their skin, mucosal surfaces, and gills. In dip vaccination, small fish are immersed for 30 seconds in a highly concentrated vaccine solution (1/10 dilution of the vaccine). In bath vaccination, larger fish are exposed for a longer period (~30 min) in a dilute vaccine solution (1/500 dilution). Dip vaccination is more widely used because it lends itself to the mass vaccination of small fish and uses a relatively small volume of vaccine solution. For example, salmonid fish as small as 2g can be vaccinated by immersion. Because the fish are not individually handled they suffer much less stress and mortality, and labor costs are much lower. Dip vaccination can also be very rapid, with up to 100 kg of fish vaccinated per liter of vaccine. It is the preferred method of vaccinating small fish or fry under 5g. Dip vaccination is impractical and cost prohibitive for larger fish.

Bath vaccination, in contrast, is less stressful on the fish and less labor intensive. Large-scale bath vaccination is used, for example, in sea bass in Europe. In this method, large groups of fish are cut off from the rest of the tank. They are sedated with a low dose of anesthetic, exposed to the vaccine while air or oxygen is pumped into the tank to prevent suffocation. However, a large volume of vaccine solution is required, which makes it expensive for the immune response induced by this method provides less protection and a shorter duration of immunity than does injection. It is somewhat effective in inducing mucosal immunity.

ORAL VACCINATION

Oral vaccination is the preferred route when fish welfare and labor costs are considered. Vaccines can be delivered at any age, stress is minimized, and the price is right. Because of the relatively low cost, oral vaccines can be delivered multiple times.

However, oral vaccination requires a very large amount of antigen and the fish need to be feeding. Additionally, like the immersion techniques, protection using these inactivated products is relatively poor and of relatively short duration. Oral vaccines generally contain heat- or formalin-killed organisms. The vaccines can be mixed with the feed or coated on the surface of the feed pellets. The major problem affecting oral vaccines is their lack of stability. The vaccine antigens have to survive the food making process and they must be stable in water and persist within the fish gastrointestinal tract. Another problem is that the dose of vaccine ingested is uncertain.

Although oral vaccines are not adjuvanted they do need to be protected against digestion and dilution in water. There are three ways of doing this. The finished feed can be "top-dressed" with powdered vaccine by adding adhesive substances such as an edible oil or gelatin. A second way is simply to spray the feed with a vaccine solution. The third way is to mix the vaccine in the feed during the feed production process. The first two methods, although simple, may result in an uneven distribution of antigen in the feed. These antigens will also be directly exposed to stomach acidity and thus may be degraded. On the other hand, mixing the antigen in the feed results in uniform distribution of antigen. However, feed is often produced by high temperature extrusion that may destroy antigens. Thus the antigen must be added at a later stage in food preparation. Vaccines may also be bioencapsulated. Once encapsulated they can then be mixed in the food. Two commercial microencapsulation processes are also used. This may involve either an "Antigen-protecting vehicle" (APV) (*Vibrio anguillarum*, *Yersinia ruckeri*, and infectious pancreatic necrosis (IPN); MSD Animal Health), or a patented MicroMatrix delivery system (*Piscinickettsia salmonis*, ISAV and IPNV, Centrovet). These processes are designed to protect antigens against gastric digestion and increase mucosal uptake. APV prevents digestion in the stomach and ensures that viral antigens are delivered to the hindgut where they are absorbed. Other approaches may include encapsulating antigens in liposomes or alginate beads.

VACCINATION PROCESS

Given the advantages and disadvantages of the different routes of vaccination described earlier, there is a clear pattern of vaccine usage designed to protect fish throughout their life. Depending on the species and production cycle, fish farmers commonly start with a dip vaccine, followed by a dip or oral boost, and finish with an intraperitoneal injection. Revaccination is not usually employed after this injection, although oral boosting against piscirickettsiosis is used in Chile.

Increasing water temperature will improve the response to vaccines and it is possible to use this to advantage. For example, vaccination in the fall leads to the immune system delaying its response until the following spring when the water temperature rises. The onset of immunity is faster in warm-water species than in cold-water species. For example, in sea bass held at 22°C antibodies appear about one week after vaccination. On the other hand, in salmon held at 10°C, antibodies only appear by four to six weeks.

Antibacterial Vaccines

Fish develop antibodies against a wide range of bacterial pathogens, and killed bacterial vaccines against gram-negative bacteria give very good protection. Oil-based adjuvants are widely employed in these injectable vaccines, although as described earlier they may produce significant injection site reactions. They are both efficacious and safe when administered correctly.

VIBRIOSIS

Listonella anguillarum (*Vibrio anguillarum*), and *Vibrio ordalli*, cause classical vibriosis, the most serious bacterial fish disease and one that causes severe economic loss. It presents as a septicemia that affects Atlantic and Pacific salmon, rainbow trout, sea bass, sea bream, turbot, cod, and eel. It is found worldwide but does not occur in very cold seawater or in freshwater aquaculture. There are at least ten different serotypes of *L. anguillarum* of which three are most significant: O1, O2a, and O2b. O1 and O2a serotypes affect salmonids and O2b affects cold-water species such as cod and halibut. As a result the salmonid vaccines cannot be used in these marine species. It is important to use the correct serotype in the bacterin.

Both injectable and immersion vaccines are available. Larvae and small juveniles need to be vaccinated by immersion. Vibrio anguillarum-ordalii bacterin (Vibrogen 2, [Elanco Aqua Health]) is administered using the same process as other dips for a 30-second exposure. The injectable vaccines are usually polyvalent adjuvanted bacterins and work well.

COLD-WATER VIBRIOSIS

The cause of cold-water vibriosis is *Aliivibrio (Vibrio) salmonicida*. The organism is most virulent between 3°C and 10°C. It is found only in seawater species. This septicemic disease was brought under control by vaccination beginning in the 1980s, for many years, but it has now reappeared. It is mainly a problem in Norwegian aquaculture, hence most Atlantic salmon and rainbow trout in Norway are vaccinated. Killed bacterins are available. They are administered by immersion or injection and appear to be very effective.

FURUNCULOSIS

Aeromonas salmonicida is the causal agent of Furunculosis, another major disease of salmonid fish. Species such as carp, cod, or flounder may also be affected. This may present as sudden death, but salmon may develop "boils" involving skin or muscle.

Both immersion and injectable bacterins are available, although oil adjuvanted injectable vaccines seem to be preferred. The injected bacterin is injected intraperitoneally to anesthetized salmonids.

WINTER ULCER

Moritella viscosa is the main causal agent of winter ulcer that affects Atlantic salmon and rainbow trout. The fish develop superficial ulcers that grow and penetrate the skin. It is economically devastating because of death losses and quality downgrading. Formalin inactivated bacterins are available. They are usually included in polyvalent vaccines so the coverage is high.

YERSINIOSIS

Yersinia ruckeri is the cause of enteric redmouth (ERM) disease. It mainly occurs in cultured salmonids such as rainbow trout. It affects very small fish, and as in so many fish diseases is attributed to stress. Trout are initially vaccinated by immersion in the hatchery. However, this only protects them for about nine months. They must therefore be revaccinated orally. Two oral vaccinations should provide sufficient protection and cause minimal stress to the fish.

PASTEURELLOSIS

Photobacterium damselae subsp. *piscicida (Pasteurella piscicida)* causes a septicemia called pseudotuberculosis. It has caused high mortality in Mediterranean aquaculture. It affects many species of marine fish. Bacterins are available for immersion or injection. Two bath immersions are used when the fish are 45 to 50 days of age. The vaccine only induces short-term immunity so this may be boosted orally or by injection

WARM WATER VIBRIOSIS

Multiple species of vibrio cause this hemorrhagic skin disease. The most important are *Vibrio alginolyticus, Vibrio parahaemolyticus,* and *Vibrio vulnificus. V. vulnificus* is an important human pathogen, causing lethal wound infections. Mixed bacterins are available. Generally fish are first vaccinated by injection and then boosted by immersion.

EDWARDSIELLOSIS

Edwardsiella ictaluri is a gram-negative bacterium that causes enteric septicemia of channel catfish, the most serious disease affecting the catfish industry in the United States. A mortality of up to 37% has been associated with *E. ictaluri* infection. The disease is associated with water temperatures over 22°C. Vaccines have not been widely employed because of the extensive methods of fish farming. Killed bacterins are of low efficacy despite inducing antibodies because this organism is a facultative intracellular organism and cell-mediated responses are probably more important. As a result, live attenuated products delivered by immersion may work better. An avirulent live attenuated vaccine (Aquavac-Esc, Merck) is used in healthy catfish by immersion. It is provided in frozen vials where each vial is sufficient to vaccinate 7.5 lbs. (3.4kg) of catfish in 5gal (20L) of water. This vaccine is efficacious in channel catfish fry as early as 7 to 30 days post hatching. A related bacterium, *Edwardsiella tarda,* causes gangrene and septicemia in other freshwater fish such as channel catfish, eels, and flounder, but there are no commercial vaccines available. It can affect humans.

FLAVOBACTERIOSIS

Flavobacterium columnare causes a significant skin disease in many different freshwater fish, especially trout, catfish, and bass. An avirulent live culture is used to vaccinate healthy catfish and largemouth bass by immersion. A killed immersion vaccine is also available.

BACTERIAL KIDNEY DISEASE

Renibacterium salmoninarum is the cause of bacterial kidney disease. An attenuated live vaccine has been licensed that relies on cross-reactivity between this organism and Arthrobacter spp. It is administered by immersion or injected intraperitoneally

PISCIRICKETTSIOSIS

Piscirickettsia salmonis is the causal agent of salmon rickettsial septicemia, a very serious disease in Chile where it may cause mortality exceeding 90% in farmed Coho salmon. Inactivated bacterins are available but of low efficacy. This lack of effectiveness may be attributed to coinfection with sea lice. A live attenuated vaccine is also available.

OTHER BACTERIAL VACCINES

Streptococcus agalactiae and *Streptococcus iniae* cause significant mortality in Nile tilapia, one of the most cultivated fish in the world after carp and salmon. These fish are farmed intensively worldwide, but the consequent increase in stocking densities has resulted in stress-induced immunosuppression, leading to an upsurge in lethal streptococcal infections. Streptococcosis is a bacterial disease that affects warm water fish in either salt or freshwater environments, typically in tropical regions. Clinical signs include septicemia, anorexia, hemorrhages, corneal opacity, and exophthalmos. Fish may also develop bloody abscesses around the mouth. High stocking densities, poor water conditions, and high temperatures are the most favorable conditions for streptococcal outbreaks. Tilapia streptococcosis affects fish from as small as 5 grams, and is present throughout the entire tilapia growth cycle. Intraperitoneal oil-adjuvanted vaccines are widely used and stimulate effective protection. Immersion, oral, and spray vaccines have also been investigated with limited success.

Lactococcosis caused by *Lactococcus garvieae*, affects saltwater fish in East Asia, especially rainbow trout, Japanese yellowtail, and gray mullet. A bacterin is available that is administered intraperitoneally.

Antiviral Vaccines

Most fish viral vaccines are inactivated products or recombinant subunits delivered by intraperitoneal injection. The nature of commercial aquaculture is such that administration of live viral vaccines will effectively result in contamination of their aqueous environment. The risks of uncontrolled spread, ecological damage, and reversion to virulence are not insignificant. As a result, few trials have been made with live vaccines in commercial aquaculture. Because of their economic value, most antiviral vaccines have been directed against salmonid pathogens.

INFECTIOUS PANCREATIC NECROSIS

Infectious pancreatic necrosis virus (IPNV) is a birnavirus mainly affecting young trout and salmon in Europe and North America. It causes a sudden mortality with abdominal swelling and anorexia. Numerous vaccines are available against IPNV. They are either subunit vaccines or inactivated products. The subunit vaccines contain the major viral antigen VP2 expressed in *Escherichia coli*. They may be delivered orally or by intraperitoneal injection. The adjuvanted vaccine is injected into pre-smolts. A combined *Aeromonas salmonicida* and IPNV oil-adjuvanted intraperitoneal vaccine is also available. Protection against IPNV has been demonstrated to last for up to 2.5 months.

INFECTIOUS SALMON ANEMIA

Infectious salmon anemia virus (ISAV) is an orthomyxovirus that affects Atlantic salmon because fish erythrocytes are nucleated they can sustain viral growth. Fish may develop pale gills but more often die suddenly so that death rates may reach 100%. Some trout may act as healthy carriers and sea lice can carry the virus. It occurs in Europe and the Americas.

Subunit and inactivated vaccines are available. The subunit vaccine contains the ISAV recombinant hemagglutinin esterase gene and is given orally. There are multiple inactivated monovalent or combined vaccines. For example there is an ISAV, *Aeromonas salmonicida-Vibrio anguillarum-ordalii-salmonicida* bacterin available. All inactivated ISAV vaccines are administered intraperitoneally.

INFECTIOUS HEMATOPOIETIC NECROSIS VIRUS

Infectious hematopoietic necrosis (IHN) is caused by a rhabdovirus. IHN affects salmonid fish on the Pacific coast of Canada and the United States where it is endemic. It is also present in Japan, Korea, and Europe. It primarily impacts farms rearing fry or juvenile rainbow trout with mortality up to 90%. Clinical signs include abdominal distention, anemia, and hemorrhage from the mouth, gills and anus, and also the yolk sac in fry. As its name implies, kidney necrosis occurs. The disease is especially interesting because the first DNA-plasmid vaccine was licensed against this disease. Studies demonstrated that only the viral glycoprotein (G) is capable of inducing neutralizing antibodies. Administered by a single intramuscular injection, the vaccine consists of a plasmid containing a cytomegalovirus promoter that drives expression of the IHN G protein. The use of a promoter from a human pathogen, cytomegalovirus, makes this vaccine "unsafe" in some countries. Encouraging results have been obtained by incorporating the vaccine into alginate microspheres and feeding it.

SALMON PANCREAS DISEASE

Salmonid alphavirus is the cause of salmon pancreas disease in Europe. It is a positive-stranded RNA alphavirus of the *Togaviridae* family. Mortality may be low but survivors fail to grow and may die months later. An inactivated vaccine given intraperitoneally is efficacious and significantly reduces viral shedding. A DNA-plasmid vaccine has been licensed in Europe for the prevention of this disease, caused by alphavirus subtype 3 (Clynav, Elanco).

VIRAL HEMORRHAGIC SEPTICEMIA

This is a highly infectious disease primarily affecting trout and flounder. It is caused by a weakly immunogenic rhabdovirus. As a result, it has been difficult to develop an effective vaccine. Several experimental vaccines have been developed including inactivated, modified live, recombinant protein, and DNA vaccines, but none have been commercialized as yet.

SPRING VIREMIA OF CARP

Spring viremia of carp (SVC) is a swim bladder infection caused by a rhabdovirus (*Rhabdovirus carpio*). Signs are similar to the other fish viral diseases including abdominal swelling, pale gills, and hemorrhage. Despite its name it affects a diverse range of cultured fish species including catfish, and trout in addition to carp. Subunit and modified live vaccines are available. The subunit vaccine is expressed as a recombinant glycoprotein in a baculovirus expression system. It is given intraperitoneally. The modified live vaccine is given orally.

KOI HERPESVIRUS DISEASE

Cyprinid herpesvirus 3 is usually found in common carp in addition to its ornamental varieties such as koi. It causes gill mottling, pale patches on the skin, and vesiculation. Mortality may reach 100%. Death may occur within 24 to 48 hours. As with the other herpesviruses, infected individuals act as healthy carriers. A modified live virus vaccine based on an attenuated carp interstitial nephritis and gill necrosis virus is available. Fish are immersed for 45 to 60 minutes. Fish may be revaccinated before stress or exposure. Because the vaccine container contains live virus, once the fish are vaccinated, the container must be sterilized by burning or immersion in bleach.

VIRAL NERVOUS NECROSIS

Viral nervous necrosis caused by a betanodovirus results in viral encephalopathy, and retinopathy and is the most important fish disease in warm waters such as the Mediterranean area. It affects many different species but is especially important in sea bass. An inactivated mineral oil-adjuvanted vaccine is available. It is given by intraperitoneal injection in a very low dose, so as a result it can be given to fish over 12 g. Immunity lasts for a year.

Antiprotozoan Vaccine

Ichthyophthirius multifiliis, is a ciliated protozoan that causes "ich" or "white spot disease." It is difficult to control by conventional methods. Patents have been awarded for an inactivated oral vaccine but it is not yet commercially available.

Adverse Events

Local injection site reactions remain an issue in aquaculture. Intraperitoneal inoculation may lead to local or diffuse peritonitis with adhesions. Multiple granulomas may also develop. The lesions contain macrophages, fibroblasts, lymphocytes, and melanomacrophages. More importantly, affected fish show reduced feed conversion and growth. Lesions in the fish result in increased condemnation and slowing of processing. Intraperitoneal oil-adjuvanted vaccines appear to induce autoimmunity in vaccinated fish. The fish produce multiple autoantibodies, and develop immune-complex glomerulonephritis, liver thrombosis, and spinal deformities. Both polyclonal IgM and antibodies to salmon red blood cells are elevated in vaccinated fish. It is possible that these antibodies are generated within the vaccine-induced granulomas.

Species Differences

Because of their high individual value, salmon are routinely vaccinated with water-in-oil adjuvanted vaccines given by injection. One commonly used vaccine is a combination product directed against furunculosis, cold-water vibriosis, winter ulcer, infectious pancreatic necrosis, and infectious salmon anemia. However there are significant differences in vaccine use in different countries based on perceived and actual threats. For example, IHN is a major cause for concern in Western Canada and a DNA vaccine is available to prevent it.

Rainbow trout vaccinations differ according to whether they are raised in seawater or freshwater. Large seawater trout are usually vaccinated by injection, whereas smaller freshwater fish tend to receive oral or immersion vaccines. The predominant vaccines employed in seawater trout include those against furunculosis, vibriosis, and winter ulcer. Freshwater trout in contrast suffer predominantly from enteric redmouth disease (yersiniosis), vibriosis (*Listonella anguillarum*), and flavobacteriosis (*Flavobacterium columnare*).

Cod raised in Norway are generally vaccinated against vibriosis and furunculosis. Sea bass and sea bream raised in Mediterranean countries suffer from vibriosis and pasteurellosis, and may receive a combination vaccine against both. Catfish are also raised worldwide. In the United States channel catfish predominate. Two attenuated live vaccines are available for use in this species against *Edwardsiella ictaluri* and *F. columnare*. Tilapia are one of the major fish species raised in aquaculture worldwide. Their major disease problem is Streptococcosis caused by *S. agalactiae*. Although vaccines are available, the low value of individual fish makes vaccination not cost-effective in many countries.

Sources of Additional Information

Bowden, T.J. (2008). Modulation of the immune system of fish by their environment. *Fish Shellfish Immunol*, 25, 373–383.

Brudeseth, B.E., Wiulsrod, R., Fredriksen, B.N., Lindmo, K., et al. (2013). Status and future perspectives of vaccines for industrialized fin-fish farming. *Fish Shellfish Immunol*, 35, 1759–1768.

Dhar, A.K., Allnutt, F.C.T. (2011). Challenges and opportunities in developing oral vaccines against viral diseases of fish. *J Marine Sci Res Development*, S1, 003.

Dhar, A.K., Manna, S.K., Allnutt, .FC.T. (2014). Viral vaccines for farmed finfish. *Virus Dis*, 25, 1–17.

Embregts, C.W.E., Forlenza, M. (2016). Oral vaccination of fish: Lessons from humans and veterinary species. *Dev Comp Immunol*, 64, 118–137.

Figueroa, C., Bustos, P., Torrealba, D., Dixon, B., et al. (2017). Coinfection takes its toll: Sea lice override the protective effects of vaccination against a bacterial pathogen of Atlantic salmon. *Sci Reports*, 7, 17817.

Gudding, R., Van Muiswinkel, W.B. (2013). A history of fish vaccination: Science-based disease prevention in aquaculture. *Fish Shellfish Immunol*, 35, 1683–1688.

Hasten, T., Gudding, R., Evensen, O. (2005). Bacterial vaccines for fish—An update of the current situation worldwide. *Prog Fish Vaccinol*, 121, 55–74.

Koppang, E.O., Bjerkas, I., Haugarvoll, E., Chan, E.K.L., Szabo, N.J., et al. (2008). Vaccination-induced systemic autoimmunity in farmed Atlantic salmon. *J Immunol*, 181, 4807–4814.

Liu, G., Zhu, J., Chen, K., Gao, T., et al. (2016). Development of Streptococcus agalactiae vaccines for tilapia. *Dis Aquat Org*, 122, 163–170.

Mutoloki, S., Munang'andu, H.M., Evensen, O. (2015). Oral vaccination of fish-antigen preparations, uptake, and immune induction. *Front Immunol*, 6, 519.

Newaj-Fyzul, A., Austin, B. (2015). Probiotics, immunostimulants, plant products and oral vaccines, their role as feed supplements in the control of bacterial fish diseases. *J Fish Dis*, 38, 937–955.

Sommerset, I., Krossoy, B., Biering, E., Frost, P. (2005). Vaccines for fish in aquaculture. *Expert Rev Vaccines*, 4, 89–101.

Tafalla, C., Bogwald, J., Dalmo, R.A. (2013). Adjuvants and immunostimulants in fish vaccines: Current knowledge and future perspectives. *Fish Shellfish Immunol*, 35, 1740–1750.

Workenhe, S.T., Rise, M.L., Kibenge, M.J.T., Kibenge, F.S.B. (2010). The fight between the teleost fish immune response and aquatic viruses. *Mol Immunol*, 47, 2525–2536.

Vaccines Against Parasites

A consistent feature of all parasite infestations is their ability to block or delay host defenses so that the parasites may survive for sufficient time to reproduce. Some parasites may simply delay their destruction until they complete a single life cycle. Other well-adapted parasites may contrive to survive for the life of their host, protected from immunological attack by highly evolved evasive mechanisms. A successful parasite will influence its host's immune responses, selectively suppressing these to permit parasite survival, while at the same time allowing other responses to proceed, and thus minimizing the problems that result from nonspecific immunosuppression.

Vaccination against parasitic diseases has therefore faced two hurdles. One is the complexity of the immune responses to these agents compounded by the fact that they, by definition, have successfully evolved to evade the immune system. Thus any antiparasite vaccine has to induce a protective immune response that is superior to the natural response. The second problem is economic. Many diverse drug treatments are available for parasite infestations, and newly developed vaccines are often much less effective. This is especially true of parasitic helminths. In addition, many parasites are only detected after an animal carcass has been processed. As a result, the farmer may have little incentive to spend money on parasite vaccines if there is no obvious economic return.

Protozoan Vaccines

GIARDIASIS

A vaccine has been available to protect dogs and cats against the intestinal parasite *Giardia duodenalis*. The vaccine contained disrupted cultured *Giardia* trophozoite extracts administered subcutaneously. It protected experimentally challenged dogs and cats against infection and clinical disease. It has now been withdrawn from the market.

TOXOPLASMOSIS

Toxoplasma gondii causes a placentitis leading to abortions, mummified fetuses, and weak lambs in sheep and goats. It is spread by cats. Because a primary infection with *T. gondii* will confer strong immunity on an animal, protective immunization is a real possibility. A vaccine containing tissue culture grown live, *T. gondii* tachyzoites attenuated by over 3000 passages in mice, the S48 incomplete strain, has been used successfully to control toxoplasmosis in sheep. This strain has lost the ability to develop bradyzoites or to initiate the sexual stages of the life cycle in cats. It induces protection against a severe challenge for at least 18 months.

This toxoplasma vaccine is available in some European countries and in New Zealand. It is made to order and is supplied as a concentrated suspension of tachyzoites plus diluent. It has a shelf life of only 7 to 10 days and must be handled very carefully to avoid human infection, especially by pregnant women. As with all such vaccines, it should be stored carefully, never frozen, or exposed to ultraviolet light. The vaccine is administered intramuscularly, but because it does not produce the cyst form (bradyzoites), vaccinated animals are not persistently infected. A single dose will provide lifetime immunity. It should be given at least four weeks before breeding.

NEOSPOROSIS

Neospora caninum is an important cause of bovine abortion. It is especially significant in the dairy industry. A killed tachyzoite vaccine was licensed in New Zealand in 2001. Its use resulted in a significant drop in the occurrence of abortions in some infected herds. It also appeared to protect against vertical transmission from cows to their calves. However, because of doubts regarding its efficacy, it did not gain widespread acceptance.

EQUINE PROTOZOAL MYELOENCEPHALITIS

This is an important neurologic disease caused by *Sarcocystis neurona* in horses. This organism's sporozoites are shed in opossum feces and contaminate horse feed. Because treatment is of limited effectiveness, prevention is very important. A killed vaccine for intramuscular use in horses is available. Studies on experimentally challenged horses have, however, failed to show protection against neurologic disease.

LEISHMANIASIS (LEISHMANIOSIS)

A disease caused by the protozoan parasites of the genus *Leishmania* transmitted by sandflies. It is endemic to the Mediterranean area, the Middle East, Central Asia, and Latin America. The most important cause is *Leishmania infantum* (also called *Leishmania chagasi*). Leishmania causes granulomatous lesions in both the internal organs and the skin of infected dogs. The disease is controlled by a combination of vector control and vaccination. Two different vaccines against canine leishmaniasis have been licensed in Brazil. Both are designed to stimulate T cell-mediated responses because this is an intracellular parasite. One such vaccine consists of a *Leishmania* component called the fucose-mannose ligand (or GP63) adjuvanted with Quil A (Leishmune, Zoetis) given in 3 doses at 3-week intervals. It induces an antibody response that blocks transmission of the organism to the sandfly vector by preventing the binding of the Leishmania to the sandfly midgut. This vaccine has been reported to have an 80% efficacy against disease and death. It may also serve as an immunotherapeutic agent, producing clinical improvement in dogs with disseminated disease. It has recently been withdrawn from the market.

An alternative vaccine containing a recombinant protein (A2) from several different Leishmania species and a saponin adjuvant appears to be 43% effective against experimental challenge, and over 70% effective in field studies (Leish-Tec Hertape Calier, Brazil). Leish-Tec may also be of benefit in treating dogs with Leishmaniasis. Another vaccine is available in Europe (CaniLeish, Virbac, France). It contains *L. infantum* excreted/secreted proteins with a saponin adjuvant (QA-21). Its efficacy is about 68%. It is used in dogs over six months of age with three primary doses given three weeks apart, and repeated annually.

Another *L. infantum* vaccine (Letifend, Leti SFU, France) contains a recombinant chimeric protein (protein Q). Four highly antigenic proteins from *L. infantum* were identified: LiP2A, Lip2B, Lip0, and a histone H2A. The genes for five antigenic determinants from these four antigens were fused and expressed in *Escherichia coli* to form the recombinant protein Q. It is given subcutaneously to dogs over six months of age. Only one priming dose is required followed by annual revaccination. The vaccine does not contain an adjuvant.

TRITRICHOMONAS

Tritrichomonas is a protozoan disease clinically similar to Campylobacteriosis. It is caused by *Tritrichomonas fetus*. Convalescent cows are usually resistant to reinfection for about two years. Whole-cell killed Tritrichomonas vaccines only confer a relatively short period of immunity and are not highly effective. As a result, they should be administered to heifers and cows immediately before the breeding season. They are not effective in bulls. This vaccine may be used in combination with Campylobacter and Leptospira bacterins.

THEILERIOSIS

Theileriae are intracellular parasitic protozoa. Tick transmitted *Theileria parva* is a major problem in cattle because it causes East Coast fever in subSaharan Africa. *Theileria annulata* occurs in southern Europe, Asia, and North Africa. *Theileria orientalis* is widespread globally but is usually subclinical. Although mainly prevented by tick control, vaccines are available against both pathogenic Theileria species.

Theileria infections, because they are intracellular parasites, must be controlled by cytotoxic T cells and these can only be induced by live parasites. For *T. annulata* a vaccine is prepared from schizonts attenuated by culture *in vitro*. This vaccine has a short shelf life and it must therefore be frozen until immediately before use. Vaccination against *Theileria parva* is based on infection followed by treatment. Cattle are infected by subcutaneous injection of a mixture of three different strains of tick-derived sporozoites, "the Muguga cocktail," and simultaneously treated with a long-acting tetracycline. As a result, the cattle get a mild infection followed by an immune response and recovery. Recovered animals develop a strong persistent immunity to homologous challenge.

BABESIOSIS

This is a tick-borne disease of cattle caused by the intracellular parasites *Babesia bovis*, *Babesia bigemina*, and *Babesia divergens*. It occurs globally, especially in tropical or subtropical countries. Animals that recover from acute babesiosis are resistant to further clinical disease.

Subunit and killed vaccines have been uniformly unsuccessful. Available vaccines consist of live, attenuated strains of Babesia produced from the blood of infected donors, especially from splenectomized calves infected with attenuated strains, or by culture *in vitro*. The spleen is important in removing infected erythrocytes so splenectomy permits very high parasitemias, and thus high parasite yields. Rapid serial passage in splenectomized calves also selects parasite populations enriched for faster growing avirulent phenotypes. This selection also narrows the diversity of the parasite subpopulations, which may affect their immunogenicity. Babesia vaccines may be stored frozen or chilled depending upon facilities available. The risk of contamination by other infectious agents from the donors of these blood-derived vaccines is significant. They also may cause reactions in older animals. Many of these live vaccines contain specially selected strains of *Babesia bovis* and *B. bigemina* and are produced in government-regulated production facilities. In addition, cattle show a significant resistance to babesiosis in the first six months of life. It is therefore possible to infect young calves when they are still relatively insusceptible to disease, so that they become resistant to reinfection. As might be anticipated, the side effects of this type of infection may be severe, and chemotherapy may be required to control them.

Protective immunity develops in three to four weeks and lasts at least four years (*B. bovis*) or less (*B. bigemina*) against local field challenges. The transfer of blood from one calf to another may also trigger the production of antibodies against the foreign red cells. These antibodies complicate any attempts at blood transfusion in later life and may provoke hemolytic disease of the newborn (Chapter 10).

Two vaccines against canine babesiosis have been marketed in Europe (Pirodog and Novibac Piro). They contain soluble parasite antigens obtained from the supernatants of *in vitro* cultures of *Babesia canis* and *Babesia rossi*. The antigens are treated with formaldehyde and then freeze-dried. The lyophilized vaccine is adjuvanted with saponin. These vaccines do not prevent infection but reduce disease length and severity. The vaccines are given around five months of age and annual revaccination is recommended.

COCCIDIOSIS

Unlike other apicomplexan parasites, coccidia of the genus Eimeria induce strong, species-specific immunity. As a result, several live and recombinant coccidial vaccines are given to poultry. These are described in Chapter 19.

Helminth Vaccines

Infection with gastrointestinal nematodes adversely impacts livestock productivity by affecting growth and fertility, in addition to meat, milk, and wool production. The financial costs of this worm burden affect almost all grazing animals. It is not surprising, considering the nature of the host response to parasitic worms and the availability of cheap and (until recently) effective broad-spectrum anthelmintics, that vaccines against helminth parasites are not widely available. Despite much ongoing high quality research and the identification of candidate vaccine antigens, parallel advances have not occurred in product development and clinical application. As a result, parasite prevention and treatment relies primarily on anthelmintic use. Nevertheless, the emergence of anthelmintic resistance and environmental concerns raised by excessive chemical use has resulted in a growing interest in the development of antihelminth vaccines. Vaccine use is predicated on the assumption that a host's immune response can be manipulated to control or prevent an infestation. This is not always obvious in helminth infestations, and traditional vaccines may be of little use.

Another issue that has impeded the development of vaccines against helminths is the tendency to develop immunoglobulin (Ig)E antibodies to helminth antigens. It has long been recognized that the biological function of IgE is to protect against helminth infestations. In many cases naturally parasitized animals make high levels of IgE. In such cases administration of irradiated larvae or helminth antigens may trigger severe allergic reactions such as anaphylaxis or generalized urticaria in previously exposed individuals. This problem was encountered when an irradiated L3 vaccine was developed for dogs against *Ancyclostoma caninum*, and humans against the hookworm *Necator americanus*.

TAENIA OVIS

A recombinant *Taenia ovis* vaccine has been produced in New Zealand that can induce protective immunity to this tapeworm in sheep. This vaccine contains a cloned oncosphere antigen (To45W) with a saponin-based adjuvant. It stimulates a response that prevents parasite penetration of the intestinal wall. Although highly effective in reducing parasite numbers by 98%, and carcass condemnation by 89%, it has not yet been marketed successfully.

ECHINOCOCCUS GRANULOSUS

Echinococcus granulosus is the causative agent of hydatidosis, an important cause of disease in sheep and humans in endemic areas. Sheep may be protected against *E. granulosus* using either oncospheres or secretory products from cultured oncospheres. Multiple antigens from *E. granulosus* were cloned into *E. coli* and then screened by the use of antibodies from immune sheep. An outer membrane protein called EG95 from activated oncospheres appeared to be highly effective as an immunogen. It was therefore cloned into *E. coli* and linked to glutathione-S-transferase (GST). (The GST assists in purifying the EG95). A commercially available vaccine (Providean Hitadil EG95 Tecnovax, Uruguay) containing recombinant EG95 adjuvanted with Montanide ISA70 and saponin has been licensed in several countries. It is administered intraperitoneally to sheep and goats and some camelid species and it is highly effective (96%–98%). The same vaccine also appears to be effective against alveolar echinococcosis caused by *Echinococcus multilocularis*.

TAENIA SOLIUM

Taenia solium is a major cause of neurocysticercosis in underdeveloped countries. It may account for as many as 29% of seizure disorders in endemic areas. These cases are caused by the presence of the larval stages of the pork tapeworm, *T. solium*, in the brain or spinal cord. Ideally vaccination may be employed in conjunction with drug treatment and education to help break the transmission cycle of this tapeworm by preventing its establishment in pigs. Immunity is antibody mediated because antibodies and complement can lyse the early development stages of the parasite. An oncosphere surface antigen, TSOL18 is highly immunogenic in pigs, where it provides more than 90% protection against experimental infection. The antigen has been cloned into *Pichia pastoris* and adjuvanted with mineral oil. This vaccine has been licensed in India (Cysvax, Indian Immunologicals Ltd).

LUNGWORM VACCINES

The lungworm, *Dictyocaulus viviparous*, causes parasitic bronchitis in cattle. Worm infestations result in a temporary immunity. As a result, a radiation-attenuated larval-based vaccine has been commercially available in some European countries for many years (Bovilis Huskvac, MSD Animal Health). Unfortunately, it has all the disadvantages of live vaccines. In this vaccine, third-stage larvae hatched from ova in culture are exposed to 40,000 R X-irradiation. These larvae are then given orally to calves over eight weeks of age. Two doses of the vaccine are given at an interval of four weeks. The residual effects of long-acting anthelmintics will interfere with the efficacy of this vaccine, so calves should not be treated with these until at least 14 days after the second vaccine dose. The vaccine can also be administered to cows at pasture as long as it is given before exposure to a strong larval challenge. The irradiated L3 larvae penetrate the calf's intestine, but because they are unable to develop to the fourth stage, they never reach the lung and are thus nonpathogenic. During their exsheathing process, the larvae stimulate the production of antibodies that can block reinfection. The efficiency of this vaccine depends very much on timing and on the size of the challenge dose, because even vaccinated calves may show mild pneumonic signs if placed on grossly infected pastures. The vaccine does not completely prevent establishment of small numbers of lungworms so pastures may remain contaminated. Likewise vaccine use is not justified in low-prevalence regions. A similar live irradiated L3 vaccine is available against *Dictyocaulus filaria* in India (Difil, Nuclear Research Laboratory, IVRI).

HAEMONCHUS CONTORTUS

Haemonchus contortus, the "barber's pole" worm, a blood-sucking parasite of the abomasum, is one of the most significant helminth parasites of sheep and goats. It is a major cause of sheep mortality in wet and tropical climates because it draws large quantities of blood from the parasitized intestine. In addition, anthelmintic resistance in *H. contortus* is a serious and increasing problem.

The major antigens produced by parasitic helminths are of two types: soluble excretory and secretory products, and antigens found on the parasite surface (somatic antigens). Some somatic antigens, such as those found in the worm gut cells, are not normally exposed to the host's immune response, and may therefore be potential candidates for vaccines.

A vaccine against *H. contortus* that makes use of antigens derived from the worm's digestive tract is now commercially available for use in sheep in Australia and South Africa (Barbervax, Wormvax Australia Pty Ltd). This vaccine is not available in the United States. As the worm feeds, it ingests the sheep's blood. Antibodies in the blood of vaccinated sheep are directed against antigens expressed on the worm's intestinal enterocytes. These antibodies interfere with the worm's digestion and growth leading to a greatly decreased egg output and a reduction in worm numbers by about 70% (Fig. 22.1). The worm vaccine antigens include two proteases: H11, an aminopeptidase expressed on the intestinal microvilli of adult worms; and H-gal-GP, a mixture of aspartyl, cysteine, and metalloproteases. Both antigens are highly protective in their native form but not if they are recombinant. This is likely caused by incorrect folding and/or inappropriate glycosylation. The vaccine is adjuvanted with saponin. This vaccine works in all classes of sheep, and worms have not evolved to cope with this challenge. However, because the antigens do not enter the sheep naturally, the protective response is not boosted by the presence of worms so repeated revaccination is necessary. These antigens can at present only be isolated from the worms extracted from infected slaughtered lambs. Three priming injections, three to four weeks

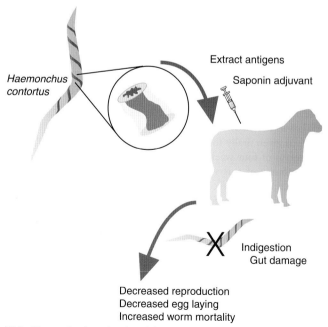

Fig. 22.1   The mechanism of action of the vaccine against *Haemonchus contortus*.

apart are required to confer immunity before the high worm-risk season. Egg production increases during lactation; this vaccine can prevent this periparturient rise. Subsequently the vaccine is administered at six-week intervals to maintain resistance.

Field trials indicate that the Barbervax induces a 75% to 95% drop in egg output. Because worm egg production is significantly reduced, the threat to unresponsive vaccinated sheep in the flock is also reduced, an example of herd immunity. Barbervax is not a substitute for good pasture management and appropriate worm control.

In general, helminth vaccines are not yet widely employed. There has been reluctance on the part of farmers to change established control procedures, especially when the major financial burden of these infestations is often borne by others. However, if highly effective, multivalent vaccines will ever become available they will revolutionize helminth parasite control.

Arthropod Vaccines

Although ectoparasites are of major veterinary importance, few commercially successful vaccines have been produced. Thus there are no available vaccines against biting flies, blowflies, or cattle grub infestations. Likewise vaccine development against mosquitoes has been disappointing. It is theoretically possible to make a vaccine against fleas (Box 6.1). There is a commercially available vaccine against aquatic sea lice, a major problem in marine aquaculture (Providean Aquatec Sea Lice [Technovax S.A. Argentina]. This is an oil-adjuvanted recombinant subunit vaccine against a protein (vitellogenin-1) of the sea louse *Caligus rogercresseyi*.

TICKS

Because many of the arthropods of veterinary importance ingest the blood of their host, they will also ingest immunoglobulins, complement components, and lymphocytes. This suggests that if an animal is immunized with internal antigens from the tick, the ingested antibodies may cause intestinal damage. These internal antigens have been called "hidden" or "concealed" antigens because under normal circumstances the host would not usually encounter them. Vaccines can therefore be made containing a gut membrane-bound glycoprotein from the intestine of the tick *Rhiphicephalus microplus*. A vaccine based on this recombinant antigen, Bm86 (and a related molecule Bm95), was available in Australia. (TickGUARD) but has been discontinued. A similar vaccine against Bm86 and Bm95 has been cloned into *Pischia pastoris* and marketed in some Latin-American countries under the name GAVAC plus. The antibodies produced bind to the brush border of tick enterocytes, inhibit endocytosis, and prevent the tick from fully engorging. Thus its digestive processes are impaired, and the tick experiences starvation, loss of fecundity, and weakness, and may disengage from its host. As a result, the number of engorged female ticks, their weight, and their egg-producing capability are reduced by 50% to 75%. Vaccination over several generations may result in a significant decline in tick burdens. After 10 years of vaccination, studies showed that there was an 80% drop in tick burden and a 67% drop in required acaricide treatments. If accompanied by appropriate acaricide treatment, tick numbers can be drastically reduced. Experimental multicomponent tick vaccines using other tick antigens show even more encouraging results. Bm86 vaccination has minimal or no efficacy against other tick species.

Encouraging results have also been obtained with experimental vaccines directed against the red poultry mite (*Dermanyssus gallinae*). Initial studies with crude mite extracts have been followed by identification of candidate vaccine antigens.

Sources of Additional Information

Bassetto, C.C., Picharillo, M.É., Newlands, G.F., et al. (2014). Attempts to vaccinate ewes and their lambs against natural infection with *Haemonchus contortus* in a tropical environment. *Int J Parasitol,* 44, 1049–1054.

Bassetto, C.C., Silva, M.R., Newlands, G.F., et al. (2014). Vaccination of grazing calves with antigens from the intestinal membranes of *Haemonchus contortus*: effects against natural challenge with *Haemonchus placei* and *Haemonchus similis*. *Int J Parasitol,* 44, 697–702.

Bassetto, C.C., Silva, B.F., Newlands, G.F., Smith, W.D., Amarante, A.F. (2011). Protection of calves against Haemonchus placei and Haemonchus contortus after immunization with gut membrane proteins from *H. contortus*. *Parasite Immunol,* 33, 377–381.

Ekoja, S.E., Smith, W.D. (2010). Antibodies from sheep immunized against *Haemonchus contortus* with H-gal-GP inhibit the haemoglobinase activity of this protease complex. *Parasite Immunol,* 32, 11–12.

Fernandez Cotrina, J., et al. (2018). A large-scale field randomized trial demonstrates safety and efficacy of the vaccine LetiFend(R) against canine leishmaniosis. *Vaccine,* 36, 1972–1982.

Florin-Christensen, M., Suarez, C.E., Rodriguez, A.E., Flores, D.A., Schnittger, L. (2014). Vaccines against bovine babesiosis: where we are now and possible roads ahead. *Parasitology,* 141,1563–1592.

Horcajo, P., Regidor-Cerrillo, J., Aguado-Martinez, A., Hemphill, A., Ortega-Mora, L.M. (2016). Vaccines for bovine neospososis: current status and key aspects for development. *Parasit Immunol,* 38, 709–723.

Lightowlers, M.W. (2013). Control of Taenia solium taeniasis/cysticercosis: Past practices and new possibilities. *Parasitology,* 140, 1566–1577.

Nisbet, A.J., McNeilly, T.N., Wildblood, L.A., Morrison, A.A., et al. (2013). Successful immunization against a parasitic nematode by vaccination with recombinant proteins. *Vaccine,* 31, 4017–4023.

Petavy, A.F., Hormaeche, C., Lahmar, S., et al. (2008). An oral recombinant vaccine in dogs against *Echinococcus granulosus*, the causal agent of human hytadid disease: A pilot study. *PLoS Negl Trop Dis,* 2, e125.

Pourseif, M.M., Moghaddam, G., Saeedi, N., et al. (2018). Current status and future prospective of vaccine development against *Echinococcus granulosis*. *Biologicals,* 51, 1–11.

Schetters, T. (2005). Vaccination against canine babesiosis. *Trends Parasitol,* 21, 179–184.

Steinaa, L., Svitek, N., Awino, E., Njoroge, T., Saya, R., Morrison, I., Toye, P. (2018). Immunization wih one *Theileria parva* strain results in a similar level of CTL strain specificity and protection compared to immunization with the three-component Muguga cocktail in MHC-matched animals. *BMC Vet Res,* 14:145.

Strube, C., Haake, C., Sager, H., et al. (2015). Vaccination with recombinant paramyosin against the bovine lungworm *Dictyocaulus viviparus* considerably reduces worm burden and larvae shedding. *Paras Vectors,* 8, 119.

Stutzer, C., Richards, S.A., Ferreira, M., et al. (2018). Metazoan parasite vaccines: Present status and future prospects. *Front Cell Infect Microbiol,* 8, 67.

Vargas, M., Montero, C., Sanchez, D., et al. (2010). Two initial vaccinations with the Bm-86 based Gavacplus vaccine against *Rhipicephalus (Boophilus) microplus* induce similar reproductive suppression to three initial vaccinations under production conditions. *BMC Vet Res,* 6, 43.

Weber, F.H., Jackson, J.A., Sobecki, B., et al. (2013). On the efficacy and safety of vaccination with live tachyzoites of *Neospora caninum* for prevention of Neospora-associated fetal loss in cattle. *Clin Vacc Immunil,* 20, 99–105.

Anticancer Vaccines

It has long been believed that one function of the adaptive immune system is to detect and destroy abnormal cells such as cancer cells. If true, it follows that the immune system may well be manipulated to enhance such immunity. On consideration, however, it is apparent that when a cancer develops in an animal it must have already defeated the immune system. For many years, immunologists have attempted to treat cancers by means of immunotherapy. Progress was distressingly slow. Successes were limited to rare cancers and even when immunotherapy worked, results were unpredictable and inconsistent. That has now changed. Vaccines against cancers are still at an early stage in their development, but new techniques involving both passive and active immunotherapy have begun to yield exciting results. Progress has not been confined to human cancers. Encouraging results are increasingly being obtained in the treatment of cancers in our domestic animals.

One reason for recent successes is that we have increasingly recognized that cancers are immunosuppressive. They employ multiple strategies to evade or suppress the host's immune system. Thus treatments that reverse this immunosuppression have the potential to "turn on" the immune system and destroy the cancer.

Preventative Vaccines

It has been estimated that about 17% of human cancers arise as a result of infection. Many different human pathogens including the bacterium *Helicobacter pylori*, hepatitis viruses B and C, Epstein-Barr virus, herpesvirus, and human papilloma virus are oncogenic. Prophylactic vaccination against these agents is therefore a practical way to prevent cancers developing.

There are established successful and effective vaccines against oncogenic viruses such as hepatitis B and human papillomavirus, the causes of hepatocellular carcinoma and cervical cancer, respectively. The most important of these in veterinary medicine are the vaccines against feline leukemia. These vaccines usually contain high concentrations of the major viral antigens, and immunity is almost entirely directed against viral glycoproteins. Other important vaccines are those directed against Marek's disease, a T cell tumor of chickens caused by a herpesvirus. The immune response evoked by these vaccines has two components. First, humoral and cell-mediated responses act directly on the virus to reduce the number of virions available to infect cells. Second, an immune response is provoked against virus-encoded antigens on the surface of tumor cells. Both the antiviral and antitumor immune responses act synergistically to protect the birds against Marek's disease.

Passive Immunization

MONOCLONAL ANTIBODIES

A major advance in cancer immunotherapy has been the development of bioengineered monoclonal antibodies that may be directed against specific tumor cell antigens or against molecules that promote tumor growth. There are now more than 75 US Food and Drug Administration (FDA)–approved, monoclonal antibodies used in the treatment of human cancers. For example, in 1987 the FDA approved rituximab, a monoclonal antibody directed against the B-cell surface antigen CD20. Rituximab has revolutionized the treatment of B cell lymphomas in humans. The anti-CD20 binds to the malignant B cells and triggers their apoptosis.

Canine B cells also express CD20 although canine monoclonal anti-CD20 does not appear to cause B cell tumor apoptosis. Canine CD20 is structurally sufficiently different from the human molecule so that Rituximab will not bind it. Caninized monoclonal antibodies against canine CD20 have been developed and some deplete B cells.

Initially these monoclonal antibodies were derived exclusively from mice. However, as monoclonal antibody technology has improved, it has proved possible to "humanize" the murine antibodies by attaching the mouse antigen-binding region to a human immunoglobulin backbone. A similar process can produce "caninized" monoclonal antibodies for use in dogs (Chapter 12).

These monoclonal antibodies can be directed against the cancer cells to destroy them through the process of antibody-dependent cellular cytotoxicity. Alternatively, monoclonal antibodies may be used to block growth-promoting factors or their receptors or they may enhance the activity of anticancer immune cells. Several caninized monoclonal antibodies directed against lymphomas have undergone clinical trials although with disappointing results to date.

Blontress (Aratana Therapeutics), is a caninized monoclonal antiCD20 antibody licensed as an aid in the treatment of dogs with B-cell lymphoma. It enhances antibody-dependent cellular cytotoxicity and promotes macrophage phagocytosis of tumor cells. The antibody is administered intravenously over a period of at least 15 minutes. Two doses on week one, at two to three day intervals, followed by one dose a week for seven weeks. Its use is accompanied by appropriate chemotherapy. Encouraging results in treating canine B cell lymphomas have been obtained by a method that combines administration of anti-CD20 with a blockade of CD47. (CD47 is expressed on tumor cells and acts as a checkpoint regulator by inhibiting their phagocytosis by macrophages.) The antiCD20 kills the tumor cells and the CD47 ensures their removal. US Department of Agriculture (USDA) has approved a DNA-plasmid vaccine directed against CD20 for the treatment of canine B cell lymphomas.

Bevacizumab is a humanized monoclonal antibody directed against vascular epithelial growth factor. Vascular endothelial growth factor (VEGF) promotes angiogenesis, blood vessel growth. This monoclonal antibody inhibits the growth of cancers by preventing the development of their blood supply. Preliminary studies suggest that this product may be effective in treating some canine sarcomas.

CHECKPOINT INHIBITION

Recent remarkable advances in the treatment of some human cancers have resulted from the use of monoclonal antibodies that prevent signaling by checkpoint molecules (Fig. 23.1). Checkpoint molecules are cell surface receptors that transmit signals, that control immune responses by suppressing T cell proliferation and cytotoxicity. The first of these molecules to be identified was CTLA-4. CTLA-4 is expressed on the surface of naïve and effector T cells. Ligands acting through CTLA-4 deliver suppressive signals to the T cells and prevent their activation. Conversely, if CTLA-4 signaling is blocked, then T cell responses are activated. CTLA-4 blockade

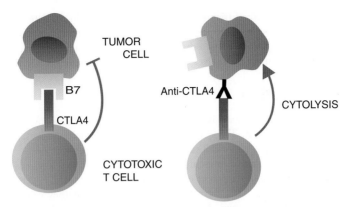

Fig. 23.1 The principles of immune checkpoint therapy. CTLA-4 is an inhibitory receptor expressed on T cells. Its ligand is B7 expressed on cancer cells. If CTLA-4–B7 binding is blocked by a monoclonal antibody (anti-CTLA4), the cytotoxic T cells are then free to attack the cancer cells and kill them.

in tumor bearing animals therefore results in a significant increase in T-cell mediated tumor cytotoxicity and the development of new antitumor T cells. Studies on humans have shown that administration of a monoclonal antibody against CTLA-4 (Ipilimumab) results in a significant increase in T cell antitumor activity and dramatic remissions in many (but not all) patients.

A second major checkpoint target is the Programmed Death-1 (PD-1)/Programmed Death-1 ligand (PD-1L) axis. PD-1 is a receptor expressed on effector T cells. Like CTLA-4, when stimulated by its ligand (PD-1L), it suppresses T cell functions. Blockade of PD-1 or PD-1L by monoclonal antibodies therefore results in a great increase in T cell cytotoxic activity and an antitumor response. (This likely works by enhancing interferon-γ production by dendritic cells and so activating cytotoxic CD8+ T cells to maximize their anticancer response.) Treatment with anti-PD-1 or anti-PD-1L monoclonal antibodies has produced dramatic and prolonged remissions in humans with melanomas, renal cell carcinomas, and non-small cell lung cancers. For example, in patients with metastatic melanoma, those treated with checkpoint therapy have a 50% survival at three years compared with 12% survival in patients receiving chemotherapy alone. (The use of these checkpoint inhibitors has been likened to taking a foot off the T cell brake pedal).

Many canine tumors such as mastocytomas, melanomas, renal cell carcinomas, and B cell lymphomas are infiltrated by T cells that overexpress PD1-L and CTLA-4. This suggests that these T cells are suppressed and are therefore potential targets for checkpoint therapy. Monoclonal antibodies have been made against canine PD-1 and PD-1L. Both molecules are present on activated canine T cells whereas PD-1L is expressed on canine dendritic cells. When treated with either anti-PD-1 alone, or a combination of anti-PD-1 and anti-PD-1L *in vitro*, T cell production of interferon γ was significantly increased. These results are of immediate relevance to the treatment of tumors in dogs.

CANINE T CELL LYMPHOMA

A caninized monoclonal antibody against CD52, a protein expressed on T cells, has been licensed by USDA as an aid to the treatment of dogs with T cell lymphoma (Tactress, Aratana Therapeutics). The product is administered intravenously over a period of at least 15 minutes. The dose is dependent on body weight. Two doses are given at two to three day intervals followed by four doses every other week. Although clinical trial results have been disappointing to date, modifications of the treatment protocol may yet produce positive results. For optimal results, monoclonal antibody therapy must often be supplemented by other treatments such as chemotherapy. Monoclonal antibodies are rarely sufficient by themselves to cause complete remissions.

Active Immunization

Therapeutic vaccination against cancer is a very active research area and many promising cancer vaccines are under development. These include adjuvanted purified antigens, DNA-plasmid vaccines, vector-based vaccines, tumor cell vaccines, and dendritic cell vaccines.

Tumor vaccines trigger adaptive immunity against tumor-associated antigens administered in such a way that they stimulate a potent cytotoxic T cell response while overcoming tumor-mediated immunosuppression. They have the great advantage that they can circumvent the resistance of tumor cells to cytotoxic drugs. Additionally, they are highly specific, have low toxicity, and have a long-lasting effect as a result of memory responses.

These tumor-associated antigens belong to two broad categories. There are tumor specific shared antigens expressed on more than one type of tumor cell and that may also be expressed on normal tissues. The other category includes unique molecules expressed by cancer cells as a result of mutations resulting from carcinogen exposure. These tumor antigens can be obtained from either autologous sources (the cancerous animal itself) or from allogeneic sources (other animals). They can include whole cell lysates or purified tumor peptides or even defined tumor cell antigens such as tyrosinase.

Many different approaches have been tested including proteins, peptides, cell extracts, and whole tumor cells. It is also possible to make DNA-plasmid vaccines expressing the genes encoding specific tumor antigens. They can be delivered directly as DNA-plasmids or inserted into appropriate recombinant viral or bacterial vectors. In theory, injected tumor antigens should induce both memory and effector T cells. As a result, immunity should persist and control tumor growth indefinitely. Unfortunately, there are few defined tumor antigens, and the recent successes of passive immunity and immune checkpoint therapy suggest that the need for such vaccines may diminish.

Many attempts have been made to produce tumor vaccines for animals. A canine lymphoma vaccine was first investigated in the 1980s. These early attempts used whole cell vaccines consisting of irradiated or lysed tumor cells together with an adjuvant. However, these whole cell vaccines were poorly defined and it was difficult to produce a standardized product. Recently some encouraging results have been obtained using autologous tumor cells.

The lack of success of these early vaccines may have resulted from immunosuppressive mechanisms acting within the tumor microenvironment, as well as the activation of regulatory T cells and the blocking of activation signals by suppressive signals. As described above, these suppressive signals are mediated by checkpoint molecules such as CTLA-4, PD-1, and its ligand PD-1L. Other checkpoint molecules that are potential targets for monoclonal antibody therapy include several found on both T cells and NK cells as well as the natural killer cell inhibitory receptor NKG2A. Checkpoint therapy is still in its infancy and results should steadily improve as experience is gained.

TELOMERASE VACCINE

The telomerase reverse transcriptase (TERT) is a subcomponent of the enzyme telomerase. Telomerase ensures that telomeres (the ends of chromosomes) do not shorten when cells divide. It is expressed at a very low level in normal cells but is highly expressed in the vast majority of neoplastic cells where it confers immortality. TERT is usually absent from normal dog tissues. Thus TERT represents a valid target for cancer immunotherapy. A current experimental vaccine consists of an adenovirus-vectored recombinant expressing TERT that is introduced into dogs by DNA electroporation. Vaccinated dogs make an antibody response against the reverse transcriptase. The vaccine appears to increase overall survival time in dogs with B cell lymphoma that also received standard chemotherapy when compared with dogs that received chemotherapy alone.

CANINE ORAL MELANOMA

Melanomas are uniquely immunogenic tumors and it has been possible to make an antimelanoma DNA-plasmid vaccine (Oncept, Boehringer Ingelheim). This vaccine contains an *Escherichia coli* plasmid engineered to express the gene encoding human tyrosinase. The plasmid also contains a cytomegalovirus promoter and a kanamycin resistance selection marker. Once inside a cell nucleus, the DNA plasmid transcribes and translates the tyrosinase gene and as a result cells produce this enzyme within the recipient. Tyrosinase catalyzes the hydroxylation of tyrosine to dihydroxyphenylalanine, a key step in melanin production. This human tyrosinase is only 85% homologous to the canine protein. This difference is such that vaccinated dogs will mount immune responses against the human protein. These responses include the production of both antibodies and T cells and result in destruction of the melanoma cells.

Four doses of this vaccine are administered transdermally to affected dogs using a jet injector (Vetjet) at two-week intervals. It is then administered at six-month intervals on the medial thigh caudal to the femur.

Oral melanomas in dogs have a poor prognosis because of their invasiveness and ability to metastasize. In untreated dogs with oral malignant melanoma the median time to death resulting from metastases or progressive disease is two months. Conventional treatments, surgery, chemotherapy, or radiation therapies lengthen median survival times from 5 to 12 months. Although surgery plus radiation has increased survival times significantly, chemotherapy has failed to demonstrate a significant benefit. Oncept aids in extending the survival times of dogs with stage II and III canine oral melanoma following local disease control (tumor-negative local lymph nodes or positive lymph nodes have been surgically removed or irradiated). In a prospective clinical trial with 58 dogs, use of this melanoma vaccine significantly increased survival times. In one retrospective study vaccinated dogs had a median survival time of 355 days. In another retrospective study, 8 of 13 dogs showed a clinical response and three dogs with oral malignant melanoma survived for 171, 178, and 288 days from diagnosis. Other investigators have failed to show benefits of Oncept treatment. Prospective, randomized controlled trials have yet to be performed. The vaccine is well tolerated with no significant adverse effects.

OSTEOSARCOMAS

Osteosarcomas are the most common primary bone tumors in dogs. Conventional treatment consists of amputation and aggressive chemotherapy. Despite this, metastasis is common. A canine osteosarcoma vaccine, Live Listeria Vector (AT-104) has been granted a conditional license by USDA (Aratana Therapeutics, Advaxis Inc.). This vaccine uses attenuated *Listeria monocytogenes* as a vector to carry a plasmid expressing a human tumor antigen called HER2/neu into macrophages. HER2/neu is a tyrosine kinase receptor overexpressed on many aggressive carcinomas and sarcomas. When injected into an animal the bacteria are rapidly phagocytosed. However, listeria is a facultative intracellular bacterium and so can enter and survive within the cytosol of macrophages. It normally uses a pore-forming lysin called listeriolysin O (LLO) to escape from the phagosome into the cytosol. The plasmids expressing the genes for HER2/neu, fused with a truncated form of LLO, transcribe and translate the chimeric antigen. This is carried to the cytosol where the fusion protein is processed as an endogenous antigen (Chapter 2), and enters the major histocompatibility complex (MHC) class I presenting pathway. The chimeric protein is also secreted so that it can also act through the exogenous antigen processing pathway. As a result, the HER2/neu is recognized by both CD4+ and CD8+ T cells and induces a potent T cell-mediated cytotoxic response. When this recombinant Listeria was administered intravenously in conjunction with amputation and chemotherapy, the median survival time of dogs with osteosarcomas was doubled when compared with amputation and chemotherapy alone. As a result, a large extended field study is currently underway.

AUTOLOGOUS TUMOR VACCINES

It is of course possible simply to excise part of a tumor and prepare an inactivated vaccine to be injected back into to the patient. The best example of this approach is the production of autologous vaccines against bovine fibropapillomas. These papillomas may develop on the teats or other inconvenient sites on cattle. They are caused by members of a large family of bovine papillomaviruses. Vaccines are available that can be used for both prevention and treatment but success depends on the specific papillomavirus involved. There are several ways of making these vaccines. For example, the papillomas can be surgically excised, and small pieces stored in 10% buffered formalin. After cleaning, selected pieces are suspended in saline and homogenized. A preservative or antibiotics are then added to inhibit bacterial growth. After filtration, more formalin may be added to ensure viral inactivation. The vaccine is administered subcutaneously in three doses at one-week intervals. Vaccination is often quite effective for the treatment of small tumors, but large papillomas may need to be surgically excised.

Although immunologists and oncologists have searched for effective, antitumor vaccines for many years, the results have been unpredictable and hence very frustrating. Occasional anecdotal successes are accompanied by many cases where no beneficial effect is seen. Even the new checkpoint blockading monoclonal antibodies do not work in every patient. As described in Chapter 6, informatics and vaccinomic studies are beginning to reveal the molecular basis of protective immune responses. Advances in generating effective vaccines against emerging diseases are being matched by the increased sophistication of anticancer immunotherapy. Individualized autologous vaccines against tumors, accompanied by careful selection of adjuvants or immunostimulants such as cytokines, will gradually improve. Such vaccines will probably be most effective when used in association with other treatment modalities. Extreme variability will also be the rule so that large, randomized, placebo-controlled studies will be required before regulatory approval can be obtained. It should also be pointed out that the costs of such individual treatments are not inconsiderable, and except in the case of individual companion animals are unlikely to be widely used in veterinary medicine.

Sources of Additional Information

A web-based database regarding current available and experimental cancer vaccines is available at http://www .violonet.org/CanVaxKB.

Ambrosius, L.A., Dhawan, D., Ramos-Vara, J.A., Ruple, A., Knapp, D.W., Childress, M.O. (2018). Quantification and prognostic value of programmed cell death ligand-1 expression in dogs with diffuse large B-cell lymphoma. *AJVR,* 79, 643–649.

Anderson, K.L., Modiano, J.F. (2015). Progress in adaptive immunotherapy for cancer in companion animals: Success on the path to a cure. *Vet Sci,* 2, 363–287.

Bergman, P.J. (2018). Veterinary Oncology Immunotherapies. *Vet Clin Small Anim,* 48, 257–277.

Gavazza, A., Lubas, G., Fridman, A., Peruzzi, D., et al. (2013). Safety and efficacy of a genetic vaccine targeting telomerase plus chemotherapy for the therapy of canine B-cell lymphoma. *Human Gene Therap,* 24, 728–738.

O'Connor, C.M., Wilson-Robles, H. (2014). Developing T cell cancer immunotherapy in the dog with lymphoma. *ILAR J,* 55, 169–181.

Peruzzi, D., Gavazza, A., Mesiti, G., et al. A vaccine targeting telomerase enhances survival of dogs affected by B-cell lymphoma. *Mol Therap,* 18, 1559–1567.

Regan, D., Guth, A., Coy, J., Dow, S. (2016). Cancer immunotherapy in veterinary medicine: Current options and new developments. *Vet J,* 207, 20–28.

Rue, S.M., Eckelman, B.P., Efe, J.A., et al. (2015). Identification of a candidate therapeutic antibody for treatment of canine B-cell lymphoma. *Vet Immunol Immunopathol,* 164, 148–159.

Suckow, M.A. (2013). Cancer Vaccines: Harnessing the potential of anti-tumor immunity. *Vet J,* 198, 28–33.

Terziev, G., Roydev, R., Kalkanov, I., Borissov, I., Dinev, I. (2015). Papillomatosis in heifers. Comparative studies on surgical excision and autogenous vaccine therapies. *Traka J Sci,* 13, 274–279.

Verganti, S., Berlato, D., Blackwood, L., Amores-Fuster, I., Polton, G.A. (2016). Use of Oncept melanoma vaccine in 69 canine oral malignant melanomas in the UK. *J Small Anim Pract,* 58, 10–16.

Weiskopf, K., Anderson, K.L., Ito D, Schnorr, P.J., et al. Eradication of canine diffuse large B-cell lymphoma in a murine xenograft model with CD47 blockade and anti-CD20. *Cancer Immunol Res,* 4, 1072–1087.

Note: Page numbers followed by "f" indicate figures, "t" indicate tables, and "b" indicate boxes.